MAYO CLINIC MONOGRAPHS

■

Thrombo-angiitis Obliterans

Thrombo-angiitis Obliterans. By George E. Brown, M. D., and Edgar V. Allen, M. D., Collaborating in Pathology with Howard R. Mahorner, M. D. 12mo of 219 pages, illustrated. Cloth, $3.00 net.

Clinical Electrocardiograms

Clinical Electrocardiograms. By Fredrick A. Willius, M. D. Quarto of 219 pages, with 368 electrocardiograms. Cloth, $8.00 net.

The Volume of Blood and Plasma

The Volume of the Blood and Plasma in Health and Disease. By Leonard G. Rowntree, M. D., and George E. Brown, M. D. With the technical assistance of Grace Roth. 12mo of 219 pages, illustrated. Cloth, $3.00 net.

Addison's Disease

A Clinical Study of Addison's Disease. By Leonard G. Rowntree, M. D., and Albert M. Snell, M. D. 12mo of 317 pages, illustrated. Cloth, $4.00 net.

Hemorrhoids

Proctoscopic Examination and the Treatment of Hemorrhoids and Anal Pruritus. By Louis A. Buie, M. D. Octavo of 177 pages, with 72 illustrations. Cloth, $3.50 net.

Neoplasms of Animals

Neoplasms of Domesticated Animals. By William H. Feldman, D. V. M., M. S. Octavo of 410 pages, with 193 illustrations.

Mayo Clinic Monographs

NEOPLASMS

of

DOMESTICATED ANIMALS

By

WILLIAM H. FELDMAN, D. V. M., M. S.

Division of Experimental Surgery and Pathology.
The Mayo Foundation, Rochester, Minnesota

With a Foreword by

CHARLES H. MAYO, M. D.

193 Illustrations

PHILADELPHIA AND LONDON

W. B. SAUNDERS COMPANY

1932

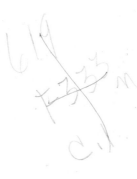

MADE IN U. S. A.

PRESS OF
W. B. SAUNDERS COMPANY
PHILADELPHIA

FOREWORD

Man has been subject to tumors, both benign and malignant, from the time of earliest recorded history. Records are in existence of early medical practitioners having watched benign tumors of the breast for signs of malignant change.

We have all noted tumors or irregular growths of plants, and especially the so-called galls found on special varieties of plants including trees. Therefore, we were ready for the many reports from the Bureau of Plant Pathology presented by the late Dr. Erwin F. Smith. He showed that cancer-like growths of vulnerable plants could be produced by injecting certain bacteria, and also that injection of certain chemical compounds would produce tumors.

It is timely to have presented, as is done in this volume, the many tumors of animals. We have long known that old dogs were subject to cancer. Other domestic animals are likely to be slaughtered before they reach the cancer age. Consequently, to assemble a large series of tumors of domestic animals is difficult. Among wild animals the struggle for existence makes it difficult to maintain life to old age; the animals go the way of all flesh, to rebuild other life in various forms, usually long before cancer would have been likely to develop. The difficulty of collecting tumors of wild animals, therefore, is extreme. This work, issued at a particularly fortunate time, when research workers throughout the world are concentrating on the conquest of cancer of man, helps to emphasize that all cellular life is subject to disease, degeneration, hyperplasia, and malignant growth. The value of studies of this type to those concerned with animal husbandry is obvious; one cannot predict the far-reaching influences they may have on the search for the cause and cure of malignant disease of human beings.

CHARLES H. MAYO

PREFACE

Little attention is given to neoplasms in the various veterinary colleges. Tumors are usually studied near the end of the course in general pathology and as a consequence adequate time for proper consideration of them is not available. The professor of pathology usually is not particularly interested in tumors, and as a result little, if any, special effort is made to collect material and obtain the necessary clinical and statistical data so essential for teaching purposes. With fuller appreciation of the subject, the pathologist may be expected to see that time is provided for proper consideration of this group of diseases. The urge of other matters of greater pedagogic and economic interest, together with an almost invariable shortage of funds in the various institutions, have retarded the development of really comprehensive collections of tumors for teaching and museum purposes. Furthermore, interest in microscopic morphologic pathology is not particularly great among many comparative pathologists. Most undergraduates have an aversion to this phase of disease and it is usually shunned entirely by the average graduate student. While this attitude obtains we cannot hope that the study of neoplasms will become popular. Lastly, the non-existence in English of a treatise devoted entirely to detailed consideration of neoplasms as they affect the domesticated mammals and fowls has constituted a serious obstacle to acquisition of knowledge concerning them. The student, in most instances, has had to depend for description of the various varieties of neoplasms on textbooks descriptive of human pathology. Many of these volumes are excellent, but they are hardly satisfactory sources of information concerning tumors of lower animals.

In an attempt to supply an obvious need of students and practitioners of veterinary medicine this volume has been prepared. Meat inspectors, physicians, laboratory workers, and others interested in the broader aspects of comparative pathology may also find the volume of interest and perhaps of value.

It is presumed that the reader possesses a knowledge of general pathology. An exhaustive treatise has been avoided, yet an attempt has been made to present the salient features of each variety of neo-

7

plasm in an understandable way. Although emphasis has been placed on the morphologic aspects of the respective tumors, the clinical phases of the subject have not been neglected. The incidence of the various neoplasms has also been considered but the paucity of statistical data that are reliable has resulted in certain portions of the text being inconclusive. The descriptive matter, pertaining to the gross and microscopic features of the respective varieties of tumors, is based, in almost every instance, on data obtained from examination of original material and not on what others have written. The amount of material examined, approximately 600 specimens, is not large compared to the material available to one interested in neoplasms of human beings, but the difficulties of acquiring a large collection of tumors of animals are rather formidable.

Practically all varieties of neoplasms were represented in the specimens obtained, but a few of the rarer forms were not secured. Inability to obtain specimens has resulted in omission of descriptions of tumors belonging to the glioblastoma, neuroblastoma, and odontoblastoma groups. Certain other conditions, such as perithelioma and cholesteatoma have not been included since in my opinion these do not represent genuine neoplasms. Teratology likewise has not been considered. With the exception of mixed tumors of the kidneys, teratomatous growths seldom occur in the domesticated animals, and my collection contained such a paucity of material as to preclude inclusion of them.

An attempt has been made to review the literature, but no claim is made for completeness and it is not unlikely that many important references have been overlooked. References have been listed at the ends of the respective chapters, and in footnotes.

With the realization of the value of illustrations in the study of morphology, a generous number has been included. I have for the most part made my own illustrations and their making has constituted a pleasurable recreation. A few illustrations were obtained through the generosity of others.

The multitudinous details necessary to the preparation of a volume of this kind enhances to a marked degree the possibility for error. Although the subject matter has been checked repeatedly it is not unlikely that errors still remain.

It is a genuine pleasure to acknowledge my deep gratitude to the many practicing veterinarians and to those veterinarians of the Meat Inspection Service of the Bureau of Animal Industry of the United States Department of Agriculture who collected a large share of the material which was studied. The ready response to my request for specimens and the appreciation of my needs have made this phase of the task less arduous. Among the veterinarians whom I wish to mention particularly are Drs. H. E. Kingman and James Farquharson, Fort Collins, Colorado; Dr. N. J. Miller, Eaton, Colorado; Dr. Herbert Lothe, Waukesha, Wisconsin, and Dr. C. F. Schlotthauer, Rochester, Minnesota. Federal employees who have been untiring in their efforts to provide me with material for this study include: Drs. Charles L. Davis, R. B. Leeper, C. M. Chase, H. L. Shorten, and William Fountain of Denver, Colorado; Dr. C. F. Payne of National Stock Yards, Illinois; Dr. E. W. Barthold, Wichita, Kansas; Dr. G. E. Totten of South St. Paul; Dr. Virgil W. Woolen of Eau Claire, Wisconsin, and Dr. D. D. Tierney of Austin, Minnesota. I am also indebted to my brother, Dr. Gordon G. Feldman and to Dr. Frank P. Mathews, who assisted materially in the collection of many of the earlier specimens.

To Dr. F. C. Mann, Chief of the Division of Experimental Surgery and Pathology of The Mayo Foundation, I am grateful for advice and counsel and to my associates at the Institute of Experimental Medicine of The Mayo Foundation who have assisted in many ways I am also grateful.

WILLIAM H. FELDMAN.

ROCHESTER, MINNESOTA,
February, 1932

CONTENTS

11

CHAPTER IX

CHAPTER X

CHAPTER XI

CHAPTER XII

CHAPTER XIII

CHAPTER XIX

CHAPTER XX

CHAPTER XXI

CHAPTER XXII

CHAPTER XXIII

Neoplasms of Domesticated Animals

CHAPTER I

THE BIOLOGY OF NEOPLASMS

A neoplasm is a biologic entity possessing certain definite characteristics by which it may be distinguished from other cellular overgrowths of tissue that are frequently the result of the body's response to specific injuries. Since the etiologic element responsible for the inception of the lawless overgrowth of cells of a tumor is as yet unknown, it is difficult to compose an accurate definition of a neoplasm, which is sufficiently flexible to embrace all forms of neoplasia and yet remain within the accepted concepts of this little understood phenomenon. Although it is convenient and permissible to use the terms "tumor" and "neoplasm" synonymously, the latter is perhaps preferable.

With certain reservations, a neoplasm may be defined as an autonomous proliferation of cells, noninflammatory, which grow continuously and without restraint, the cells resembling those of the parent cells from which they are derived, yet serving no useful function, and lacking orderly structural arrangement. Hyperplastic proliferations, cysts which develop as a consequence of retention of fluids, and infectious granulomas such as occur in tuberculosis, actinomycosis, and infection of wounds must be separated from the true tumors since each of these processes possesses features foreign to neoplasms, although grossly they may sometimes be confused with genuine tumors.

Historically, tumorous growths are as old as civilization. Carcinoma of human beings is frequently mentioned in the older literature of Egypt and the far East and the ancients even advanced theories as to its cause, a favorite one being that the disease developed from a concentration of black bile. Elaborate methods of treatment were sometimes used to combat the malady and the use of escharotics is frequently mentioned. Incisions were also practiced, and some of the ancient wise men recommended a vegetable diet, but walnuts were forbidden. In medieval times, enlargements due to the bacillus of tuberculosis, as well as those resulting from syphilis, were commonly confused with, and often diagnosed as, carcinoma. During this period, it was the popular opinion that the elements of carcinoma were fluid, and were transported to the various sites in the body by way of the veins. In the early part of the nineteenth century, carcinoma was defined as an organized exudate from the blood, resulting from overnutrition and overgrowth. It was only after the development of the achromatic microscope in 1824 that scientists discovered that tumors were growths of tissue, resulting from proliferation of new cells. Since that time a great deal has been learned concerning the morphology and clinical behavior of new growths, but as yet the character of the essential element within the protoplasm of the tumor cell that enables the cell to overcome the normal influences of growth restraint, and to enter on a career of continuous proliferation, has not been determined. In other words, the fundamental reason why certain cells of the body suddenly assume a more or less independent existence, and prosper by the flagrant disregard of the laws governing normal tissues, is unknown. The problem is one of the most profound enigmas of all time.

THEORY OF ETIOLOGY

The elusiveness of the cause of tumor and the failure of the earlier observers to agree on a common etiologic agent, together with the remarkable strides made in the knowledge of bacteriology resulted in a great variety of microörganisms being regarded as the cause of tumorous growths, particularly of carcinoma. At various times, bacteria, protozoa, yeast, and molds have all been considered the specific etiologic elements in the inception of neoplasms. One observer even went so far as to describe the complete life cycle of what he considered to be the parasite of carcinoma, which on subsequent investigation was found to be particles of cork in the various stages of disintegration. Cork had been employed in the preparation of sections of the tumor that was studied. Many tumor cells, and particularly those of the malignant varieties, are more or less prone to degenerative changes which become most evident in the cytoplasm of the cells, in the form of vacuoles, or of droplets of fat or mucin. All of these have been mistaken for parasites of etiologic significance when they were in reality nothing more than the products of abnormal cellular metabolism.

Most tumors, especially those of softer consistence, such as the highly cellular malignant forms, are excellent culture mediums for the growth and multiplication of bacteria, and if the growth becomes eroded through trauma or ulcerates as a consequence of necrosis, portions of the surface of the mass are likely to become the residence of considerable numbers of bacteria. Although these represent nothing more than parasites subsisting on the cellular débris of the neoplasm, in the past much has been written in an attempt to fix the responsibility for the tumor's inception on these microörganisms. The very nature of neoplasms makes such an hypothesis untenable, and although the exact causative factor responsible for the inception of a tumor is not known, it is generally agreed that whatever the cause or causes, bacteria in themselves are of no significance.

The biology of tumors fails to indicate that neoplasms are in any way analogous to infectious diseases. They are neither infectious nor contagious* in the bacteriologic sense, for tumors do not occur in epidemic forms and, with the possible exception of the transmissible lymphosarcoma of dogs, contact with victims of neoplastic growths is not attended with danger to the nonaffected. In the exception noted, contact not uncommonly brings about transference of some of the tumor cells from the dog bearing the tumor, to the tissues of the nonaffected individual. This, however, is an example of transmission by the mechanical transplantation of definitely formed cells of the parent tumor into the tissues of a susceptible recipient. It is not accomplished by a growth-exciting element, from the animal bearing the tumor, initiating a separate and unrelated growth of neoplastic cells entirely from the tissue elements of the second animal.

The fact that there are so many different species of animals affected with such a large variety of tumorous growths constitutes further evidence that bacteria are not responsible for the genesis of the process. Again, if tumors were due to bacteria the disease should spread throughout the body as such. Instead, neoplastic disease is usually a local entity unless passed along to other tissues and organs by the dissemination of living tumor cells.

Furthermore, specific antibodies have not been demonstrated in individuals possessing tumors, and proof of the development of a specific immunity as a consequence of the existence of tumors is lacking.† The presence of one tumor does not successfully protect the body against the appearance of a second or even a third tumor and in certain subjects, particularly old dogs, a dozen or more tumors may be present simul-

---

* The words "infectious" and "contagious" should not be confused with the word "transmissible." Some neoplastic tissues, if implanted in healthy tissue, will grow; this is an example of transmissibility but not of contagion or infection.

† Exception must again be noted in the instance of the transmissible lymphosarcoma of dogs. The tumor spontaneously disappears from some animals and they exhibit marked resistance to subsequent exposure to the disease.

taneously in the same animal. (See multiple neoplasms, Chapter II, page 51.)

The knowledge extant does not justify a belief that neoplasms are infectious. The attack on the problem of the ultimate cause of tumors must be in other directions.

It was Cohnheim's belief that some time in early embryonic life a disturbance occurs in the orderly development of certain tissue cells, and that they become established in foreign situations, where they remain latent and sooner or later grow in an unrestrained manner; subsequently they assume the characteristics of neoplasia. It is well known that gross congenital defects such as moles, branchial clefts, and undescended testis are not uncommon, and that tumors may arise from such. Cohnheim stated that microscopic misplacements or malformations of cells also occur in the various tissues from which tumorous growths arise. Although Cohnheim's theory is useful in the interpretation of an occasional tumor the situation and cellular constituents of which clearly suggest developmental delinquency, it fails to supply an acceptable explanation for the genesis of the great majority of neoplasms. The most serious objection to this theory is that if it fails to reveal why the embryonically misplaced cells eventually begin to grow, and why, after growth has started, the cells produce tumors instead of normal structures.

Ribbert's theory of the origin of tumors embraced the idea that cells became dissociated from their normal tissue relationships, either in uterine existence as a result of embryonal misadventure, or in extrauterine life, as a consequence of certain external agencies, such as trauma, inflammation and other irritating processes. Ribbert contended that the misplaced cells started to grow as a consequence of their inherent capacity to regenerate, and proceeded to proliferate in a continuous and lawless manner because of the absence of the normal growth-restraining influence, exerted by the tissue tension of their normal associations. This is neither a complete nor a satisfactory theory and does not explain the genesis of all tumors.

Irritative influences.—There seems to be a significant correlation between nonspecific chronic irritation and the appearance of certain neoplasms, particularly epithelial malignant growths. An example of this is the so-called pipe-smoker's carcinoma, which develops on the lip, following prolonged and repeated smoking; another is the carcinoma of the mouth, common among those natives of India and the Philippines who make a practice of chewing betel-nut. The carcinoma develops where the betel-nut is held in contact with the cheek. Again, in cattle, carcinoma of the liver is often associated with biliary cirrhosis, which is usually due to the presence of a parasite which supplies constant irritation to this organ. Also carcinoma of the skin overlying the abdomen is not uncommon among the natives of Kashmir, who wear baskets of glowing charcoal under their robes for warmth. Another example is the chimney-sweep carcinoma of the scrotum. This develops among boys, about the age of puberty, who have been more or less continuously exposed to dirt and soot which accumulates about the scrotum. Workers in dye and paraffin industries often have carcinoma of the bladder, and repeated and prolonged exposure to roentgen rays may produce a fatal type of carcinoma. The possible irritative effect of the acinic rays of sunshine is suggested in certain carcinomas of the skin of cattle. Drabble observed a large number of cattle in Australia with carcinoma of the skin which developed following severe keratosis, induced by sunlight, in the skin of light-colored animals that previously had become photosensitized by ingestion of a certain plant. Carcinoma may also develop in old scars, years following injury, particularly scars that occur as a result of a burn; an example is the so-called brand cancer of cattle.

The literature pertaining to the cause of neoplasms contains many references to tumors which have seemed to arise following a single episode of trauma, but as Knox has pointed out, after careful and comprehensive examination of the literature, causative relationship between a single episode of trauma, and the subsequent appearance of a neoplasm, never has been completely established. Further evidence that trauma is neither a direct nor a contributory cause of neoplasm is found in the fact that it never has been possible to produce a malignant growth experimentally in animals by a single episode of trauma. Trauma must therefore be dismissed as unworthy of serious consideration in the etiology of tumors.

Experimentally, it was shown, by Yamagiwa and Ichikawa, that carcinoma could be produced in the skin of the ears of rabbits by applications of coal tar for variable periods. The malignant character of the growths was proved in several instances by the development of metastasis to lymph nodes. The nonspecific carcinogenic nature of the tumor-inciting element of tar is indicated by the fact that carcinomas of the skin of animals have been induced experimentally by application, at high temperatures, of various substances, including yeast, acetylene, and petroleum. Carcinomas have also been produced by exposure of the tissues to solutions of hydrochloric acid or sodium hydroxide. Evidently there exist many agents that possess the capacity of inciting previously normal cells to form neoplasia through the medium of chronic irritation.

Fibiger was perhaps the first to achieve the experimental production of carcinoma. Having observed in the rat spontaneous carcinoma of the mucosa of the stomach, in which he identified a nematode parasite, Fibiger planned what was to be a brilliant experiment. The parasite, which he eventually designated Spiroptera neoplastica, passes a portion of its life cycle in the muscles of the cockroach (Periplaneta americana). Therefore, a supply of infested cockroaches was obtained, and the insects were fed to a series of rats, with the result that in twelve of the sixty-two animals that survived the experiment for more than sixty days carcinoma of the stomach developed. The parasites were numerous throughout the primary tumors but none was to be found in the few metastatic growths that occurred.

The age of the rats had little effect on the resultant tumor; the significant factor was the length of time the irritant was permitted to act. Neither was there any apparent relation between the degree of inflammation and the subsequent development of the tumor. Fibiger was of the opinion that the active substance in the production of the neoplastic process was some sort of poisonous secretion from the nematode rather than a specific virus of carcinoma.

Another parasite that has been used extensively in experimental production of tumors is the cystic stage of a cat tapeworm, Taenia crassicollis. That the larval stage of the tapeworm (Cysticercus fasciolaris) could be used as the agent of irritation in the production of neoplasms, was reported by Bullock and Curtis.[1, 2, 3] Infestation was accomplished as a consequence of the ingestion by the rat of feces of the cat, containing the ova of the tapeworm. The primary tumors, which were practically all malignant, were invariably of mesoblastic character and occurred in the liver in association with the parasitic cyst (Figs. 1 and 2). Extensive metastasis was frequently observed. Neoplastic proliferation of the parenchymatous cells of the liver did not occur. In a series of several thousand rats exposed to infestation with cysticercus, sarcomatous neoplasia was observed in from 19 to 20 per cent of the animals. The tumors occurred more frequently in certain strains of rats than in others. The work of Bullock and Curtis has demonstrated the inherent capacity of the mesoblastic tissue to undergo neoplastic transformation as a consequence of chronic irritation and has emphasized the variable character of the irritative substance that may influence normal cells to enter on a lawless career of proliferation.

Relation of age to neoplasia.—It has long been the popular belief that the occurrence of tumors was in some way influenced by age, and that the conjectural incidence of different kinds of tumors varied in the different age periods. The mesoblastic malignant tumors (sarcomas) were supposed to affect young individuals much more commonly than those in advanced years, whereas the malignant epithelial tumors were thought to exhibit a definite predilection for individuals of advanced age.

Observations indicate that although age in itself is not a barrier to the inception of neoplasia, certain kinds of new growths do occur with

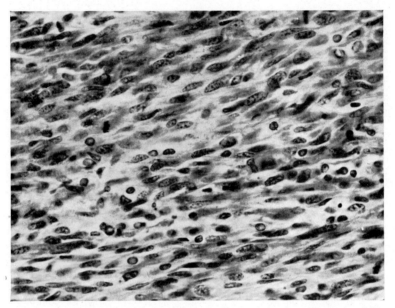

Fig. 1.—Experimentally induced sarcoma of the liver of a rat. The tumor followed the infestation of the liver by Cysticercus fasciolaris. The spindle-shaped cell predominates. Photomicrograph × 525, prepared from a slide obtained from Dr. F. D. Bullock, Institute of Cancer Research, Columbia University.

greater frequency at certain periods of life than others. Data pertaining to the malignant epithelial tumors are particularly impressive.

Ninety horses affected with carcinoma in Sticker's series, in which the age was known, revealed data as follows:

Two horses (2.2 per cent) were aged four years; four (4.4 per cent) were aged from five to six years; nine (10 per cent) were aged from seven to eight years; fourteen (15.5 per cent) were aged from nine to ten years; eight (8.8 per cent) were aged from eleven to twelve years; ten (11 per cent) were aged from thirteen to fourteen years; sixteen (17.7 per cent) were aged from fifteen to sixteen years; eleven (12.2 per cent) were aged from seventeen to eighteen years; thirteen (14.4 per cent) were aged from nineteen to twenty years, and three (3.3 per cent) were aged from twenty-three to twenty-five years.

Although the foregoing data are in no sense comprehensive, they indicate that the tumors were definitely more common in those animals which had passed the young age period; the highest percentage of frequency was in animals which were between the ages of ten and twenty years.

Detroye observed seventy-seven new growths of cattle in a meat inspection service covering twelve years. Seventy-three of the tumors

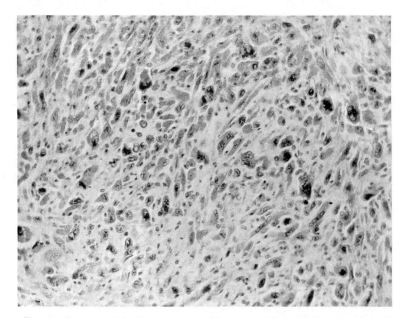

Fig. 2.—Sarcoma of the liver of a rat. The tumor followed infestation of the liver by Cysticercus fasciolaris. Polymorphic cell-forms are numerous. Photomicrograph × 225, prepared from a slide obtained from Dr. F. D. Bullock, Institute of Cancer Research, Columbia University.

occurred in adult cattle, and only four in calves. In relation to the entire number of cattle slaughtered, the incidence among adult animals was 1 : 1,000, whereas the incidence among calves was 1 : 6,000. These figures agree with the experience of veterinarians of America who have occasion to examine large numbers of cattle at necropsy. There is no question but that the greater number of neoplasms is found among adult cattle with perhaps the greatest number among older cattle commonly referred to as "canners."

In Trotter's series of 300 bovines affected with neoplasms, of which 91.47 per cent were carcinomas and 8.52 per cent were sarcomas, three of the animals were aged three years or less, and 297 were considered as aged. Although the exact age of the old animals was not determined, Trotter considered that 25 per cent were aged less than fifteen years, and that the remainder were between fifteen and twenty years of age.

The greater incidence of neoplasia among older cattle is also brought out in the report of the Bureau of Animal Industry of the United States Department of Agriculture for the year ending June 30, 1930. Of approximately 8,200,000 cattle that came to necropsy, lymphoblastoma was the cause of the condemnation of 1,265, whereas only forty-three calves (cattle aged one year or less) among approximately 4,400,000 were rejected as a consequence of this disease. The ratio of frequency of occurrence among adult cattle is 1 : 6,500 and that among younger cattle 1 : 102,325.

With reference to dogs, some interesting statistics are available concerning the relation of age to neoplasms, although most of the data pertain to carcinoma. Sticker listed a total of seventy dogs that were affected with carcinoma of the integument in which the various age groups were as follows:

Ten dogs (14.3 per cent) were aged from two to three years; eighteen (25 per cent) were aged from five to six years; twenty (28.5 per cent) were aged from seven to eight years; fourteen (20 per cent) were aged from nine to ten years; four (5.7 per cent) were aged from eleven to twelve years, and four (5.7 per cent) were aged from twelve to fifteen years.

Sticker also recorded the respective age groups in an additional series of forty-nine dogs affected with carcinoma which died as a consequence of the disease or were killed for humane reasons:

One dog (2 per cent) was aged one and a half years; four dogs (8.1 per cent) were aged from two to four years; five (10.2 per cent) were aged from five to six years; eleven (22.4 per cent) were aged from seven to eight years; seventeen (34.7 per cent) were aged from nine to ten years; seven (14.2 per cent) were aged from eleven to twelve years, and four (8.1 per cent) were aged from thirteen to fifteen years.

The foregoing data from German sources are comparable to those compiled from French sources by Cadiot and Almy. The carcinomas of 100 dogs were distributed through the various ages as follows:

Six dogs (6 per cent) were aged from one to three years; eighteen (18 per cent) were aged from three to five years; thirty-three (33 per cent) were aged from six to nine years; twenty-six (26 per cent) were aged from nine to twelve years; fourteen (14 per cent) were aged from twelve to fifteen years, and three (3 per cent) were aged from fifteen to twenty years.

Although these data are in no sense exhaustive, they seem sufficient to indicate rather definitely that the great majority of epithelial tumors occur in older adult dogs and that they occur infrequently in those aged less than three years; they seem to be most numerous in the aged period of six to ten years.

The occurrence of neoplasms in fowls also indicates definite relationship to age; most of the new growths are observed in fowls aged more than one year. Curtis reported finding seventy-nine tumors among 880 chickens and expressed the opinion that there is a significant positive correlation between age and the occurrence of neoplasia. Of the 880 chickens that were aged less than twenty-seven months, only 7.37 per cent possessed neoplasms, whereas they were present in 19.17 per cent of the chickens aged more than twenty-seven months.

Among 472 young chickens on which necropsy was done for diagnostic purposes during one year at the New York State Veterinary College of Cornell University at Ithaca, three (0.6 per cent) were affected with tumors. In the same period 964 adult chickens were examined and a total of 207 neoplasms was discovered including seventy-seven cases (21 per cent) of so-called leukemia. Although the striking difference revealed in the incidence of tumors in common domestic fowls of these two age groups was probably due in part to the large number of deaths among the younger fowls as a consequence of specific infectious diseases, the susceptibility of the older chickens to neoplasms is none the less apparent.

The explanation of the higher frequency of carcinoma in animals of advanced age groups may not be related to increased susceptibility of the organism to neoplasia on account of age in itself. Without question, the chances for the occurrence of carcinoma are enhanced the longer the animal lives. Extension of the duration of life may well increase the percentage of probability for the development of neoplasia in the same manner that long life provides greater probabilities for fracture of a leg, or for accidental death from any cause. On the other hand, there are certain biologic changes which are ushered in with the advent of senescence that may exert a definite contributory influence on the inception of carcinoma. Such factors as senile atrophy, fibrosis, and structural changes of the blood vascular system may, under some circumstances, favor the development of malignant lesions. Such factors, however, are perhaps of minor importance, and the real reason that carcinomas are most often observed in older animals is probably due to the fact that the lapse of time brings about the maturity of a process that had its inception earlier in life. The genesis of this process is, in all probability, related to, and perhaps dependent on, certain complex, intrinsic elements, the most significant of which is possession by the individual of an hereditary predisposition to the development of neoplasia.

Heredity.—The existence of inheritable resistance or susceptibility to the growth of tumor has been apparent to many observers for a long time. By the application of the principles of genetics in the breeding of animals it is possible to develop strains in which susceptibility to tumor is dominant, whereas other strains may be produced in which the resistance to neoplasia is so pronounced that tumors never occur. Virchow pointed out the hereditary influence in the development of melanotic tumors of horses (see Chapter XVI, page 267) and Warthin contributed convincing evidence of the influence of heredity in the occurrence of epithelial malignant growths in certain so-called cancer families of man. Also, there is considerable evidence that would lead one to believe that the occurrence of certain forms of leukosis of fowls are probably influenced by heredity.

Slye's[12, 13] extensive researches have shown, by appropriate genetic procedures, that heredity plays a significant part in the origin of tumors of mice, but the exact influence of heredity on the appearance of spontaneous neoplasms in higher mammals and fowls is difficult to estimate. Under experimental conditions the ancestral history of the various animals is definitely known, and the subsequent crosses likewise can be accurately controlled and a given result prophesied with confidence. Under ordinary circumstances so little is known of the ancestral history of the lower animals and of man that tangible evidence of the influence of heredity in the etiology of a given tumor, is usually absent. Nevertheless, the summation of clinical and experimental observations indicates rather definitely that heredity is not without significance in the genesis of neoplasia. Heredity alone is not responsible for the inception of a new growth, but hereditary influences may so affect the germ plasm of an individual that the cells, when exposed to proper irritative stimuli, will become neoplastic.

Fortunately the majority of animals seems to possess a natural immunity against tumors rather than a hereditary susceptibility to them. To intensify the degree of susceptibility to tumor by the injudicious mating of individuals with tumors should be avoided if neoplasia is to be controlled at its source.

Briefly it may be stated that aside from the occasional tumors that may arise as a direct consequence of some developmental mischance there are at least two factors necessary for the inception of most tumors, particularly of carcinomas. These include, first, an intrinsic predisposition or susceptibility to neoplasia that is in all probability influenced by heredity, and second, the potential neoplastic cells must be exposed to some form of chronic irritation. The irritative element is nonspecific and may be mechanical, chemical, thermal, actinic, or parasitic.

Although the foregoing summary of the most important facts concerning the nature of neoplasia may enable one to understand some of the more obvious aspects of the process, one is as yet denied the secret of the biologic mechanism that operates within the protoplasm of a cell, as a consequence of which the cell assumes a state of autonomy which is characterized by an ever increasing propensity for growth. This quality is passed along to the succeeding generations of cells, so that functional and morphologic resemblances to the parent tissue may be entirely lost, and a new structural and physiologic entity established.

CLASSIFICATION AND NOMENCLATURE

The description of various types of tumors should be prefaced by a scheme of classification. In the absence of exact knowledge pertaining to the specific cause of neoplasms, any attempt to provide a systematic arrangement of the new growths is likely to lead one into difficulties. Of the many schemes of classification that have been suggested, that of Mallory seems both logical and practical. Mallory's classification is based on the embryogenesis and histologic identity of the respective cells constituting normal tissues, and takes cognizance of the fact that tumors may arise from any of the sixteen or more distinct varieties of cells that are normally concerned in the structural or functional welfare of the body. Most cells of normal tissue in their mature state possess characteristics by which they can be recognized readily but unripe or immature cells frequently exhibit so little differentiation that recognition may be difficult or uncertain. All gradations of cellular differentiation may be observed in tumors. Those that progress slowly and remain localized are composed of cells that bear a close resemblance to cells of normal tissue of the same kind; whereas those that grow rapidly and are inclined to destroy tissues and to spread to distant parts of the body, may resemble only remotely the parent cells from which the tumor arose. These variations in rate of progression of a tumor must be provided for in any systematic grouping of the different varieties of new growths that may be attempted.

By following the classification suggested by Mallory, a specific and understandable nomenclature for tumors is possible. By adding the word "blastoma," which means true tumor, as a suffix to the name of the type cell from which a given tumor originates, a simple, yet distinctive and significant title results. For example, a tumor of which the type cell is the fibroblast becomes a fibroblastoma, and one composed of epithelial cells is properly designated epithelioblastoma. This is of much value in referring to a given variety of neoplasm in a general way or as a group, but certain clinical and histologic considerations frequently make it desirable to use terms that are somewhat more specific. For this reason such words as sarcoma and carcinoma have long been retained in the nomenclature of tumors. Sarcoma refers to a tumor consisting of immature connective tissue elements that is clinically or histologically malignant. The word sarcoma should not be used alone, but rather as a suffix, in combination with the name of the type cell responsible for the growth; that is, fibrosarcoma, myxosarcoma and so forth. To designate a growth simply as a sarcoma is to acknowledge one's inability to recognize the identity of the cellular constituents of the tumor in question. Carcinoma is preferable to the older term "cancer" as designating tumors of epithelial origin that are malignant. The use of clinical terms such as benign and malignant should be avoided if possible. The use of the word malignant is permissible, however, in referring to the malign form of such a tumor as melanoblastoma, the character of the type cell of which is undetermined. The use of the suffix "oma," indicating a neoplasm, joined to the specific designations of the respective type cells usually indicates a benign tumor. An example would be the word, "fibroma."

In the classification of tumors which follows (Table 1) a few additions and modifications have been made to Mallory's original scheme.

Tumors also arise from undifferentiated embryonic cells of varied potencies and as a consequence new growths may occur that contain two or more kinds of tissue; the greater the multipotency of the cells giving rise to the tumor, the more complex the structure of the neoplasm. Among the tissues that may be recognized in tumors of this type are fibrous connective tissue, bone, cartilage, and smooth and striated muscle. Mixed tumors are commonly referred to as teratomas, although the rather common mixed tumor of the kidney may be conveniently designated "embryonal nephroma."

TABLE 1

CLASSIFICATION OF SIMPLE TUMORS

Type cell.	Normal product.	Tumor.
1. Fibroblast.......	Connective tissue	Fibroblastoma, including fibroma, and fibrosarcoma
2. Myxoblast.......	Mucous connective tissue	Myxoblastoma, including myxoma and myxosarcoma
3. Chondroblast.....	Cartilage tissue	Chondroblastoma, including chondroma and chondrosarcoma
4. Osteoblast.......	Bone tissue	Osteoblastoma, including osteoma and osteogenic sarcoma
5. Lipoblast........	Fat tissue	Lipoblastoma, including lipoma and liposarcoma
6. Leiomyoblast.....	Smooth muscle tissue	Leiomyoblastoma, including leiomyoma and leiomyosarcoma
7. Endothelioblast...	Blood and lymph vessel endothelium	Endothelioblastoma,* including hemangio-endothelioma and lymphangio-endothelioma
8. Lymphoblast.....	Lymphocyte	Lymphoblastoma, including lymphoma and lymphocytoma, leukemic, and aleukemic
9. Myeloblast.......	Myelocyte	Myeloblastoma, including myelocytoma and chloroma
10. ?..............	?	Myeloma
11. Mesothelioblast...	Mesothelium of serous surfaces	Mesothelioblastoma, including mesothelioma
12. Melanoblast......	Pigment cell	Melanoblastoma, including melanoma and malignant melanoma
13. Rhabdomyoblast..	Striated muscle	Rhabdomyoblastoma, including rhabdomyoma and rhabdomyosarcoma
14. Glioblast........	Neuroglia cells	Glioblastoma, including glioma and gliosarcoma
15. Neuroblast.......	Nerve cell	Neuroblastoma, including neuroma
16. Epithelioblast....	Epithelium	Epithelioblastoma, including papilloma, adenoma, and carcinoma

    * Mallory included under endothelioblastoma tumors arising from the dura mater, designating these "dural endothelioma." Since the histogenesis of the cells of this structure is unsettled, it seems best for the present not to assign tumors arising from them to a definite place in the classification. Some pathologists refer to such tumors as "meningiomas." This term is permissible until the embryogenesis of the type cell is settled.

BIBLIOGRAPHY

    1. Bullock, F. D. and Curtis, M. R.: The experimental production of sarcoma of the liver of rats. Proc. New York Path. Soc., **20:** 149–175, 1920.

2. Bullock, F. D. and Curtis, M. R.: A study of the reactions of the tissues of the rat's liver to the larvæ of *Tenia crassicollis* and the histogenesis of Cysticercus sarcoma. Jour. Cancer Res., 8: 446–481 (Dec.), 1924.

3. Bullock, F. D. and Curtis, M. R.: Types of cysticercus tumors. Jour. Cancer Res., 9: 425–443 (Dec.), 1925.

4. Cadiot and Almy: Quoted by French, Cecil. In: Surgical diseases and surgery of the dog. Chicago, Alexander Eger, 1923, p. 383.

5. Cohnheim: Quoted by Ewing, James. In: Neoplastic diseases. Ed. 3. Philadelphia, W. B. Saunders Co., 1928, pp. 97–119.

6. Curtis, M. R.: Frequency of occurrence of tumors in the domestic fowl. Jour. Agr. Res., 5: 397–404, 1915.

7. Detroye: Cancers et tumeurs chez les animaux. Bull. soc. centr. de méd. vét., 60: 390, 1906.

8. Drabble, J.: Skin cancer in cattle. Australian Vet. Jour., 5: 71–76, 1929.

9. Fibiger, Johannes: Untersuchungen über eine Nematode (Spiroptera sp. n.) und deren Fähigkeit, papillomatöse und carcinomatöse Geschwulstbildungen im Magen der Ratte hervorzurufen. Ztschr. f. Krebsforsch., 13: 217–280, 1913; Weiter Untersuchungen über das Spiroteracarcinom der Ratte. Ztschr. f. Krebsforsch., 14: 295–326, 1914.

10. Knox, L. C.: Trauma and tumors. Arch. Path., 7: 274–309 (Feb.), 1929.

11. Mallory, F. B.: The principles of pathologic histology. Philadelphia, W. B. Saunders Co., 1914, 270 pp.

12. Report of the New York State Veterinary College of Cornell University for the year 1929–1930, p. 49.

13. Ribbert: Quoted by Ewing, James. In: Neoplastic diseases. Ed. 3. Philadelphia, W. B. Saunders Co., 1928.

14. Slye, Maud: The inheritance behavior of cancer as a simple Mendelian recessive. Jour. Cancer Res., 10: 15–49 (April), 1926.

15. Slye, Maud: Some observations in the nature of cancer. Jour. Cancer Res., 11: 135–151 (June), 1927.

16. Sticker, Anton: Ueber den Krebs der Thiere. Arch. f. klin. Chir., 65: 616–696, 1902.

17. Trotter, A. M.: Malignant diseases in bovines. Jour. Comp. Path. and Therap., 24: 1–20, 1911.

18. Virchow, R.: Quoted by Williams, W. R. In: The natural history of cancer. London, W. Heinemann, 1908, p. 363.

19. Warthin, A. S.: The further study of a cancer family. Jour. Cancer Res., 9: 279–286 (June), 1925.

20. Yamagiwa, Katsusaburo, and Ichikawa, Koichi: Experimental study of the pathogenesis of carcinoma. Jour. Cancer Res., 3: 1–21 (Jan.), 1918.

CHAPTER II

GENERAL CHARACTERISTICS OF ANIMAL NEOPLASMS

A tumor consists of protoplasmic units which are subject to factors similar to those that influence the well-being of normal cells. However, the behavior of the cells of a neoplasm is quite unlike that of the structural elements of normal tissues. The propensity for growth is exaggerated, and a growth-restraining mechanism which is operative against normal cells of the body is absent or ineffective in limiting the growing proclivities of the cells of a tumor. The tissue constituting a neoplasm is a specialized entity, growing at the expense of the remainder of the body. The perverted cells do not perform a useful function, and the accelerated metabolism which obtains for many of them predisposes to the early advent of retrogressive changes.

COMPARISONS WITH NORMAL TISSUE

Independence of growth.—MacCallum wrote: "The really essential difference between tumors and normal tissue is not the increased energy of growth, but the emancipation of the tissue from obedience to the laws that govern the growth of normal tissues." Normal cells grow according to a well-defined architectural plan for a given species, and when a part is perfected in accordance with that scheme, growth ceases and the cells are concerned in the functions of maintenance until they are overtaken by death or senility. Tumor cells are bound by no such laws of conduct. They are purely anarchic in their behavior and are dependent for their well-being on the continuance of the blood supply and room for their extension.

Vitality.—Tumors as a rule exhibit considerably more vitality than normal tissue of the same cellular constituents. Although the patient may waste away and the immediate tissue become atrophied and disappear, the cells of the tumor usually will prosper and show every indication of adequate nutrition. Unless removed or overtaken by retrogression, tumors usually continue to grow until the host finally dies due to their destructive or mechanical influence on some vital part. Occasionally, however, a tumor is observed to undergo spontaneous regression and eventually to disappear.

Fortunately certain agents exist, in the presence of which tumor cells show less resistance than normal tissue cells. Two of these are roentgen rays and radium. By the intelligent application of these agents, it is often possible to modify or reduce the tendency of the cells to proliferate without injury to the normal tissues, and, as a result, to cause regression.

Functional capacity.—Although a tumor may consist of cells capable of contributing to the functional efficiency of an organ or part under normal circumstances, as tumor cells they are usually handicapped by the body's inability to utilize the products of their activity. Carcinomas of the intestinal mucosa may secrete a large amount of mucus, but, as excretory channels are lacking, the secretion can be of no value to the host. Again, the cells of adenocarcinoma of the oviduct of a hen may produce a certain amount of secretion which cannot be evacuated, and its continual manufacture eventually results in the formation of large cysts. A fibroma or a leiomyoma does not add strength or usefulness to a part; it fails to fit into the scheme of things, and, as a consequence, becomes disfiguring and occasionally actually dangerous, due to its size and situation. In hogs large tumors of the kidney of the type of embryonal nephroma occur. The structure of these tumors varies; often it is closely allied to that of the normal kidney, yet the functional efficiency of the organ decreases with the increased size of the tumor, due, of course, to the replacement of renal tissue by the neoplasm. This continues until the kidney, as such, has given way to a tumor many times its size, and its function must be assumed by the other kidney, for function is not assumed by the tumor, even though it may contain elements similar to those of the kidney. Another example of a parenchymatous type of tumor which is unable to contribute its functional assistance to the cells from which it arises, is the primary hepatic cell carcinoma or hepatoma. Although the cells of a hepatoma may secrete bile, the structural make-up of the tumor is such as to make it difficult, if not impossible, to carry on activities peculiar to normal hepatic tissue. However, in several instances I have demonstrated the presence of glycogen within many of the cells of tumors of this character.

In one instance[8] I observed a large adenocarcinoma from the neck of a bovine. The tumor contained large cavities filled with a colloid substance, and the structure resembled that of the thyroid gland. Such material, needing no duct for its escape, could, perhaps, be absorbed directly, and although in case of thyroid deficiency this might be of use, it is more likely to be harmful than beneficial. As an example of a tumor disturbing the metabolic equilibrium by virtue of its functional ca-

3

pacity, the case of a human being, reported by Wilder, Allan, Power, and Robertson is of unusual interest. They studied a clinical case of carcinoma of the pancreas, the type cell of which had a striking morphologic resemblance to the cells of the islands of Langerhans. The patient had required frequent doses of glucose to prevent convulsions from spontaneous hypoglycemia, and this, together with the fact that alcoholic extracts prepared from metastatic carcinoma in the liver acted like insulin on injection into rabbits, constitutes impressive evidence that the cells of the tumor in this instance were endowed with specific functional capacity not unlike that of their parental type. All-in-all, it is hardly conceivable that a neoplasm ever contributes to the physiologic well-being of the affected individual.

STRUCTURE

Like the more specialized tissues, tumors consist of a framework, or stroma, supporting the type cells, or parenchyma. The respective elements vary greatly in amount, from that seen in highly cellular structures, such as lymphocytomas and rapidly growing carcinomas, to the dense make-up of a hard fibroma, or the abundant stroma of a regressive carcinoma. Although in most tumors the stroma may be distinguished easily, yet in a few, such as the fibroblastomas, such distinction is often difficult.

The stroma.—The stroma appears to be of secondary importance in the growth of neoplasms. It usually originates from the surrounding tissue and not from the cells of the parenchyma of the tumor. Apparently, the slower a tumor grows the more stroma is developed; whereas the parenchyma of certain rapidly growing neoplasms appears to prosper with minimal framework.

Cells of the parenchyma.—The cells which constitute the parenchyma of tumors have a remarkable tendency to exhibit the distinctive characteristics of the parent cells. A squamous-cell carcinoma of the skin consequently undergoes cornification, due to the production of keratin, which, being beneath the surface, cannot escape as it normally would when this substance is formed from the epithelium of the skin. The cells of a thyroid carcinoma produce colloid material, and tumors of the intestinal tract frequently produce mucus. As a rule, the tendency toward differentiation is most marked in slowly growing tumors; in those that grow with considerable rapidity, differentiation is often difficult, if not impossible. Broders, in an extensive study of squamous-cell epithelioma, concluded that the degree to which carcinoma cells become differentiated has a direct bearing on the ultimate results of the process. He maintained that the less the tendency of a tumor (carcinoma) cell to differentiate, the more dangerous it is.

Tumor cells individually often depart considerably from the parent type in both size and shape. Again, they often suffer marked alterations, due to pressure and the influence of various retrograde changes.

INNERVATION OF TUMOR TISSUE

Up to the present little attention has been given to the possible innervation of tumors. Since the ordinary histologic methods fail to reveal nerve tissue in tumors, it has been generally accepted that neoplasms are devoid of nerves.

The recent work of Oertel in this regard is interesting and suggestive. By a modification of the Bielschowsky stain for nerves he was able to demonstrate what he considered to be nerves in several forms of carcinoma and sarcoma. The material represented well-developed tumors of man, and the nerves were found to constitute a definitely connected system, with equally definite relations to the parenchyma of the tumor, blood vessels, and stroma, in which could be recognized some resemblance to the innervation of normal tissues.

The significance of the presence of nerves in the make-up of a tumor must, for the present, remain problematic, since information on this phase of structure is limited and somewhat contradictory. Whether the nerves which may be present, function in a trophic capacity or simply represent a secondary accompaniment which follows the carcinoma cells cannot be definitely stated at this time. Although the morphologic studies of Oertel indicate a specific physiologic rôle for these fibers, the observations of Herzog support the latter view. Herzog studied approximately 100 cases of benign and malignant tumors also using a modification of Bielschowsky's method. He found that most of the tumors possessed nerve structures provided that the tumors were not circumscribed or encapsulated, and that nerves were a natural constituent of the tissues into which the tumors were growing. If the tumors were primary, and were strictly limited in their infiltrative propensities, nerves were consistently absent. The same was true of metastasis from the circumscribed tumor. Although Herzog's observations would indicate that neoplasms can grow without specific innervation, the entire subject concerning the innervation of tumors is worthy of continued study, and much more information will be necessary before the exact status of the question is established.

GROWTH

Cell multiplication.—In many rapidly growing tumors indirect division of the cells can often be seen. If the growth is extremely vigorous, many mitotic figures depicting different phases of the phenomenon, may occur in a single field and occasionally multiple mitosis takes place. The nuclear material always is basophilic, and, as a consequence, nuclei undergoing this change appear larger than the nondividing forms. In some rapidly growing tumors mitosis is so abundant, and the dividing cells so large, as to render them clearly visible under low magnification.

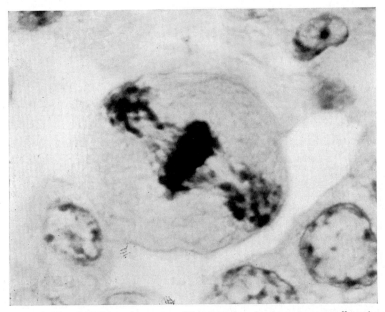

Fig. 3.—Mitotic division of a cancer cell in a lymph node of a squamous-cell carcinoma of the bovine. The division is in the metaphase stage with the chromosomes lying in a single plane to form the so-called equatorial plate. The spindle fibers have a lateral attachment and indistinctly connect with the opposite spindle poles. The strongly basophilic staining reaction is characteristic of this phase of the phenomenon ($\times$ 2,000).

Usually the middle power (high dry) of the microscope is necessary to see and study mitotic figures satisfactorily. It is in this phase of the study of tumors that one must exhibit patience and persistence, for in some material a mitotic figure is found only after long and diligent search (Fig. 3).

Although mitosis is usually one of the characteristics of a malignant lesion and a valuable aid in distinguishing between fibroma and fibrosarcoma, or between adenoma and adenocarcinoma, one should not put absolute dependence on its presence or absence. Mitosis is commonly seen in excessively proliferating granulation tissue (keloid), and is often the cause of error in calling such formations malignant tumors. Experience teaches that one must consider all phases of a given case. The history and clinical data are extremely important and must be given equal weight with the microscopic data before a diagnosis is made. Again, in some tumors that are clinically unmistakably malignant, it may be extremely difficult to demonstrate mitosis. Yet, from the type cell and its relation to the stroma, together with its attitude

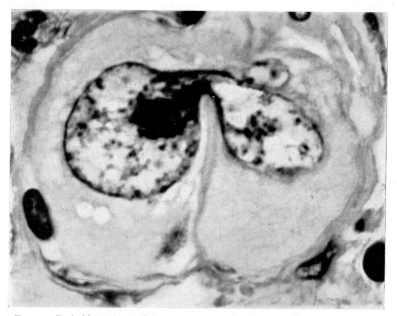

Fig. 4.—Probable amitotic division in a case of squamous-cell carcinoma of an ox. The hour-glass shape of the nuclear mass and the dividing membrane incompletely separating the cytosome may be noted (× 2,000).

toward the adjacent tissue, one cannot help being impressed by an aggressiveness suggestive of malignancy.

In certain malignant tumors, more particularly carcinomas, infrequently cells are seen which appear to be undergoing direct division or amitosis (Fig. 4). The cells of such a tumor are usually large and irregular. Many possess two or more distinct nuclei, each complete with a nucleolus. Some of them can be seen sending out protoplasmic prolongations, which will become separate cells, but which as yet are incompletely separated from the parent cell. Many of the cells have a vacuolated cytoplasm, and hyaline droplets may be present.

The exact significance of amitotic division of tumors is not clear. My opinion is that this process represents a desperate effort to reproduce on the part of cells which are gradually being overtaken by retrogressive influences. Since it seems to be a rare phenomenon for direct division of the nucleus to be followed by severance of the cytoplasm, it is improbable that this method of cellular division contributes appreciably to multiplication of cells in neoplasms.

Gross development.—Tumors increase in size by multiplication of their own cells. "Like begets like," and tumor cells of one variety are never transformed into cells of a different variety. The growth of a

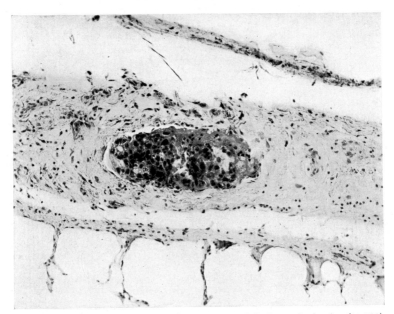

Fig. 5.—Carcinomatous cells in pleural lymphatic of the lung of a bovine ($\times$ 130).

tumor may be very slow, so that a small nodule is years in developing, or it may be so rapid as to produce huge masses within a comparatively short time. Most of the slow-growing tumors enlarge expansively and encroach on the surrounding tissues, causing pressure which is distributed along the line of contact. Rapidly growing tumors, such as many of the carcinomas, infiltrate the adjacent tissue and push their way into and along blood and lymph channels and into preëxisting cavities, usually following the line of least resistance. Growth may continue until the tumor weighs more than its host, and the individual, because of the size of the tumor, may find it difficult or impossible to move about. As a rule, the more rapidly a tumor grows the more dangerous it is. The more slowly growing tumors frequently become encapsulated by layers of fibrous tissue, but the more aggressive forms discourage encapsulation by the speed of their growth and their invasive character; fibrous tissue and even bone yield to their advances.

Mode of direct extension of tumors.—Simple benign tumors seldom extend beyond the immediate zone of their origin. Of the malignant types, however, the contrary is true, and columns or groups, or even single cells, may be seen pushing into the adjacent tissues, and into the lymph or blood channels, in a menacing manner (Fig. 5). Although the invaded channels and spaces may become occluded by solid cords of

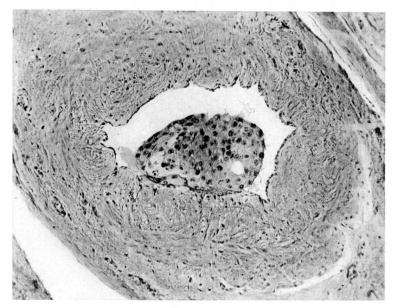

FIG. 6.—An accumulation of cancer cells within the lumen of a blood vessel of a bovine (× 130).

tumor cells, growth continues, and new foci, which are constantly enlarging, are common. Tumors may also extend along mucous and serous surfaces by continuity, where they are usually adherent to the underlying tissues. For the most part, sarcomas extend by way of the blood vessels and lymphatic vessels, whereas carcinomas extend most frequently by means of the lymph channels, and only occasionally through the blood vessels (Fig. 6).

REACTION OF THE BODY TO GROWTH OF TUMORS

In most instances the presence of tumor cells initiates a reaction on the part of the adjacent, nontumorous elements. The intensity of the reaction varies, and is dependent on various factors, the most important of which are the type of neoplasm, the nature of the tissue containing the growth, and the inherent weakness or resistance of the tissues to neoplastic growth. Neoplasms of pronounced malignancy, with an excessive capacity for growth, seem to overwhelm the visible protective elements of the body, and complete their destruction with the greatest dispatch. This is well exemplified by certain lymphoblastomas of dogs, cattle, and fowls, which rapidly institute widespread generalization, and death occurs within a comparatively short time.

The cells of some tumors recognize no barriers to their advancing movements; they are seen invading and destroying skin, muscle, and even bone with equal facility. The natural protective agencies of the body are wholly inadequate to provide sufficient inhibitory influences noticeably to impede the progress of such tumors, and they continue their career of wild growth and destruction practically unopposed, so far as can be judged by the usual evidence of resistance of tissue.

In most cases of tumor there is a definite reaction on the part of the surrounding tissue. Here, as in many other situations in which the normal tissues are being encroached on, and are in need of a protective substance, fibrous connective tissue is often utilized in an attempt to wall off the advancing tumorous elements. If the neoplasm grows slowly, complete encapsulation by connective tissue frequently occurs. This has the result of localizing the deleterious effects of the presence of the tumor. Many of the benign tumors of the soft tissues become encapsulated early. Even in an occasional carcinoma the fibrous stroma may outgrow the parenchyma and so encroach on it as to cause atrophy and complete regression. In most malignant tumors, however, the reverse is true, and the fibrous elements are usually reduced to a minimum, sufficient only for a stroma, and encapsulation does not occur.

Eosinophilic leukocytes are present in many tumors. They may vary in quantity from one to 100 or more in a microscopic field. The exact part these cells play in the reaction against tumor is not fully understood, although it is generally believed that they are related to the protective or inhibitory mechanism. Pavlovsky and Widakowich have expressed the belief that they exert a definite disintegrating influence on the tumor cells, in a manner similar to the action of phagocytes against bacteria. The presence of eosinophiles in tumors is explained by Battaglia on the basis of a positive chemotactic substance which is the product of the tumor cells. Battaglia, as a result of an experimental study, concluded that the eosinophilia of malignant tumors is to be regarded as a defensive measure against the excessive production of lactic acid produced by the cells of some tumors.

Lymphocytes and endothelial leukocytes may likewise be attracted to the site of tumor, and the presence of such cells at the periphery of the growth is considered by some observers as evidence of lessened vitality on the part of the neoplastic elements (Fig. 7).

The significance of the lymphocyte in the resistance of the body to neoplastic growth has long remained controversial, and much experimental work has been done in an attempt to solve the problem; the work of Murphy and Morton has been of particular importance.   By

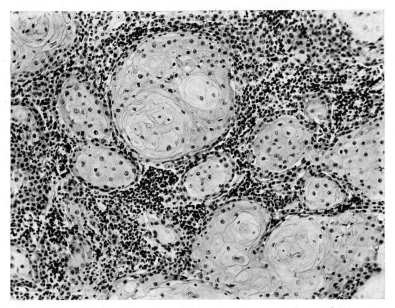

FIG. 7.—Leukocytic infiltration of an epidermoid carcinoma of the membrana nictitans of a bovine (× 120).

injecting defibrinated blood of mice into ten mice preliminary to their inoculation with transplantable carcinoma, a resistant state, accompanied by marked lymphocytosis, was induced; the mice were accorded 100 per cent protection.   In the ten control mice lymphocytosis was absent, and the grafts were successful in 60 per cent.

Knowing that repeated small doses of roentgen rays destroy the lymphoid system of the mouse, Murphy and Morton reasoned that if the lymphocyte is an essential part of the protective mechanism its destruction should be accompanied by loss of immunity.   In an attempt to demonstrate this hypothesis twenty mice were given injections of defibrinated blood, and ten of these were subjected to successive exposures to roentgen rays. Studies of the blood revealed marked reduction in the circulating lymphocytes following exposure to the roentgen rays. All the mice were then inoculated with transplantable mouse carcinoma as were ten additional normal mice, as controls. The same number of successful takes was noted in those injected with defibrinated blood and exposed to roentgen rays, as in the control mice. This experiment seemed to indicate that by preventing the usual lymphoid reaction, the immunity that would otherwise have existed was abolished.

Contradictory to the evidence supporting lymphocytic immunity to neoplasia, the observations of Sittenfield[25, 26] must be considered. At the conclusion of a series of experiments with rats inoculated with the Flexner-Jobling carcinoma he was convinced that "neither the increase nor reduction of the lymphoid elements in the blood has any influence on either resistance or susceptibility to tumor growth."

Wood[30, 31] has been foremost among those who are opposed to the theory of lymphocytic inhibition of tumors. On the basis of extensive experimental studies he concluded that "the lymphocyte is in no way correlated with cancer immunity." He mentions metastasis of tumor cells to lymph nodes as of much significance in refuting the contention that lymphocytes are particularly antagonistic to neoplastic growths. His conclusions were drawn from the following experimental results:

Mice with lymphatic leukemia or high leukocyte count did not appear to be immune to tumor.

A preliminary reduction of the total leukocyte count was produced by the roentgen rays or by radium, but it was impossible to demonstrate an increase in the percentage of takes of normal thyroid grafts.

Attempts were made to increase the growth potentiality of a slow-growing fibrosarcoma of the guinea pig by destroying the lymphocytes by roentgen rays before and after inoculation of the tumor, the site of the tumor being protected by lead. No increase in the number of takes was noted.

An immune strain of rats was treated by roentgen rays, but no change in the susceptibility was observed.

Half of a series of animals possessing transplanted tumors were treated by roentgen rays, and the other half remained untreated; no difference could be observed between the two groups.

Obviously, such contradictory views lead one into a dilemma and make it extremely difficult to obtain from the experimental facts presented, a definite understanding of the question. However, the small number of animals used in Murphy and Morton's work furnishes a basis for the most serious criticism; moreover, their work was done largely with animals of one variety. Wood's conclusions, on the other hand, were based on an experimental series consisting of thousands of animals, and several different varieties of tumors were used.

After examining the evidence propounded by Murphy and Morton, and others in support of the hypothesis that lymphocytes have a part in resistance to tumor, Woglom was disinclined to say that the lymphocyte was without immunologic significance. Although unwilling to accept Murphy and Morton's conclusions in their entirety, Woglom, nevertheless, felt that "there is something to be said for the lymphocyte." He felt that any resistance extended by the lymphocyte for carcinoma cells might possibly be dependent on some connecting factor between the lymphocyte and the neoplastic cells, the exact nature of which is unknown.

MacCarty,[18-20] from data obtained from a large amount of clinical material from human sources, found that patients having tumors in which there was lymphocytic infiltration lived longer after operation, on an average, than those having tumors in which there was no lymphocytic infiltration. MacCarty also stressed the importance of differentiation, fibrosis, and hyalinization in the phenomena of resistance to neoplasia. On the other hand, Lacassagne has objected to such interpretation concerning the presence of leukocytic infiltration in the tissues adjacent to tumors. He suggested that such infiltrations might indicate a local inflammatory condition which antedated the tumor, and he mentioned, in support of this, the absence of similar infiltrations in metastatic foci. He also directed attention to the susceptibility of certain tumor cells to spontaneous necrobiosis, and under such conditions local leukocytic infiltration is a physiologic phenomenon.

The suggestion that the presence of one tumor protects against another tumor, by virtue of the presence of immune substances elaborated by the first, cannot be accorded much substantiation. The incidence of multiple primary neoplasms in certain species tends to make such a hypothesis untenable. The failure of such immunity to be established is offered by some as added proof against the infectious origin of neoplasia.

However, in contradiction to the general denial of the production of immunity by tumors, the observations of Beebe on venereal or transmissible lymphosarcoma of dogs is of interest. He noticed that a few dogs recovered spontaneously from the tumor and were then immune to further implantation of a tumor of like virulence. Beebe also noted evidence that the blood of an immune dog confers passive immunity on a susceptible animal. It seems unusual that such reactions should be peculiar to this particular tumor only. Wade, in studying this variety of lymphosarcoma of dogs, noted that their development was accompanied by increase of lymphocytes in the blood.

Failure successfully to transplant a tumor from one species to another might be considered additional evidence that the tissues possessed a certain refractory or protective substance. Whatever their nature may be it has long been known that heterogeneous transplants usually fail by virtue of inability of the transplanted cells to adapt themselves to an unfavorable environment. This, however, is not peculiar to neoplastic cells, but is generally true of cells from normal tissues, of which it is extremely difficult to obtain transplantation takes even in the same animal, or in another animal of the same species. Since this obtains for practically all nonneoplastic tissues, it is not surprising that tumor cells, with few exceptions, fail to proliferate when artificially transferred from their point of origin.

Woglom, after a critical review of the entire subject of bodily resistance to transplantable tumors, concluded in part as follows: "Immunity to transplantable tumors is a generalized refractory condition which appears to be entirely unrelated to other forms of immunity. No single organ has yet been proved responsible for its elaboration, nor is it affected by physiological conditions such as age or pregnancy."

GROSS APPEARANCE OF TUMORS

Although no two tumors are ever exactly alike, there are a few features possessed in common by tumors of the same type and by these features the experienced observer often can classify a given specimen with a fair degree of accuracy. If the clinical history reveals the origin of the growth it is not difficult in many cases to correlate these facts with the gross appearance, and to arrive at a correct diagnosis.

Size.—This is one of the most variable characteristics of tumor, and is dependent on a number of factors, such as position, blood supply, type of tumor, rate of growth, and duration of the disease. A tumor may vary from a microscopic focus of cells up to a mass larger than the host. Jordan described an ovarian tumor weighing 370 pounds which was found in an old cow at slaughter.

Hewitt mentioned a tumor weighing 106 pounds which involved and completely surrounded the kidney of a mare. Barthold observed a 66-pound tumor of the kidney in a hog. In experimental studies with mice it is not uncommon for tumors to become so huge as to make it difficult for the mice to move, and the growth may actually weigh more than the mouse.

External tumors are seldom permitted to attain maximal size, and because of early recognition and early removal, extremely large tumors are less frequently seen than formerly. Internal tumors are rather inaccessible, are usually inoperable in lower animals, and sometimes become very large. On the average, however, tumors of animals vary in size from nodules a few centimeters in diameter, and weigh from a few to several ounces, up to masses weighing several pounds. Extremely large specimens are rare. The size of many diffusely growing tumors is difficult to determine with accuracy, due to irregularity of shape and the intimate manner by which they are attached to the surrounding tissues.

Shape.—Most tumors assume an irregular, nodular shape, but no two are ever identical in this respect. Occasionally they are flattened; others are almost spherical. As a rule, the benign, encapsulated and pedunculated tumors are inclined to be nodular or spherical, whereas those that proliferate rapidly and are invasive, are often practically shapeless and difficult to describe.

Color.—The color of tumors varies considerably and is dependent on a number of factors, such as blood supply, type cell, pigment, and fluid content. Extremely vascular tumors are likely to have a bloody color, whereas those with a minimal amount of blood usually appear pale and blanched. Most nodules are grayish-white, and when present in the kidney, liver, or lung they appear in sharp contrast to the surrounding tissue. Tumors of the liver are frequently greenish-yellow, due to bile pigment, and pigmented melanoblastomas are easily recognized by their dark brown or black color, that is due to the melanin produced by their cells. Lipomas are dirty white to yellow; the surface of suppurating tumors may be greenish-yellow to black, owing to the type of bacteria present and to the amount of coagulated blood present. Tumors of the adrenal gland are usually yellow, and malignant lymphoblastomas are often pinkish-gray. Many large carcinomas, particularly those of the squamous cell variety, often exhibit irregular yellowish areas, indicating the presence of necrosis.

Consistence.—This is another characteristic that is extremely variable, and that depends on the type of tumor and the relative proportions of stroma and parenchyma. Ordinarily, the more abundant the stroma the firmer the growth; on the other hand, highly cellular tumors, with a minimal amount of stroma, usually are soft to the touch and of a delicate consistence. The presence of secondary changes, such as calcification and hyalinization, makes for denseness, and tumors that have undergone amyloid degeneration are much firmer than similar tumors without this substance. As a rule malignant tumors are softer than benign tumors, and although the tissue in a malignant growth may be closely knit, it is often soft and friable. Naturally the histologic character of the tumor has some influence on its consistence, and a chondroma or an osteoma will, of course, be much firmer than a fibroma or a rapidly growing carcinoma. Tumorous tissue undergoing necrosis is always of a soft, friable character, and the presence of much fluid often exerts a "water soaked" effect on the tissue.

SPECIAL PROPERTIES OF TUMORS

Recurrence.—One of the characteristics of many tumors is their capacity to recur after surgical removal. The only tenable explanation of such recurrence is that all the neoplastic cells were not removed, and the remaining ones served as a focus of growth for the recurring mass. Many difficulties stand in the way of complete removal of all the cells of a tumor, and one should not be overly critical of the surgeon who fails in this regard. Especially difficult is it to affect complete removal of an infiltrating growth. Here the cells are likely to permeate the adjacent tissues in every direction, and even to invade the lymphatic structures in such an intricate fashion as to make it impossible to completely extirpate the cells.

Whereas, the earlier operation is performed the less likelihood there is of recurrence, yet clinical experience has taught that occasionally a tumor will recur even though radical operation is performed almost immediately after the growth is discovered. This fact emphasizes the hopelessness in some cases of malignant tumor, and justifies the use of radium and roentgen rays following the operation. Unfortunately the use of these agents has not received the attention from veterinarians that their usefulness warrants. Little is among the few who have appreciated their effectiveness in the treatment of selected cases. If the animal is valuable enough to warrant the necessary expense, the veterinarian who does not embrace these newer forms of treatment is denying his patient the benefits of remedial measures that are frequently efficacious. Of course, few practicing veterinarians are equipped to administer radium or roentgen rays, and the development and practice of this form of treatment must remain for the time being with those who possess or can secure the necessary equipment.

Another factor in recurrence, that should be recognized, is the possibility of transplantation occurring when loose neoplastic cells are permitted to fall into the fruitful soil of the wound during manipulation incidental to operation.

The possibility of recurrence of malignant growths is far greater than the possibility of recurrence of benign growths. In fact, it is only occasionally that a benign growth is observed to recur. Many benign growths are encapsulated, and because of this the tumor cells find it difficult to infiltrate the surrounding tissue to any extent. If such a tumor is removed, with the capsule intact, the chance of recurrence is slight.

The recurrent tumors are, as a rule, more aggressive than the original growths, and what may have been a small, innocent swelling before the operation, may recur with all the vicious destructiveness characteristic of marked malignancy. Most of the recurrent tumors have the same general histopathologic characteristics as the parent growth, and usually develop in the wound or in the tissue immediately adjacent to it.

Metastasis.—The appearance of metastatic tumors at a distance from the primary tumor is a frequent sequel of many malignant growths. This capacity to grow in situations entirely foreign to the initial growth is one of the most feared features of malignant tumor, and results from the transference of cells from the primary growth, through the blood or lymphatic vessels, or over the membranous surfaces, to secondary sites favorable to their growth (Fig. 8).

The different kinds of tumors favor certain routes for their metastatic movements. Carcinomas extend most commonly by way of the lymphatic structures, and infrequently by way of the blood vessels. Lymphoblastomas also frequently become distributed by way of the lymphatic channels, which may be due to the fact that they probably originate from lymphoid tissue. Lymphoblastomas also metastasize by the blood stream; Ewing remarked that certain forms of lymphoblastoma, when spread by the blood "yield the most abundant and widely disseminated metastasis seen with any type of neoplasm." This is well illustrated in certain cases of lymphoblastoma of cattle.

The other sarcomas usually travel by way of the blood vessels; the lymphatic channels are comparatively immune to their invasive attacks. The frequency of invasion of the blood stream by sarcomas can be accounted for, I believe, by the intimate relationship of the vessels to the parenchyma in this type of neoplasm. In many highly cellular, rapidly growing sarcomas, it is difficult, if not impossible, to demonstrate tissues separating the blood cells and the tumor cells. I have seen sarcomas in which large "lakes" of blood were in direct contact with the cells of the tumor for a considerable extent. With such a relationship it is not surprising that metastasis by the blood stream should occur.

In human beings dissemination of tumor cells over the peritoneal serosa and the pleural surfaces is sometimes observed, but such a condition is rarely described in veterinary literature. I have observed, however, in several cases of adenocarcinoma of the intestine of chickens, wide dissemination of tumorous nodules over both the parietal and visceral serosa, the occurrence of which could be explained only on the basis of spread of the tumor cells over the surface of the peritoneal membranes. Similar metastasis often occurs from carcinoma of the ovary

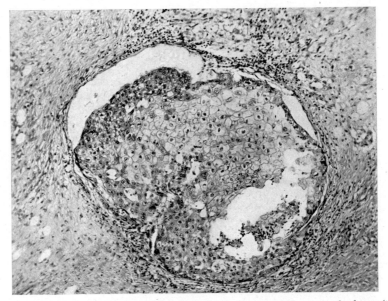

Fig. 8.—Tumor cells occupying a blood channel. Carcinoma of the penis of a horse (× 100).

and from the adrenal gland in the bovine. In man a number of instances of extension of tumor by way of the thoracic duct have been described. This usually results in generalized metastasis by way of the blood and lymph channels. In the majority of such cases, the growth has been carcinoma, the invasion usually coming from tumors of the stomach and uterus.

Of the cells which enter the blood or lymph stream from a tumor, not all survive. Their exact fate is not known, but undoubtedly many are disposed of as other foreign material which may by chance enter these channels. In the blood spaces the cells are carried along to a point at which they are larger than the lumina of the vessels, and if conditions are favorable they may divide and start a focus of growth which may be extended for considerable distance along the interior of the vessels. Within the lymphatic channels they find their way to lymph nodes, where their growth and multiplication may obliterate the lymphoid tissue entirely, and may often form swellings as large as or larger than the primary lesion. From the involved lymph nodes, further metastasis to other nodes and organs may result, and generalization is not uncommon (Fig. 9). Malignant cells possess a certain restlessness favorable to a migratory existence, and it is not unusual for a secondary focus of tumor cells within an organ to give rise to further metastasis in other

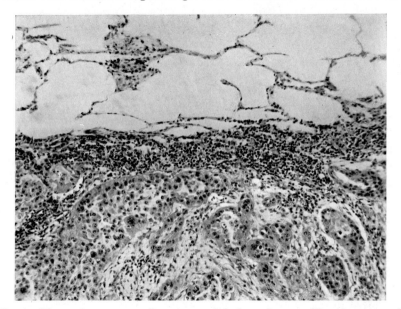

Fig. 9.—Metastatic squamous-cell carcinoma of the lung of a cow. The primary growth was in the eye (× 100).

organs and parts. Metastasis may occur soon or late in the course of the disease, the rapidity varying with the different kinds of tumors and with individual differences in tumors of the same general type. For instance, some external carcinomas may attain considerable size and may be very destructive locally, but show little, if any, tendency to metastasize; in others, metastasis may result so early that the secondary tumor will be of considerable size when the primary tumor is discovered.

Malignancy.—From the standpoint of their clinical behavior and microscopic anatomy, tumors can be classified as benign or malignant. The determination of malignancy, however, often calls for all the knowledge that can be assembled in the case at hand. Not only must one be

4

thoroughly familiar with the miscroscopic appearance of tumors, but one should assemble as many of the clinical facts as possible before venturing a prognosis.

Clinically, there is a sharp distinction between various kinds of tumors, based on their ability to endanger the life of their host. Some persist as more or less harmless nodules, disfiguring and troublesome perhaps, due to their size and position, but growing slowly, and with no tendency toward actually menacing life by infiltrating the surrounding tissue or extending to vital parts by metastasis. Malignancy is usually revealed by one or all of the following features: (1) Rapidity of growth; (2) ability to infiltrate and destroy the adjacent tissue, and (3) development of metastasis.

It is obvious that all of these features cannot be determined by the study of one, or even of several microscopic sections from the primary growth. Careful examination of all clinical aspects is essential, if logical and proper conclusions are to be reached.

Rapidity of growth is best determined by microscopic examination of the tumorous tissue. Cells of a malignant tumor present certain abnormalities that aid materially in estimating their propensities for growth. Mitosis has long been considered of value in this regard; the more malignant forms show abundant and even multiple mitosis. The appearance of the cells themselves is important, and one can usually see marked differences between adult and immature forms. In the rapidly growing tumors, as a rule, are the most immature types of cells. The immature cells are inclined to be larger than the more adult forms, and their nuclei usually contain an excessive amount of chromatin, as a consequence of which they stain intensely. Conspicuous nucleoli are often present. A minimal amount of supportive stroma also characterizes the more malignant forms of neoplasm. Again, the more the tumor cells differ from the parent tissue from which they arise, the greater is their potential malignancy.

Infiltrating tumors are seldom encapsulated, and although I have seen several malignant tumors that were encapsulated, the majority of them are not. Infiltrating tumors do not "shell out" at operation but must be dissected away, often with considerable difficulty. Many possess more or less irregular margins and a like irregular destruction of the invaded tissue. Microscopically, the infiltrating tumor cells can be seen pushing along sinuses; crowding out and destroying normal tissue, and, in general, presenting an unrestrained, anarchistic type of growth (Fig. 10).

Metastasis may be so evident as to constitute the most striking feature of many cases of malignant disease, as in generalized malignant lymphoblastoma, or the evidence may be so slight as to render the microscope necessary for its demonstration. However, metastasis is the one unfailing criterion of malignancy. One may be mistaken in the diagnosis of the primary growth, and may consider a given tumor benign, but if metastatic foci appear, any other diagnosis than malignancy would be untenable. Finally, there can be no hard and fast differences between many benign and malignant growths, for there are unquestionably borderline forms. Some are definitely malignant but positiveness of

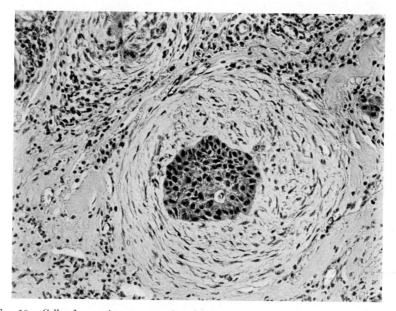

FIG. 10.—Cells of a carcinoma occupying the central portion of a nerve in the eye of a bovine (× 160).

diagnosis should be avoided with regard to others. Particularly is this true if opinion is based on histologic examination only.

Multiple primary tumors in the same individual.—In an animal of advanced age, and particularly in an old dog, it is not uncommon to observe two or more primary heterogenous neoplasms. Betke reported a fibromyoma of the uterus and two large papillary adenocarcinomas in the mucosa of the cervix of a captive wild rhinoceros aged forty years. Fox mentioned a jaguar with fibro-adenoma of the uterus, fibro-adenoma of the bile ducts, and lymphangioma of the mesentery.

Multiple neoplasms appear to be the rule among old dogs. Goodpasture in a study of fifty old dogs found 228 tumors of which 215 were

benign and thirteen were malignant.   Cohrs, in a series of 737 postmortem examinations of dogs, found tumors in seventy; two or more
primary tumors were present in twenty-six.   All but one of these dogs
were aged more than ten years, thus emphasizing the influence of age.
In one of Cohr's cases, that of a dachshund fourteen years old, eleven
neoplasms, several of which were malignant, were found.   In one of my
cases, that of a shepherd dog thirteen years old the following tumors
were found: Recurrent squamous-cell carcinoma of the mouth, with
metastasis to the submaxillary lymph nodes, hemangioma of the liver,
leiomyosarcoma of the cecum, tumor of the interstitial cells of the testis,

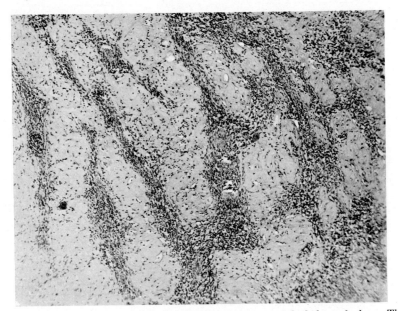

Fig. 11.—Hyalinized collagen areas in embryonal tumor of the kidney of a hog.   The
excessive retrogression has markedly reduced the amount of the tumor's parenchyma
($\times$ 90).

and papillary cystadenoma of the prostate gland.   Multiple lympho-
matous nodules were also present in the spleen.[9]

It has been suggested that with the advent of senility the various
cells are more prone to unrestrained growth, and that many true tumors
develop as a consequence.   However, the reason for this is not clearly
understood.   The hypothesis of Goodpasture, that cells which have
been injured because of old age and have, as a consequence, lost spe-
cificity and assumed increased power of growth, likewise appears insufficient to explain such widespread tendencies toward tumorous
proliferation.

The general occurrence of multiple primary neoplasms among old dogs would suggest the possibility of the existence of a similar tendency among the other species of domestic animals. However, of the domestic animals, the dog is the only one which is generally permitted to attain what might be considered old age. The majority of the others are killed at a comparatively early age for food, and thus prevent the development of tumors.

The predilection for the formation of multiple tumors in old age suggests that every animal has within its tissues the latent possibility

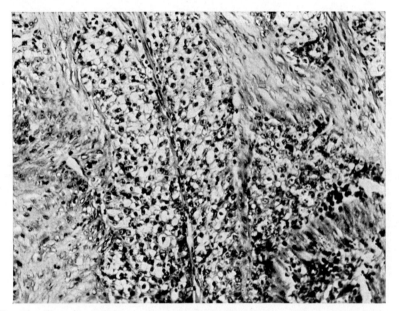

Fig. 12.—Retrogressive changes in a squamous-cell carcinoma of the prepuce of a horse (× 180).

of self-destruction if sufficient age is attained to permit neoplasms to develop.

Retrogressive changes.—Tumors are susceptible to the same retrograde influences as normal tissue, and within them extensive necrosis, calcification, accumulation of fat, hemorrhages, and occasionally amyloid degeneration are commonly seen. I have found amyloid in a lymphoma from the lumbar region of a bovine and have also observed hyaline degeneration of the stroma of connective tissue mentioned by Mallory. Atrophy of the parenchyma is common in some tumors because of overproduction of the fibrous stroma (Fig. 11).

The individual tumor cells are subject to many regressive changes,

such as hyaline and fatty degeneration; the latter is commonly observed
in squamous-cell carcinoma (Fig. 12).   I have seen extensive colloid
degeneration in an adenocarcinoma resembling the thyroid gland from
the neck of a bovine.

Necrosis of tumors is frequently associated with suppuration, and
is the result of a number of causes such as trauma, infection, and lack of
nutrition.   The loss of blood supply to a part of a tumor often results in
a lesion similar to an infarct.   Pedunculated tumors are likely to suffer
a twist, as a consequence of which the blood supply may be entirely cut
off.   The cells of a rapidly growing carcinoma commonly outstrip the

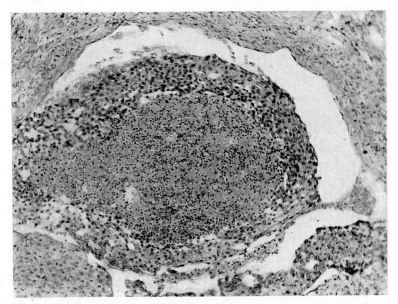

Fig. 13.—Caseation necrosis of a squamous-cell carcinoma of the penis of a horse (× 100).

stroma containing the blood channels, and death of portions of the
tumor ensues (Fig. 13).   Hydrops may occur both in the parenchyma and
in the stroma of tumors.   According to Ewing this is most likely to
occur in a tumor the cells of which are more or less constantly bathed
in fluids.   In some specimens an excess of serous fluid between rows or
strands of tumor cells may so modify the morphology that the growth
resembles an angiomatous structure.   If the neoplasm encroaches on
blood vessels, or interferes with the elimination of urine, marked edematous infiltration of the tumor and of the adjacent structures may ensue.
This is particularly noticeable in tumors of the lungs and of the kidneys
(Figs. 14 and 15).

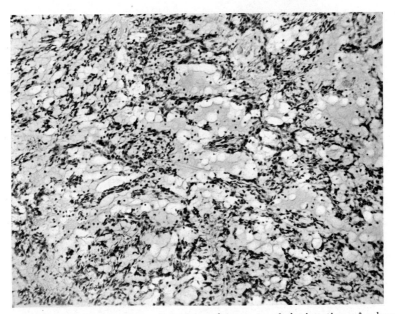

FIG. 14.—Excessive accumulation of fluid in a leiomyoma of the intestines of a horse (× 120).

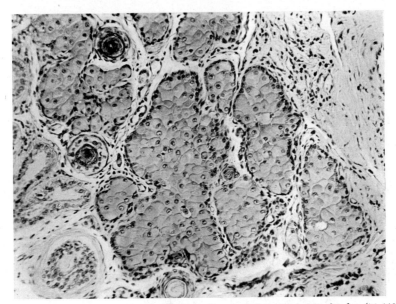

FIG. 15.—Swollen cells in a squamous-cell carcinoma of the anal region of a dog (× 440).

Hemorrhage is often profuse, and the dried, dark, clot which may appear on the surface may cause one to mistake a nonpigmented tumor for a pigmented one. Following hemorrhage within the substance of the tumor, the usual hemic by-products, such as hemoglobin, hematoidin, and hemosiderin are likely to be found. Hemosiderin, the product of cellular activity, is usually found within endothelial leukocytes.

The various inflammatory reactions are noted to occur in tumors, and serous exudation, leukocytic infiltration, and congestion may appear to such a degree as to obscure the cells of the tumor. Among the leukocytes commonly seen are polymorphonuclears, particularly in surface ulcerations, lymphocytes, and eosinophils. Eosinophils are sometimes present in such numbers as to constitute a considerable

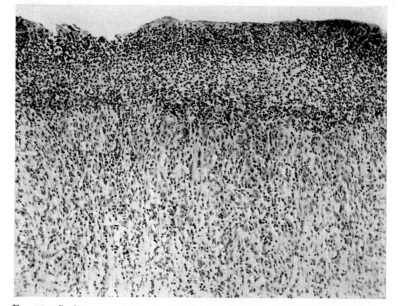

Fig. 16.—Surface zone of infection. Fibroma of the glans penis of a bull (× 100).

part of the microscopic picture, but as a rule only an occasional one is seen. Giant cells are not infrequently present.

Ulceration is common in tumors of the skin and mucous membranes, especially in carcinomas. In fact it is very uncommon to find carcinoma of the penis of a horse or of the eye of a bovine or equine that is not ulcerated to some degree. The ulceration usually results from trauma and the entrance of pyogenic bacteria. Suppuration soon follows, and the tumor becomes repulsive in appearance and odor (Fig. 16).

Pathologists hold that the onset of ulceration frequently transforms a relatively benign tumor into a dangerously malignant process because of toxic absorption, and general infection. However, evidence of this is seldom seen in lower animals, perhaps because of the early destruction of animals affected with hopelessly inoperable malignant growths.

Effects on the host.—Tumors vary greatly in their effect on the animal organism, and there are even considerable differences in the effect of the same type of tumor in different organisms and tissues. This would suggest that relative immunity is possessed by certain individuals and tissues and possibly that others lack it. As a rule the effect of tumors depends first on the type or kind, and second on the site of the growth, with the assumption that the rapidity and nature of the growth, whether infiltrative or encapsulated, and the occurrence of metastasis, are all important factors.

Benign tumors produce their effect largely by mechanical interference with function; the more vital the part involved, the more serious the interference. As an example of the relative significance of position, one may compare a simple fibroma of the shoulder or neck with a tumor of the heart or lungs. The tumor of the neck or shoulder may at times prove annoying and perhaps disfiguring but it would not menace life as do the tumors situated in vital tissues. It might be said that a histologically benign tumor in a vital situation is more dangerous to life than a histologically malignant growth in a position of relatively less importance to the host. Also, malignant tumor cells may affect the body directly, by infiltrating and destroying normal tissue. It is this fact, together with the capacity of malignant tumors to metastasize, that makes malignant tumors as a class potentially more dangerous than benign tumors.

Many of the retrograde changes of tumors also have an indirect bearing on the affected individual, and, if ulceration is associated with necrosis and suppuration, toxic absorption and even septicemia may result. Then again, fatal hemorrhage may result from a tumor's presence. Chickens suffering from lymphocytoma frequently die suddenly, due to rupture of the liver as a consequence of the increased friability of the organ and the increased pressure exerted by the tumor. Rupture of cysts, and even abscesses, may occur; these are serious or not, depending on the character of the evacuated material and the anatomic situation.

In man the emaciation accompanying the growth of tumor is often a striking and significant feature, and is thought to be due chiefly to inanition. The starvation is attributed to lowering of the digestive capacity, psychic influences, and interference with nutrition combined with the action of toxic products derived from degenerating portions that may or may not be infected. In man a neoplastic disease, if inoperable, is permitted to run its course so that the full measure of such influences becomes evident. If, however, the disease of animals is inoperable, they are usually killed, and, as a result, cachexia from tumors is seldom seen in animals. Again it is possible that animals are spared the mental depression and other psychic disturbances that so much influence the human sufferer affected with neoplasms.

Animals with malignant tumors usually tire more easily and fail to show the ordinary vitality common to the normal animal. A universal dislike for food does not appear to obtain in animals suffering from tumor, unless it involves the digestive tract.

BIBLIOGRAPHY

1. Barthold, E. W.: Quoted by Feldman, W. H.: A study of the histopathology of the so-called adenosarcoma of swine. Am. Jour. Path., **4**: 125–138 (March), 1928.

2. Battaglia, F.: Sul significato dell eosinofilia locale nei tumori malign. Tumori, **13**: 191–208, 1917.

3. Beebe, S. P.: The growth of lymphosarcoma in dogs: Summary of recent observations. Jour. Am. Med. Assn., **49**: 1492–1493 (Nov. 2), 1907.

4. Betke, R.: Multiple Tumoren bei einem Nashorn. Frankfurter Ztschr. f. Path., **6**: 19–26, 1911.

5. Broders, A. C.: The grading of carcinoma. Minnesota Med., **8**: 726–730 (Dec.), 1925.

6. Cohrs, Paul: Über primäre Multiplizität von Geschwülsten bei Haustieren. Ztschr. f. Krebsforsch., **24**: 156–221, 1927.

7. Ewing, James: Neoplastic diseases. Ed. 3. Philadelphia, W. B. Saunders Co., 1928, pp. 44 and 82.

8. Feldman, W. H.: An adenocarcinoma resembling the thyroid gland. Am. Jour. Path., **1**: 281–284 (May), 1925.

9. Feldman, W. H.: Multiple primary neoplasms in lower animals; report of a case. Am. Jour. Path., **4**: 497–506 (Sept.), 1928.

10. Fox, Herbert: Disease in captive wild mammals and birds: incidence, description, comparison. Philadelphia, J. B. Lippincott Co., 1923, p. 478.

11. Goodpasture, E. W.: An anatomical study of senescence in dogs, with especial reference to the relation of cellular changes of age to tumors. Jour. Med. Res., **38**: 127–190 (May), 1918.

12. Herzog, Ernst: Beitrag zur Frage der Innervation der Geschülste. Arch. f. Path. Anat. u. Physiol., **268**: 536–565, 1928.

13. Hewitt, S. J.: Enormous tumor of a horse. Abstract. Am. Vet. Rev., **42**: 568 (Feb.), 1913.

14. Jordan, J. A.: Enormous ovarian tumor. Abstract. Am. Vet. Rev., **43**: 95 (April), 1913.

15. Lacassagne, A.: The direct and indirect action of radiation on cancer tissues. Radiology, **2**: 393–402 (Nov.), 1928.

16. Little, G. W.: Some studies in the behavior of malignant growths in dogs and horses. Jour. Am. Vet. Med. Assn., **71**: 171–188 (May), 1927.

17. MacCallum, W. G.: A textbook of pathology. Ed. 3. Philadelphia, W. B. Saunders Co., 1924, p. 1099.

18. MacCarty, W. C.: A cytologic key to the diagnosis and prognosis of neoplasms. Jour. Lab. and Clin. Med., **13**: 354–365 (Jan.), 1928.

19. MacCarty, W. C.: The cancer cell in the practice of medicine. Radiology, 11: 379–387 (Nov.), 1928.

20. MacCarty, W. C. and Mahle, A. E.: Relation of differentiation and lymphocytic infiltration to postoperative longevity in gastric carcinoma. Jour. Lab. and Clin. Med., 6: 473–480 (June), 1921.

21. Mallory, F. B.: The principles of pathologic histology. Philadelphia, W. B. Saunders Co., 1914, p. 264.

22. Murphy, J. B. and Morton, J. J.: The lymphocyte in natural and induced resistance to transplanted cancer. II. Studies in lymphoid activity. Jour. Exper. Med., 22: 204–211 (Aug.), 1915.

23. Oertel, Horst: Innervation and tumour growth. A preliminary report. Can. Med. Assn. Jour., 18: 135–139 (Feb.), 1928.

24. Pavlovsky, A. J. and Widakowich, V.: La eosinofilia local en el cáncer. Semana méd., 33: 1265–1278 (June 10), 1926.

25. Sittenfield, M. J.: The significance of the lymphocyte in immunity to cancer. Jour. Cancer Res., 2: 150–157 (April), 1917.

26. Sittenfield, M. J.: Further studies on the importance of the lymphocyte in cancer immunity. Jour. Med. Res., 38: 465–468, 1918.

27. Wade, Henry: An experimental investigation of infective sarcoma of the dog, with a consideration of its relationship to cancer. Jour. Path. and Bacteriol., 12: 384–425 1908.

28. Wilder, R. M., Allan, F. N., Power, M. H., and Robertson, H. E.: Carcinoma of the islands of the pancreas, hyperinsulinism and hypoglycemia. Jour. Am. Med. Assn., 89: 348–355 (July 30), 1927.

29. Woglom, W. H.: Immunity to transplantable tumours. Cancer Rev., 4: 129–214 (March), 1929.

30. Wood F. C.: Immunity in cancer. Tr. Assn. Am. Physicians, 33: 128–132, 1918.

31. Wood, F. C.: Tumors. Nelson Loose-leaf Surgery. New York, Thomas Nelson & Sons, 1927, 2: 3–133.

CHAPTER III

INCIDENCE

Statistical data pertaining to the occurrence of tumors of lower animals are meager and fragmentary. Veterinarians are far behind physicians in this regard, owing, perhaps, to the greater interest manifested by physicians and laymen in malignant neoplasms of human beings.

A conservative estimate places the annual number of deaths of human beings in the United States of America, as a result of carcinoma, at well over 100,000. This fact, together with the system of registration of deaths, and the increase in the number of postmortem examinations, makes it possible to determine with some degree of accuracy the incidence of tumors in human beings.

Owing to the lack of a central agency where causes of spontaneous deaths of animals can be analyzed, much of statistical value with regard to tumor is not available. Further, as has been pointed out, most of the meat-producing animals are slaughtered before the age at which malignant tumors are most likely to develop; thus the incidence of neoplastic disease if these animals were permitted to attain a longer life cannot be estimated.

That relatively few neoplasms are found in animals killed for meat is shown by the figures compiled from the report of the chief of the Bureau of Animal Industry of the United States Department of Agriculture for 1930. In the report of the inspection of carcasses in abattoirs supervised by federal meat inspectors an attempt is not made to differentiate condemnation made for true tumors and for abscesses. In other words, all swellings, whether neoplastic or inflammatory, are listed as tumors. Consequently, the percentage of neoplasms encountered in packing-house material is much lower than the figures in Table 2 would indicate.

In the same period the neoplastic condition listed in the federal reports as leukemia occurred in the respective species as follows: (1) Among 8,221,243 cattle there were 1,265 cases of so-called leukemia; (2) among 4,482,129 calves there were forty-three cases of so-called leukemia; (3) among 15,283,989 sheep and lambs there were fourteen cases of so-called leukemia; (4) among 46,553,438 swine there were 274

TABLE 2

COMBINATIONS FOR TUMORS AND ABSCESSES

Animals.	Carcasses examined.	Condemned for tumors and abscess.	
		Carcasses.	Parts.
Cattle	8,221,243	3,186	8,527
Calves*	4,482,129	82	3,229
Sheep and lambs	15,283,989	430	203
Swine	46,553,438	2,852	422,871
Horses	135,984	152	2

* Bovine animals aged one year or less.

cases of so-called leukemia, and (5) among 135,984 horses there were no cases of so-called leukemia.

These figures are somewhat difficult to interpret on account of the prevalence of localized abscesses in cattle, calves, and particularly swine. It is regrettable that the federal meat inspection authorities do not provide means for determining the actual incidence of tumors in the millions of meat-producing animals that are examined under supervision every year. The separation in the records of definite abscesses from neoplastic new growths should be possible in most instances, and although there are many instances in which the true character of a neoplasm can be determined only by microscopic examination, if the custom of listing abscesses and tumors in a common total were discontinued, much valuable information on the occurrence of neoplasia among the various species could be compiled.

With few exceptions the larger veterinary clinics in America have contributed little data to the problem of incidence of tumors as it affects the common domesticated animals and one is required to turn to foreign sources for much of the information that is available.

The susceptibility of the different species of animals to neoplastic diseases cannot be accurately gauged by data showing the number of live animals in veterinary clinics in which there is demonstrable evidence of neoplasia. Tumors of the interior of the body are generally not detected except at necropsy, and the question of whether a neoplastic disease will develop can be definitely determined only if animals are permitted to live out what would be their natural span of life, or at least are permitted to enter on what would generally be considered as old age. In the majority of dogs between the ages of ten and fifteen years, as has been pointed out, some form of tissue overgrowth and different varieties of genuine malignant growths may be observed.

As a matter of fact in order to determine the susceptibility of a given species to tumor, it would be desirable to permit the entire animal population to attain old age and to perform necropsy carefully in each case in order that tumor may not be overlooked. The impracticability of such a procedure is obvious, except when large numbers of small animals, such as rats and mice, can be kept under experimental observation for a period of years.

HORSE

Most of the reported studies on the occurrence of neoplasms in horses have been concerned with carcinoma only; relatively few data are available concerning incidence of neoplasms in general, so far as horses are concerned. This is probably due to the greater interest incited by the malignant lesions of the epithelium, on account of the ubiquity of these growths and their capacity for destruction.

Fölger compiled statistics from the annual reports of the Prussian-Würtemberg army and of the Army of Saxony, and noted that in 559,163 horses 648 tumors had been observed. This is a very low incidence (0.116 per cent), but it should be pointed out that the animals represented a selected group so far as general physical condition and age are concerned. No doubt the incidence of tumor in the general horse population of the respective German states, from which these data were compiled, was much higher. The varieties of neoplasm represented by the 648 specimens were as follows: Fibroma 343 (52.8 per cent); papilloma 159 (24.3 per cent); sarcoma eighty-seven (13.4 per cent); lipoma twenty-two (3.39 per cent); carcinoma ten (1.54 per cent); adenoma seven (1.08 per cent); chondroma six (0.92 per cent); osteoma three (0.46 per cent); myoma three (0.46 per cent); myxoma two (0.31 per cent); neuroma one (0.15 per cent); hemangioma one (0.15 per cent), and teratoma four (0.61 per cent).

The compiled statistics of the various clinics of the Royal Veterinary High School of Berlin, as reported by Fölger, show that during a period of fourteen years, beginning with the year 1896 a total of 175,748 horses was treated from which 2,141 neoplasms (1.21 per cent) were obtained.

In the ambulatory clinic of the New York State Veterinary College during the year 1929–1930, five cases of neoplastic disease were noted among 443 horses. One of the tumors was a carcinoma. In the surgical and consulting clinics of the same institution during this period, twelve tumors were found among 433 horses. Five of the growths were malignant.[28]

Sticker[33] mentioned the dissection of a series of 4,183 horses in a period of nineteen years, among which were found six cases of carcinoma (0.14 per cent). Cadiot reported that 218 horses were affected with carcinoma among 18,100 (1.02 per cent) examined during a period of four years. From the dissection of 3,877 horses Schütz reported six cases of carcinoma (0.15 per cent). Sticker[31] noted that 103 horses with carcinoma were treated in the course of twenty-two years at the clinic of the Royal Veterinary High School at Berlin. The tumors occurred among 215,137 horses (0.046 per cent). These cases were observed clinically and not at necropsy. With this in mind it is evident that although the foregoing data no doubt represent rather accurately the frequency of occurrence of carcinoma of the exterior of the body of horses, the figure undoubtedly would have been much higher if carcinoma of the interior of the body could have been added. In examination at necropsy of 768 horses Crocker found eight tumors (approximately 1 per cent). Six of the growths were carcinoma and two were sarcoma.

The use of horse flesh for human food has provided an opportunity to obtain information concerning the occurrence of neoplasms of the interior of the body of many of these animals. Data secured by this means are much more comprehensive than those obtained from veterinary surgical and medical clinics, since each carcass is subjected to rather complete examination. Of much interest, therefore, is the report of Martel,[10] chief of the Sanitary Veterinary Service of Paris, who compiled statistics on the incidence of carcinoma of horses from material secured from a total of 38,800 horses slaughtered in the abattoirs of that city. The majority of the animals were aged more than fifteen years, and consisted of mares, 20,000; geldings, 16,200, and stallions, 3,600.

Animals found to be affected with carcinoma numbered 184, distributed as follows: Eighty-six in mares, forty-three in geldings, and fifty-five in stallions; thus, malignant epithelial tumors were present in about 0.5 per cent of the animals. The melanotic tumors were not counted, because of their common occurrence, nor was information given pertaining to other varieties of neoplasms encountered. In the 184 cases the following organs and tissues were affected: Kidney, sixty-two; testis, fifty; mammary gland, forty-five; intestine, nine; urinary bladder, six; ovary, two; lungs, two; uterus, one; sheath, one, and region of jaw, one. Generalization was noted in six of the affected animals and in five the situation of the tumor was not established. Multiplicity of involvement was not uncommon. Both testes were involved in ten of the fifty cases in which the testes were affected, and of the forty-five cases of carcinoma of the mammary gland the condition was bilateral in six.

The incidence of new growths of the intestinal canal of horses was reported by Achilles who obtained material from 3,500 horses that were slaughtered in a period of two and a half years at the abattoir at Dresden. Neoplasms were found in the intestines of seven of the animals, and of the ten new growths encountered, nine were sarcomas of the serosa, muscularis or submucosa, usually of the large bowel. One carcinoma only was found in the series reported by Achilles.

Küst studied tumors of the external genitalia of 195,239 mares, examined at the Berlin Polyclinic in a period of twenty-two years. Tumors of the vagina, clitoris, and vulva were found in thirty-six of the animals (0.019 per cent). In the same period four among 20,226 animals (0.018 per cent) presented in a Berlin surgical clinic, had tumor of the external genitalia. Twenty-one of the series of thirty-six tumors were in the vagina and seven of them were carcinomas. Four of the tumors involved the vulva and these consisted of one papilloma, one carcinoma, one sarcoma, and one malignant melanoma. Of the eleven tumors of the clitoris nine were carcinomas and two were sarcomas.

The nature of the statistical data makes it difficult and perhaps unwise to draw definite conclusions as to the incidence of neoplasms of horses. Although tumors are by no means rare in this species, the evidence does not indicate that new growths develop in any considerable percentage of horses even in those of advanced age. Exceptions must be made in the case of melanotic tumors which are so strikingly prevalent in old white or old gray horses (chapter on melanoblastoma, page 247). Aside from the melanoblastoma of gray or white horses of advanced age the horse is perhaps one of the more resistant species so far as the development of neoplasms is concerned, and it is probably correct to conclude that neoplasms are much less common in the horse than in the dog, and that they are less common in horses than in cattle.

BOVINE

Considering the enormous numbers of cattle slaughtered annually for food under federal supervision, and subjected to rather complete necropsy, it is surprising that so few reliable statistical data are available on the incidence of neoplasm in this species. Although the greatest percentage of bovines is slaughtered within the first few years of life, the abattoir is the final destination for most old dairy cows that eventually become unprofitable as milk producers and are consequently sent to slaughter in order that something may be salvaged. In this group, neoplasm is not infrequently present although there is no definite information as to what percentage of the animals is likely to be affected. The data are limited largely to the incidence of malignant tumors, and in only a few instances has a sufficiently large group of animals been observed to yield data that are comprehensive and trustworthy.

Trotter reported that in 1903, in Glasgow, 47,362 cattle of all ages including 1,549 calves were slaughtered and at necropsy a total of 131 cases of malignant neoplasms was found. Sticker noted seven cases of carcinoma among 5,795 cattle presented for treatment at the Berlin veterinary clinics in a period of ten years. Trotter[2] made a comprehensive analysis of 300 cases of malignant neoplasms of bovines. The animals were presented for slaughter and were consequently submitted to careful examination. Two of the animals were steers (oxen) and 298 were cows. With the exception of three of the animals the ages of which were fifteen months, eighteen months and three years, respectively, about 75 per cent of the cattle were considered to be aged between fifteen and twenty years; the remainder were less than fifteen years. The physical condition of seventy-four (24.6 per cent) was given as poor, of 202 (67.3 per cent) as fair, and of twenty-four (8 per cent) as good. The majority of the animals (268) came from Ireland.

From the 300 animals with malignant neoplasm, 305 specimens of primary malignant tumor were obtained (Table 3). Four of the cattle examined were affected with more than one primary tumor; in one instance three primary growths were found, and in three, two primary tumors were obtained from each animal.

The tumors primary in the liver and in the rumen were carcinomas and those of the thymus were sarcomas. Of the eight tumors of the small intestine, seven were carcinomas and one was a sarcoma. One carcinoma involved the ileocecal valve and one was in the rectum. Eight tumors of the lung were carcinomas. Four of the five tumors of the ovary were carcinomas and one was a sarcoma. The tumors of the eye and of the vulva were carcinomas. The tumors of the lymph nodes were sarcomas. Carcinomas were also found in the kidneys, gallbladder, uterus, and skin. A tumor of the eighth rib was a spindle-cell sarcoma and one of the parotid gland was a mixed-cell sarcoma.

Besides the malignant neoplasms encountered in the 300 cases, Trotter mentioned that the suprarenal glands were affected with some

5

TABLE 3

ANATOMIC DISTRIBUTION OF THE TUMORS OF TROTTER'S SERIES*

Organ or tissue affected.	Number.	Per cent.
Liver	222	74.0
Rumen	25	8.3
Thymus	16	5.3
Intestines	10	3.3
Lung	8	2.6
Ovary	5	1.6
Eye	4	1.3
Vulva	3	0.9
Lymph nodes	3	0.9
Kidney	1	0.3
Gallbladder	1	0.3
Uterus	1	0.3
Bones	1	0.3
Skin	1	0.3
Fascia	1	0.3
Salivary glands	1	0.3
Undetermined	2	0.6
Total	305	

* There were 279 (91.47 per cent) carcinomas and twenty-six (8.52 per cent) sarcomas.

form of neoplasm in twenty-seven instances. Whether Trotter meant twenty-seven different animals or twenty-seven separate glands is not clear. It was Trotter's belief that the rate of frequency of neoplasia in bovines is comparable to that in man, although a difference in the site of the lesion is exhibited in the two species.

Although sufficient data to justify definite conclusions are not available, it is my opinion that neoplasms are more common in cattle than in horses, or perhaps than in any of the other ruminants, but this species is not as susceptible to development of the tumor as the dog.

DOG

Several factors have made it possible to obtain perhaps more information on the occurrence of neoplasms in dogs than in most of the other animals. The dog is one of the more numerous of the domestic animals, and on account of the place it holds in man's affection, a larger number attain old age than any of the other species; thus, the maximal opportunity is permitted for the development of neoplasia. The difficulty of performing necropsy is much less than with a large animal, such as a horse. Furthermore, a considerable percentage of dogs receives veterinary attention sufficiently often to insure the detection of neoplastic diseases that might escape the notice of a layman. The practice of placing the sick canine in a veterinary hospital for observation and treatment also provides a circumstance that enhances the probability of necropsy in case the animal dies. Large animals, and even dogs dying on the farm, on the contrary, are seldom examined, and as a consequence internal neoplasms of such animals are seldom demonstrated and identified.

Although the foregoing factors are responsible, to a considerable extent, for the large number of tumors of dogs that has been reported and described, there is still another element of no little significance, although of an uncertain character, and difficult to define. This is the inherent tendency to the development of neoplasia of animals of the canine species. This fact is well brought out in the studies of Goodpasture, and of Goodpasture and Wislocki, who recorded the finding of tumors in every one of fifty old dogs examined. In many old dogs two or more primary tumors may be found; 228 were found in the series of fifty dogs, thirteen of which were classified as malignant and 215 as benign. Although there might be some question about accepting the entire 228 tumors as true neoplasms, the observations of Goodpasture and Wislocki emphasize the latent possibilities of the tissues of dogs for proliferative overgrowths that are often definitely neoplastic. The loss of restraint on growth seems to be more evident with the advent of senescence.

The majority of observers who have contributed information pertaining to the incidence of tumors in dogs have based their data on the tumors in animals treated in veterinary clinics and not on necropsy. A few reports are available, however, in which necropsy data have been recorded. Schütz, during a period of fourteen years, when a total of 1,241 dogs was examined at postmortem found carcinomas in sixty-nine (5.4 per cent). Anatomically the carcinomas in this series were distributed as follows: Integument, 20.8 per cent; urogenital apparatus, 26.6 per cent; digestive tract, 25.8 per cent, and respiratory tract, 26.6 per cent. Sticker mentioned that 1,306 dogs were examined at necropsy at the Pathological Institute in Berlin in a period of fifteen years. Carcinoma was present in seventy-two (5.5 per cent) of the animals. Since carcinoma only was mentioned in Sticker's report, the total incidence of tumors, if all types had been considered, would have been much higher. Cohrs reported on necropsy of 737 dogs; neoplasms were present in seventy (9.5 per cent). Of a total of fifty-two dogs examined at necropsy in one year at the New York State Veterinary College, four (7.6 per cent) had tumors. Three of the growths were carcinomas, and one was a lymphoblastoma. In the clinic of the New York institution for small animals there were treated, in the same period, approximately

2,000 dogs, among which twenty-five (2.5 per cent) were observed to have tumors. Sixteen of the growths (0.8 per cent) of the total number of animals observed) were carcinomas affecting the exterior of the body. From necropsy of 1,548 dogs, Crocker reported the occurrence of tumors in twenty-seven (1.7 per cent). Twenty of the growths were malignant, twelve of which were carcinomas. The ages of the animals were not given.

From foreign countries, particularly Germany, one may obtain rather comprehensive data on the incidence of malignant lesions of the epithelium of dogs presented for treatment, and one interested in this phase of the carcinoma problem should consult the valuable publications of Sticker[31] in the original. He reported from the hospital clinic at Berlin that among 15,455 dogs there were 465 (3 per cent) affected with carcinoma. During eight years at the Polyclinic in Berlin, Sticker also reported that of a total of 75,818 dogs there were 491 (0.6 per cent) affected with carcinoma. Sticker estimated the incidence of carcinoma in dogs to be at least thirty-seven to every 10,000 dogs. His estimate was made from 29,044 dogs in Berlin in 1897. Since Sticker based his conclusions on clinical evidence rather than on necropsy, one must conclude that the actual incidence of the disease was much greater.

Ortschild quoted Semner's figures that tumors were present in 354 (about 8 per cent) of 3,525 dogs presented for treatment. Fröhner compiled data for a period of eight years, on 60,471 dogs observed at the Berlin Veterinary High School. Of this number, 2,871 (approximately 4.7 per cent) had some form of tumorous growth. Since the tumors observed did not include growths that may have been present in the interior of the body, the exact incidence of neoplasia was no doubt much greater. In one series of 8,897 dogs examined at the hospital clinic in Berlin in the course of the years 1886 to 1894 inclusive, 643 animals were operated on for some form of neoplasm, and of this number 262 (approximately 40 per cent) were carcinomas.

Cadiot, who found 854 cases of carcinoma among 22,450 dogs (3.8 per cent), considered the occurrence of tumors of the dog to be two to three times that of herbivora.

To recapitulate: Available information indicates rather definitely that dogs are frequently affected by neoplastic diseases, and that a considerable percentage of new growths are epithelial in character. It was shown elsewhere (Chapter I, page 25) that the tumors, and particularly carcinomas, occur with greatest frequency in later years of life. A conservative estimate places the percentage of older adult dogs affected with tumors between 8 and 10 per cent, of which carcinoma represents 40 to 50 per cent. The evidence strongly suggests the dog as the most susceptible to neoplastic proliferations of the domestic mammals.

CAT

There are only a few reports pertaining to the frequency of occurrence of tumors in cats. Sticker's[31] statistics show that during a period of ten years (1891 to 1901) fifty-four cats were treated in the hospital clinic of Berlin, and carcinoma was present in two (3.7 per cent), whereas during eight years 1,688 cats were examined at the Polyclinic and nine of these (0.53 per cent) had carcinomas. Schütz, from observations over a period of years, concluded that 6 per cent of all cats examined had carcinoma. A comparable rate of incidence was observed at necropsy of thirty-four cats at the Pathological Institute of Berlin, in which two (5.9 per cent) were found to be affected with carcinoma.

At the New York State Veterinary College at Ithaca there was treated, in 1929 and 1930, a total of 582 cats, and only one tumor, a carcinoma, was found. Crocker at the University of Pennsylvania found four neoplasms at necropsy of 401 cats. None of the tumors in Crocker's series was carcinoma.

Murray listed ten cats affected with neoplastic diseases. One animal harbored two primary neoplasms; a squamous-cell carcinoma of the tongue, and a "small round sarcoma" of the small intestine. Seven of the eleven tumors were carcinomas and four of these involved the mammary gland. There was also recorded a spindle-cell sarcoma of the humerus and a myxosarcoma of the axilla. There was no information as to what percentage of a given feline group the ten cases in Murray's series represented.

It would seem that although tumors are rather uncommonly present in young cats, a considerable number may be disclosed by necropsy of old cats. The majority of neoplasms of cats are malignant, carcinoma constituting the greatest proportion.

OTHER DOMESTIC MAMMALS

Tumors are less frequently observed in sheep, swine, rabbits, and goats than in horses, cattle, dogs, and cats. Although the inference is that the former species is more resistant to the development of neoplasia than the latter, at least the fact that the majority of the former animals are slaughtered relatively early, whereas many of the latter are permitted to live relatively long must be considered before a conclusion can be reached. This circumstance undoubtedly accounts for the apparent insusceptibility of certain species to tumorous growths, but is insufficient in my opinion to provide an entirely adequate explanation. Although the greater number of sheep is slaughtered as lambs or as young adults it is equally true that a large number of old ewes are examined at necropsy each year, and that the frequency of tumor is less than that which obtains for dogs and cattle of comparable ages. The evidence seems fairly conclusive, therefore, that the sheep possess marked racial insusceptibility to new growth. Tumors are seen so infrequently in adult goats and rabbits as to suggest that these animals are less susceptible than many of the others. With the exception of embryonal nephroma of the region of the kidney of swine, tumors are not commonly seen in this animal. Since embryonal nephroma probably originates as a consequence of some congenital mishap, the inception of the growth is unlike that concerned in the genesis of the majority of tumors. Embryonal tumors of the kidney originate as a consequence of a faulty developmental mechanism, and are frequently well established at an early age, whereas most other tumors arise as a consequence of factors that are vague and little understood, and that require the lapse of much time before they become discernible.

By far the greater number of swine killed is aged less than two years, and although early death prevents development of neoplasms in the majority of these animals, there is little evidence that tumors are as prone to develop in swine as in dogs or cattle. However, to my knowledge a large number of swine of an age comparable to that not uncommonly attained by old dogs has not been observed. Certainly hogs of advanced age have not been examined at necropsy in numbers large enough to permit comparison with the rate of incidence of neoplasia in the other domestic species that frequently do attain old age.

Among Sticker's[31] compiled data on approximately 1,200 carcinomas of animals, only twelve carcinomas were obtained from hogs. Two of these affected the integument; three, the digestive apparatus, and seven, the kidney. Although the renal neoplasms were listed as carcinomas, I am inclined to believe that the majority of them at least were embryonal nephromas, since genuine primary carcinoma of the kidney of swine is extremely rare. Fölger cited the observations of Gaylord and Zink, who noted four (0.2 per cent) malignant growths among 2,000 swine slaughtered at Buffalo. The tumors affected the liver, kidney, and skin.

In the surgical and consulting clinics of the New York State Veterinary College at Cornell University at Ithaca during the year 1929 to 1930, five tumors were found among approximately fifty-two sheep examined. However, this incidence must be regarded as very unusual and not as indicative of the true incidence of neoplasia in this species.

The failure to observe many tumors among goats may be due in part to the relatively small numbers of these animals examined. Some idea of the number of goats present in the United States may be gathered from the fact that during the year ending June 30, 1930, federal meat inspectors made postmortem examinations of more than 8,000,000 cattle, approximately 15,000,000 sheep and lambs and only 21,887 goats. Of these goats, tumors or abscesses were the cause of the condemnations of only two carcasses and in no instance did the presence of tumors make the disposal of parts of carcasses necessary.

Eggling observed a carcinoma of the mammary gland of a goat, which was the only case of carcinoma encountered among 238 goats examined. In my collection of approximately 550 neoplasms of the domestic species, only one is from a goat. This was a lymphoma that seemed to have originated in a lymph node in the anterior thoracic cavity of a male goat aged six or seven years.

Few tumors have been reported as occurring in rabbits. Polson reviewed the cases published prior to 1927, and found a total of fifty-two, to which he added fourteen, making a total of sixty-six. Polson commented on the difficulty of making an accurate estimate of the incidence of tumors in rabbits and gave statistics which showed that eleven tumors were obtained from approximately 1,100 animals. Polson considered the uterus the most frequent site of tumors of the rabbit; this organ was affected in thirty of the sixty-six cases reported. Practically all of the uterine tumors were epithelial, and the majority were malignant; five had metastasized. Seven of the sixty-six tumors mentioned by Polson involved the kidneys, and apparently had their origin in embryonic renal tissue. Among the benign tumors of the rabbit included in Polson's series were nine adenomas, eight of which occurred in the uterus. Of the fifty malignant tumors fourteen were listed as sarcomas. The only tumor of the rabbit I have encountered in a total of approximately 550 animal tumors was a malignant lymphoblastoma with tumorous foci in the omentum and in the lungs.

FOWLS

The one animal for which it should be possible to assemble more or less reliable data on the occurrence of tumors is the common fowl. The poultry industry has attained such an important position commercially, that the owner of poultry is keenly interested in every condition which may affect the well-being of his flock. The average normal death rate among chickens is relatively high, and consequently large numbers of fowls come to necropsy and many tumors are revealed.

Curtis reported on the frequency of tumors among domestic fowls which had been found at necropsy over a period of eight years at the Maine Agricultural Experiment Station. Of the 880 fowls examined, tumors were found in seventy-nine (8.96 per cent), approximately ninety neoplasms in each 1,000 birds. Most of the fowls were hens, and many of the tumors involved the ovary and the oviduct. In fact, 37.76 per cent of all the tumors occurred in the ovary, and 18.36 per cent affected the oviduct and the broad ligament. In fowls that died a natural death the neoplastic process was considered to be the direct or indirect cause of death in from a third to a half of the cases. The majority of the tumors were confined to one organ, but in fifteen cases metastasis was observed.

The report of Curtis, although it contained much of significance on the incidence of the occurrence of tumors in fowls, unfortunately loses some of its possible value to the pathologist since histologic studies were not made. Curtis arbitrarily divided the tumors encountered into two classes on the basis of gross characteristics: Cystic tumors constituting 22.78 per cent, and tissue tumors, 74.68 per cent. The failure in this instance to examine the material microscopically might justify skepticism in accepting the entire seventy-nine cases as instances of neoplasm.

In contradistinction to the high percentage of tumors in fowls reported by Curtis, are the observations of Bürger, who concluded that tumors in fowls are relatively seldom seen. Bürger quoted figures obtained from one of the statistical reports of the Institute of Animal Diseases of the University of Leipzig which showed that among 852 fowls examined in one year, only twelve (1.4 per cent) tumors were found, seven of which affected the ovary. Klee's figures, as given by Fölger, are comparable to those of Bürger. In a period of ten years, during which 6,111 fowls were examined, tumors were encountered in eighty-nine (1.28 per cent). The tumors in Klee's series were classified as follows: Sarcoma, thirty-four (38.2 per cent); carcinoma, seventeen (19.9 per cent); lipoma, nineteen (22 per cent); angioma, one; cystoma, one; myxosarcoma, one; leiomyoma, one; myxochondroma, one; lymphoma, one, and undetermined, twenty-three. The report of Ehrenreich also suggests the relative infrequency of tumors of fowls, since only seven malignant neoplasms were found among 2,000 adult hens dressed for food at a hotel. It should be noted, however, that Ehrenreich's material was not selected at necropsy by one trained in pathology, but was obtained through the coöperation of the hotel employe assigned to prepare the carcasses for cooking. This circumstance may have resulted in failure to detect certain neoplasms that might have been demonstrable by one especially skilled in the recognition of disease.

Malke also attempted to determine the incidence of tumors of fowls by observing during one year the number of fowls affected with tumors presented for necropsy at the Institute of Animal Diseases of the University of Leipzig. Of 858 fowls aged more than three months, tumors were found in thirty-three (3.8 per cent). They were grouped as follows: Sarcomas, twenty-one; carcinomas, three, and endotheliomas, two. The ovary was the organ most often affected, and metastatic dissemination was frequently observed.

The report of the Department of Poultry Husbandry of the New Jersey State Agricultural Experiment Station for the year ending June 30, 1924, shows that at necropsy of 142 adult hens, tumors were found in seventeen* (approximately 11 per cent). In the report of the same institution for 1925, seven tumors were found in a total of 106 hens examined (6.6 per cent), and in a series of 861 pullets sixty-five tumors (7.5 per cent) were found.

During the year 1929 to 1930 at the New York State Veterinary College at Cornell University at Ithaca, at necropsy of 1,436 fowls, neoplastic diseases, including seventy-seven cases of so-called leukemia, were present in 210 (16 per cent). At the Farmingdale, Long Island Laboratory of the same institution, fifty-seven cases of tumor, including twenty-two cases of so-called leukemia, were found among a total of 1,350 fowls (4.2 per cent). The marked difference in the incidence of the disease of these two groups may have been due in part to the differences in age of the respective series. In the group examined at Ithaca, approximately 60 per cent of the fowls were adults whereas about 40 per cent of those examined at the Farmingdale Laboratory were adults. The influence of advanced age on the inception of neoplasms of fowls is particularly significant, and the percentage of incidence may be expected to exhibit a striking acceleration with the advent of adult life.

Perhaps the most noteworthy attempt to determine the frequency of spontaneous tumors of the domestic fowl was that reported by Schneider. Data were obtained on about 11,000 pullets, aged approximately six to eighteen months, during the period of observation. The fowls were from many different states, as well as from England and Canada, and

* Five of the cases that I have included with the total of seventeen were classified in the report as examples of leukemia.

most of the common breeds were represented. No distinction was made between benign and malignant neoplasms; examination of the respective carcasses was concerned with the presence or absence of gross evidence of tumor. The groups of birds under observation were subject to the same general conditions of management and all received optimal care. Data were obtained over a period of four years.

Electric lights were used during the winter months to force production of eggs among a portion of the fowls observed. In this group the highest incidence of tumor occurred in March and April, and then diminished rapidly, whereas under normal conditions the frequency reached its peak in May and June, and continued at approximately the same level throughout the summer and autumn months. Since the peak of frequency of tumor came two or three months earlier when methods were used to force production of eggs, Schneider believed that the spring increase in frequency is definitely associated with production of eggs; the inference is that reproductive overwork predisposes the tissues to neoplastic proliferation. Schneider concluded that the normal annual incidence of tumor for fowls between the ages of six and eighteen months is about 2 to 3 per cent.

Besides the 11,000 fowls from which the foregoing data were obtained, Schneider mentioned 500 pullets that had been hatched and reared at the Storrs Agricultural Experiment Station, Connecticut, from which the incidence of tumor was 3.24 per cent.

Schneider found evidence to indicate that tumors of fowls not infrequently appear in an endemic form. In about thirty of 100 pullets that died tumors were found on gross examination, an incidence of about 10 per cent based on the whole flock of 300 pullets, which was strikingly high compared to the usual rate of 2 to 3 per cent. A pathologic analysis of the material obtained from the fowls observed in Schneider's study would have been of great value.

It is obvious, from a summary of the different data, that much variation exists pertaining to the incidence of tumor for the common domestic fowl. Such factors as age and methods of recognition, whether gross or microscopic, may have contributed significantly to the evident inconsistencies in published statistics. To draw correct conclusions from such data is difficult if not impossible. However, from the available facts, if one makes allowances for factors influencing the variation in the frequency rates given, it would seem that chickens less than six months of age are seldom the victims of neoplasia, but that between the ages of one and two years an incidence of tumor often surprisingly high may be expected. An annual incidence of tumor of from 2 to 3 per cent in fowls aged one year or less is perhaps approximately correct, with the frequency increasing markedly in the second year of life. If fowls are aged more than one year, the lymphoid neoplastic entity known conveniently, but erroneously as leukemia is common, and among the older adult fowls the various neoplastic diseases may be expected to affect from 6 to 10 per cent of a given flock. All factors considered, neoplasm is perhaps more common in the domestic hen than in any of the other domestic species.

Little is known of the incidence of tumor among fowls other than those which are domesticated, although some information may be obtained from the figures of Sticker[32] who reported on the occurrence of carcinoma among fowls in the clinics of the Veterinary High School of Berlin during a period of thirteen years:

Among 2,144 chickens there were thirteen cases of tumor (0.6 per cent); among 2,335 parrots there were sixty-eight cases of tumor (2.8 per cent); among 444 doves there were twenty-two cases of tumor (5 per cent), and among 1,600 small birds there were forty-seven cases of tumor (3 per cent).

In the summary of 180 cases of tumors of birds contributed by Joest and Ernesti, the distribution of neoplasia among the different species is apparent. The numbers were as follows: Hens, 147; parrots, eleven; doves, six; ducks, five; canary birds, two; gobblers, two; partridge, one; capon, one; crow, one; finch, one; buzzard, one; ostrich, one and Spanish pepper eater, one. Seventy-four of the tumors were sarcomas, and fifty-seven were carcinomas. Fifty-eight of the sarcomas occurred in hens, and these animals also possessed forty-eight of the tumors diagnosed as carcinomas.

CAPTIVE WILD ANIMALS

The keeping of wild mammals and fowls for exhibition in permanent institutions has provided an opportunity to gather data on the occurrence of neoplasms of many of the wild species. Fortunately the administration of many of the collections have provided comparative pathologists to supervise the health of the animals and to ascertain the cause when any died. Careful necropsy is had, and neoplastic growths, if present, are disclosed.

Brooks reported on observations that were made on the animals of the New York Zoological Society and stated that of 2,645 living animals observed in a period of five years a case of true neoplasm was not found. Among 744 that died and were examined, only one tumor was encountered, a myxosarcoma of the ovary of a white racoon dog, an animal of which the purity of species is questioned. Brooks was of the opinion that neoplasms are extremely rare in wild animals living under natural conditions, and felt that abnormal conditions, such as inbreeding, increased the incidence of new growths in the common domestic and experimental animals.

The scarcity of neoplasms in the animals reported by Brooks is considerably at variance with the data of Fox, of the Zoological Society of Philadelphia, who has contributed what is perhaps the most comprehensive study of tumor obtained from captive wild animals. Among 5,356 animals, in a period of nineteen years, ninety-four tumors were obtained from ninety-two animals (1.7 per cent) giving a rate of incidence of about one in every sixty animals. As Fox stated, this is not a low percentage. The lesions in this series were sixteen sarcomas, nineteen adenomas, and twenty-five carcinomas. The most common sites affected were the kidney in fourteen cases; the liver in nine, and the uterus in eight. Forty-four of the tumors were in fowls, the greatest number occurring in parrakeets. Of all avian tumors, 27 per cent affected the kidney.

For one interested in neoplasms of captive wild mammals and birds, the valuable treatise by Fox should be consulted. Suffice to say that tumors do occur in wild animals not infrequently, and it is perhaps not incorrect to conclude that the frequency of neoplasms in wild animals is comparable with that for the domesticated species in general.

WILD RATS

Campaigns for the eradication of rats waged by the federal authorities in the furtherance of plague control have made it possible to ascertain something of the development of neoplasms in the ordinary wild rat (Mus norvegicus). In this regard, the observations of McCoy are of interest and significance. During a period from June 1, 1908 to May 15, 1909, about 100,000 rats were examined at the federal plague laboratory at San Francisco, California, and among this number were 103 rats with tumors in suitable condition for study. A few specimens were decomposed and were discarded as unfit for microscopic examination. A considerable number of the growths was adenomatous; the majority were adenomas, and very few were adenocarcinomas.

A summary of the tumors obtained by McCoy shows that the varieties of growths affecting the subcutaneous tissues were as follows: Fibromas, sixteen; lipomas, one; sarcomas, five; mixed fibrous and adenomatous tumors, nine; adenomas, nineteen; carcinomas, four; cystic adenomas, two. Those of the liver included fibromas, two; angioma, one; sarcomas, eighteen, and adenofibroma, one. Eleven of the tumors affected the kidney; four of these were adenomas, three were adeno-carcinomas, one was a papilloma, and three were carcinomas. Other growths included adenoma of the vulva, a round-cell sarcoma of the pelvis, and angiosarcoma of the testis, an endothelioma of the uterus, two sarcomas of the omentum, a cystic adenoma of the mesentery, and three sarcomas of the mesentery.

The possible etiologic influence of parasitism on the inception of sarcomatous growths of the livers of rats is suggested by McCoy's statement: "The sarcomas of the liver were of especial interest as they were usually associated with the presence of a parasite, Cysticercus fasciolaris." This parasite, which is the cystic stage of a cat tapeworm, Tænia crassicollis, has been used for many years, particularly at the Institute of Cancer Research, Columbia University, in the experimental production of sarcoma of the liver of rats on a large scale (Chapter I, page 22).

Confirmatory of McCoy's observation concerning the presence of sarcoma of the liver associated with parasitic cysts were the observations of Bridre and Conseil, who examined about 2,000 wild rats and found primary sarcoma of the liver in five, four of which contained the cystic stage of Tænia crassicollis.

SUMMARY

The data on the occurrence of neoplasms, fragmentary though it may be, should convince one that tumors probably occur in all species of mammals and fowls, domestic and wild, and that habits of diet, domestication, and environmental influences are of little if any significance on the etiology of neoplasms or in the degree of susceptibility exhibited by any one species. The explanation of the inception of neoplasia is vague to say the least, and the factors underlying apparent resistance manifested by individuals to tumorous growths are ill defined and difficult to formulate in a convincing way.

BIBLIOGRAPHY

1. Achilles, A.: Quoted by Fölger.
2. Age incidence in cancer. Vet. Rec., 18: 164–165, 1905–1906.
3. Bridre and Conseil: Quoted by Trotter.
4. Brooks, Harlow: Tumors of wild animals under natural conditions. Proc. Soc. Exper. Biol. and Med., 3: 39–40, 1906.
5. Bürger, Max: Untersuchungen über das Huhnersarkom (Peyton Rous). Ztschr. f. Krebsforsch., 14: 526–542, 1914.
6. Cadiot: Sur le cancer chez les animaux. Rec. de méd. vét., 84: 5–25, 87, 1907

7. Cohrs, Paul: Über primäre Multiplizität von Geschwülsten bei Haustieren. Ztschr. f. Krebsforsch., 24: 156–221, 1927.

8. Crocker, W. J.: Three thousand autopsies. Cornell Vet., 9: 140–161 (Jan.), 1919.

9. Curtis, M. R.: Frequency of occurrence of tumors in the domestic fowl. Jour. Agr. Res., 5: 397–404, 1915.

10. Editorial. Cancer in horses. Am. Vet. Rev., 44: 299–300 (Dec.), 1913.

11. Eggling: Quoted by Sticker.

12. Ehrenreich, M.: Weitere Mittheilungen über das Vorkommen maligner Tumoren bei Hühnern. Med. Klin., 3: 614–615 (May), 1907.

13. Fölger, A. F.: Geschwülste bei Tieren. Ergebn. d. all. Path. u. path. Anat., 18: 372–676, 1917.

14. Fox, Herbert: Disease in captive wild mammals and birds, incidence, description, comparison. Philadelphia, J. B. Lippincott Co., 1923, p. 462.

15. Fröhner: Statistische und casuistische Mittheilungen über das Vorkommen und die chirurgische Behandlung der Geschwülste beim Hunde. Monatschr. f. prakt. Thierh., 6: 1; 79; 111, 1894–1895.

16. Goodpasture, E. W.: An anatomical study of senescence in dogs, with especial reference to the relation of cellular changes of age to tumors. Jour. Med. Res., 38: 127–190 (May), 1918.

17. Goodpasture, E. W. and Wislocki, G. B.: Old age in relation to cell-overgrowth and cancer. Jour. Med. Res., 33: 455–473, 1916.

18. Joest, E. and Ernesti, S.: Untersuchungen über spontane Geschwülste bei Vögeln. Ztschr. f. Krebsforsch., 15: 1–75, 1915.

19. Klee: Quoted by Fölger.

20. Küst: Kasuistische Beiträge zur Kenntnis der Tumoren an den äusseren weiblichen Geschlechtsorganen; Vagina, Klitoris, Vulva, des Pferdes. Monatsh. f. prakt. Tierh., 23: 145–178, 1911–1912.

21. McCoy, G. W.: A preliminary report on tumors found in wild rats. Jour. Med. Res., 21: 285–296 (Sept.), 1909.

22. Malke, Erich: Geschwulstbildung beim Haushuhn. Ztschr. f. Krebsforsch., 31: 47–66, 1930.

23. Murray, J. A.: The zoological distribution of cancer. Third scientific report on the investigation of the Imperial Cancer Research Fund, 1908, pp. 41–60.

24. Ortschild, J. F.: A report of eight cases of canine neoplasm. Bull. Johns Hopkins Hosp., 16: 186–196 (May), 1905.

25. Polson, C. J.: Tumours of the rabbit. Jour. Path. and Bacteriol., 30: 603–614, 1927.

26. Report of the Department of Poultry Husbandry of the New Jersey State Agricultural Experiment Station for the year ending June 30, 1924.

27. Report of the Department of Poultry Husbandry of the New Jersey State Agricultural Experiment Station for the year ending June 30, 1925.

28. Report of the New York State Veterinary College at Cornell University for the year 1929–1930.

29. Schneider, Margaret: On the frequency of spontaneous tumors in the domestic fowl. Jour. Exper. Med., 43: 433–441 (March), 1926.

30. Schütz: Ueber Vorkommen des Carcinoms bei Thieren, 1901, 240 pp.

31. Sticker, Anton: Ueber den Krebs der Thiere. Arch. f. klin. Chir., 65: 616–696; 1023–1087, 1902.

32. Sticker, A.: Quoted by Wolff, Jacob. Die Lebre von der Krebskrankheit. Jena, Gustav Fischer, 1913, 3: 274.

33. Sticker, A.: Quoted by Fölger.

34. Trotter, A. M.: Malignant diseases in bovines. Jour. Comp. Path. and Therap., 24: 1–20, 1911.

CHAPTER IV

FIBROBLASTOMA

The class, fibroblastoma, embraces fibromas and fibrosarcomas.

FIBROMA

Definition.—Fibroma is a benign growth composed of connective tissue consisting largely of fibroblasts and their products. The fibroblast produces three kinds of fibrils: Fibroglia fibrils, collagen fibrils, and elastic fibrils. In fibroblastoma the greater number of fibrils is of the collagen variety, and there are few elastic fibrils. By using special stains recommended by Mallory and Wright fibroglia may be demonstrated distinctly, but by the hematoxylin and eosin stain they are observed with difficulty.

Incidence.—Fibroma is far more common among animals than reports in the literature would indicate. In fact, these tumors are so common as to be considered ordinarily unworthy of report by the average observer. Casper quoted Fröhner's statistics, in which it was shown that 643 dogs were operated on for tumor in a period of eight years, and ninety-seven (13 per cent) of the tumors were fibromas. During a period of seven years 150 tumors were obtained from 5,000 horses, and twenty of them were fibromas, a ratio of one fibroma to every 250 horses. In the Prussian army over a period of seven years, 115 fibromas were observed among 335 tumors of horses. Casper also gave Johne's figures on the incidence of fibroma from material examined in the course of twenty-five years at the Pathological Institute of the Veterinary High School of Dresden:

Among 250 tumors of horses twenty-seven (10.8 per cent) were fibromas; among 417 tumors of cattle eighteen (4.3 per cent) were fibromas; among ninety-two tumors of swine four (4.3 per cent) were fibromas, and among 209 tumors of dogs sixteen (7.6 per cent) were fibromas.

According to these statistics, fibroma is more common in horses and dogs than in other animals.

In 510 tumors in my collection seventeen were fibromas affecting the respective species as follows:

Of 214 tumors of cattle nine (4.2 per cent) were fibromas; of forty tumors of horses five (12.5 per cent) were fibromas; of seventy-eight tumors of dogs one was a fibroma; of thirty-nine tumors of sheep one was a fibroma, and of six tumors of mules one was a fibroma.

Figures of the occurrence of fibroma, as compared to that of other tumors, would indicate that they constitute a considerable share of all neoplasms.

Situation and points of origin.—Potentially, fibromas may develop from any situation where fibrous connective tissue normally occurs. Clinically, however, the majority of these new growths arise from the integument; the skin of the head, neck, shoulder, and leg are sites of predilection (Fig. 17). Many of these tumors seem to occur following chronic irritation, which may account for their frequency in the regions mentioned since they are particularly subject to trauma.

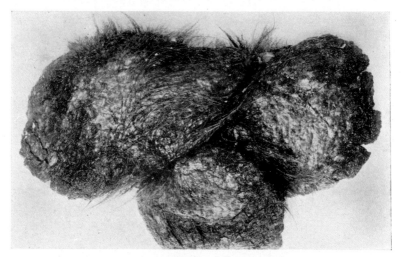

Fig. 17.—Multiple fibroma of the skin of a bovine.

Although fibromas are usually single, occasionally they are multiple, and may be distributed over much of the external surface of the body. This condition is considered to have some relation to the peripheral nervous system and is known as cutaneous neurofibromatosis. Although the structure of these tumors may be somewhat complex, the predominating cell is the fibroblast, which has its origin in the various connective tissue elements of the peripheral nerves. As a consequence of the fibroblastic overgrowth, the specialized nerve tissue usually undergoes atrophic retrogression.

Besides arising from the integument, fibromas may occasionally originate elsewhere. Thompson observed a growth of this kind which involved the mitral valve of a mare nine years old, which died suddenly.

Parker reported a fibroma weighing 1.4 kg. that was removed surgically from the cervix of a mare. Petit observed two rather unusual fibromas in stallions. The spermatic cord of one animal was affected, and in the other, multiple tumors were found on the surface of the left testis. Law has noted that pedicled fibromas may occur between the mucous and muscular coats of the rectum of the horse. In one of my cases the tumor affected the eyeball.

A large fibroma of the neck of the urinary bladder, which interfered with urination, was described by Fumagalli as occurring in a cow, and Noack observed a fibroma of the heart of an eight-year-old cow which had died suddenly. The tumor was in the endocardium of the right auricle, immediately under the orifice of the vena cava. Fibromas may also occur on the tongues of cattle. Fibroma of the uterus of cows is sometimes seen, although a study by Fuchs indicates that they are by no means common. In an examination of the uterus of 5,000 cattle Fuchs twice found what he considered to be fibroma. One of these was in an eight-year-old animal, and was probably a true neoplasm; the other, from the description given, may have represented a tuber-culous process. Fölger quoted Ratigan's case of polyp-like fibroma of the cervix. The tumor weighed 7.8 kg. and was removed surgically. Casper noted, in the older literature, records of an enormous fibroma of the uterus of a cow which weighed 100 kg. My collection of fibromas ob-tained from cattle includes a large tumor from the wall of the vagina, which weighed 9.8 kg., a small tumor from the vulva, and one from the frontal sinus. Four tumors were from the glans penis of bulls.

In the dog, it has been reported that fibromas occurred in the va-gina, the mammary gland, and in the mouth. In one case which I observed, the tumor occurred in the midlateral region of the back, over the last five ribs (Fig. 18), and weighed 590 gm.; it was situated in the loose tissues over the intercostal muscles.

Ribbert obtained from the right side of the abdomen of a dog a hard fibroma, portions of which he used for a series of transplantation ex-periments. Fragments of the original tumor were inoculated subcu-taneously into the same animal. The transplants developed slowly to about 4 cm. in diameter at the end of four months. Autotransplanta-tion from the secondary tumors was also successful, but attempts to obtain growths from grafts inoculated into another dog failed. Mann attempted a series of transplantations from a fibroma that occurred in the structures over the lateral aspect of the tibiotarsal articulation of the left leg of an adult male cat. A total of twenty-five cats was inoculated with portions of the original tumor, none of which grew. However, four

6

of the five transplantations made into the tissues of the animal possessing the original tumor were successful.

Casper quoted Kitt as having observed a fibroma of the uterus of a hog; the mass weighed 13 kg. One of the fibromas in my series was obtained from the apex of the heart of a four-year-old sheep, and weighed 240 gm. Two cases of fibroma of the testis of donkeys were described by Galli. Crocker mentioned the finding of a fibroma of the cerebellum in the course of 401 postmortem examinations of cats. The tumor was not described. In the captive wild mammals and birds, the observations of Fox would indicate that fibromas are not common.

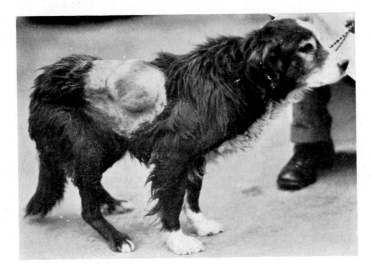

Fig. 18.—Fibroma.

Multiple primary fibroblastic tumors of the integument are sometimes observed. This condition, which is designated cutaneous neurofibromatosis because of its relation to the peripheral nerves, occurs most frequently in horses. Kitt quoted Siedamgrotzky as having observed more than 100 fibromas of the skin of a thirteen-year-old stallion. The tumors occurred in the pectoral region, abdomen, neck, and face. I observed a similar condition in a two-year-old black mule; the tumors, which varied in size from 1 to 10 cm., occurred in the skin of the forearm, shoulder, over the right eye, around the anus, and at the base of the tail. The tumors of the forearm extended down the anterior surface of the limb to the knee; those of the anus involved the ventral surface of the tail for a distance of 15 cm. Multiple neurofibromas of the skin also have been observed in dogs.[1, 6] I observed one case, that of a deer, in which large numbers of tumors were distributed over practically the entire surface of the body.

Nasal polyps.—A somewhat common variety of fibroma is the polypoid growth of the nasal passages and the nasopharynx known as nasal polyp. The statistics of Karnback, as quoted by Fölger, on the occurrence of nasal polyps in horses show only forty-one of these neoplasms in a total of 234,569 horses treated in Berlin clinics during a period of twenty-two years. The majority of nasal polyps occur in horses, and although they are usually unilateral in the nasal passage, they are sometimes bilateral. The nasal polyps are significant because of the respiratory embarrassment which they frequently cause. The tumor originates from the submucous fibrous connective tissue and gradually pushes into the lumen of the nasal passage. The polyps frequently become pedunculated, and vary in size from a few centimeters in diameter up to masses which may entirely occlude the nasal passage and weigh as much as 1 kg. They are rather characteristic in appearance, for they are smooth, glistening, ovoid masses, slimy to the touch. When incised they are found to be covered with a deflection of the mucous membrane, which may become roughened or even ulcerated. Infection and hemorrhage occur not infrequently. The tumor proper consists of an interlacing of fibrous connective tissue elements which are often rather loosely arranged and somewhat edematous. Numerous small blood vessels are usually present. Associated with the tumor elements are variable quantities of lymphocytes, monocytes, and eosinophiles. They vary from dull white to flesh pink in color (Figs. 19 and 20).

Nasal polyps which are true fibromas should not be confused with certain nodular hyperplasias of the nasal passages of horses which sometimes occur usually bilaterally, in the lower third of the nares. This condition appears in the form of multiple, dome-like, yellowish red enlargements, the surface of which often appears lacerated. The nodules vary from 0.5 to 3 cm. in diameter. According to Kitt these nodules represent hyperplasia of the glandular and connective tissue elements of the nasal mucosa, and therefore are not true tumors.

Effects.—Since fibromas are benign they must depend on their size, shape, and position to exert a harmful influence on their host. As a rule exterior tumors are disfiguring, and by their position may interfere with the normal function of the part affected. If they are on the shoulder of the horse or mule, they prevent the proper placing of the collar; if on the penis or within the vaginal passage, they make sexual contact impossible. The external forms are more or less susceptible to trauma, and

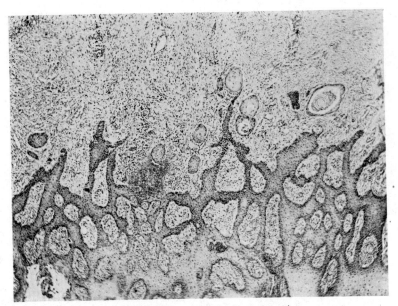

FIG. 19.—Nasal polyp of a horse (× 50).

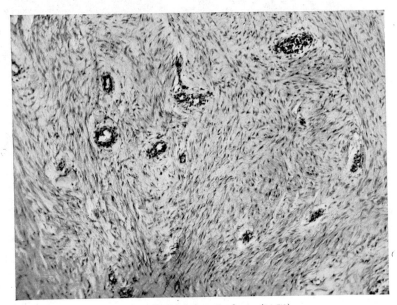

FIG. 20.—Nasal polyp of a horse (× 70).

accompanying infection and hemorrhage, although seldom serious, are frequently offensive. The involvement of vital tissue by a tumor is always serious, and if fibroma should occur in the larger cavities of the body, the effect would be significant, depending on the size attained by the tumor and its exact situation.

Metastasis or malignancy.—In the strict sense fibromas are not malignant. They do not metastasize but remain localized. The occasional development of multiple fibromas may suggest metastasis, this usually can be explained on the basis of their relationship to the connective tissue structures of the peripheral nervous system.

Gross characteristics.—Although fibromas vary considerably as individual specimens, they have many features in common. They consist, usually, of somewhat flattened or nodular, dome-like swellings,

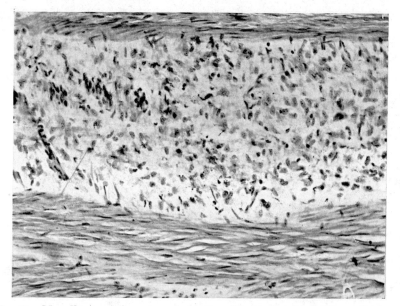

Fig. 21.—Myxofibroma of the rectum of a bovine. Myxomatous tissue between the dense strands of collagen (× 150).

possessing a capsular investment. They are commonly well embedded in the surrounding tissue, but may be pedunculated. Those of the exterior surfaces are usually covered by skin which is frequently ulcerated, and extensive infection with subsequent suppuration often leads to more or less necrosis of the underlying tumor. If the tumor is unusually large, parts of it may suffer regression due to lack of nutrition. Cysts may form and myxomatous degeneration may occur (Fig. 21).

If permitted to grow without interference fibromas sometimes become very large, but their average growth ranges in weight from a few grams to an occasional specimen weighing 5 kg. Lobulations are not common. The tumors are a grayish-white to a pink, depending on the consistence and the amount of blood present. Ordinarily they are not particularly vascular, but sometimes hemorrhage after removal is considerable.

Microscopic description.—Structurally, fibromas are simple, and consist of fibroblasts and strands of collagen fibrils often running in every conceivable direction. The fibrils of collagen may be tangled and twisted, which makes it impossible to trace them any great distance. The fibroblasts present their longitudinal axes parallel to the strands of collagen, and the nuclei are often spindle-shaped (Fig. 22). The type cell varies in size and number, depending on the rate of growth. In the

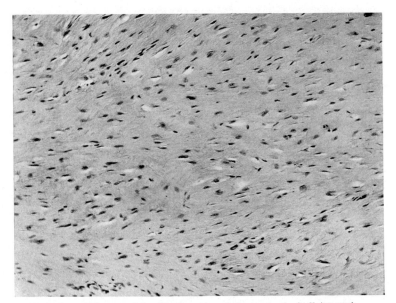

FIG. 22.—Fibroma of the distal portion of the penis of a bull ($\times$ 120).

more rapidly growing tumors the cells are larger and more numerous than in those which grow slowly. By special stains, fibroglia can be seen running longitudinally through the nuclei. A separate stroma is difficult to perceive. It consists of connective tissue derived from the elements of the tumor and blood vessels, which may be present. The vessels may be large or small, immature or well developed. Erythrocytes may even exist in direct contact with collagen, without a discernible separating membrane. Eosinophiles are often seen in the substance of the tumor and in areas of infection, and necrosis and polymorpho-nuclear leukocytes are usually present.

Fibromas which are compactly knit, and which appear hard and

nodular, are called fibroma durum, whereas those more loosely con-
structed and of a soft, flabby consistence, are known as fibroma molle.

Diagnostic characteristics.—Diagnosis is not, as a rule, difficult if
acceptable sections of the tumor have been prepared and the clinical
aspects are given due consideration. One must, however, guard against
the error of confusing with true fibroma certain nodular masses of
granulation tissue called keloids (Fig. 23). Keloids, which consist of
rapidly proliferating fibroblastic tissue, arise only as a result of definite
injuries, as from trauma, heat, and chemicals. They also tend to recur
when removed, but do not metastasize. Furthermore, if one takes into

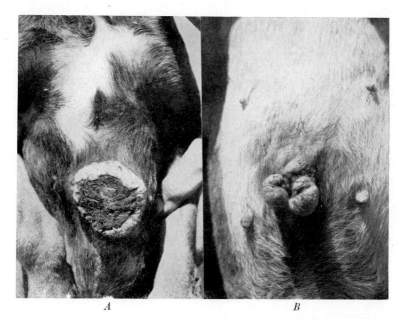

A   B

Fig. 23.—Keloids of the skin of dogs. *A*, sessile form of attachment; *B*, lobulated, pedunculated type of growth.

consideration the fact that keloids present a picture of richly vascular-
ized granulation tissue, with infection and polymorphonuclear leukocytes constituting the greater portion of the material, the proper diagnosis should not be difficult (Fig. 24).

It may also be necessary to distinguish fibroma from the closely
related malignant form of fibroblastoma known as fibrosarcoma. Although the clinical data may be helpful, the only dependable evidence
is that obtained from microscopic study of prepared sections. Fibrosarcomas consist of immature, vigorously growing fibroblasts, characterized by frequent mitosis, a minimal amount of collagen, and an

infiltration type of growth. Such tumors also exhibit a tendency to recur when removed but they rarely metastasize.

Clinical considerations.—Fibromas as a class are amenable to successful surgical treatment providing they occur in accessible situations. In case of doubt as to the character of a tumor of this kind, biopsy should be done and a diagnosis obtained from microscopic study of the material. Surgical removal is not ordinarily attended with technical difficulties if one is prepared to control the resultant hemorrhage, which in some

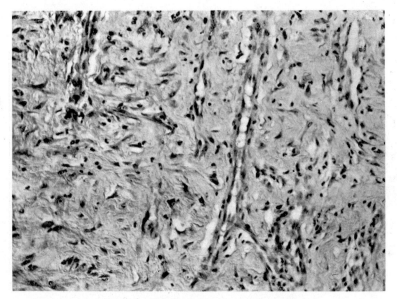

FIG. 24.—Keloid of skin of a dog (× 220).

instances may be profuse. This should be kept in mind, particularly in surgical removal of nasal polyps.

FIBROSARCOMA

Definition.—A fibrosarcoma is a malignant tumor made up of connective tissue consisting of immature fibroblasts and their products.

Incidence.—Reliable statistics pertaining to the incidence of fibrosarcoma in lower animals are not available, largely because of the unfortunate use of the term "spindle-cell" sarcoma in older literature on the subject. The term was used in a morphologic sense to denote any sarcomatous growth in which the type cell was considered to be spindle shaped. Under this designation were recorded tumors the histogenesis of which may have been connective tissue, bone, cartilage, or smooth muscle. It is not uncommon to find fibrosarcomas in horses, dogs, and cattle. I noted fifteen in a total of 510 neoplasms in my collection. They were distributed among the respective species as follows:

Six fibrosarcomas in 214 cattle; three in seventy-eight dogs; two in five mules; one in forty horses; one in thirty-nine sheep, and two in fifty-three chickens.

Occurrence and points of origin.—Since a fibrosarcoma consists of the same tissue elements as those which constitute benign fibroblastomas,

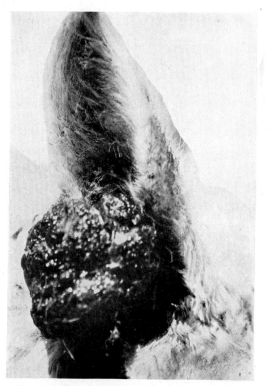

Fig. 25.—Fibrosarcoma of the concha of a horse.

it would be correct to assume that it can arise from any situation where fibromas develop. In other words, a fibrosarcoma may originate from any place where fibroblastic connective tissue is found. In this regard, it should be emphasized that the essential difference between a fibroma and a fibrosarcoma is that the latter is malignant, whereas the former is benign. Fundamentally the same cellular constituents are present in each.

Kinsley stated that fibrosarcoma is common in the eyelids and labial commissures of horses and mules, and that several cases have been observed in which the growth occurred in the region of the withers. Specimens have also been obtained from the facial sinuses of horses and cattle (Fig. 25).

The six fibrosarcomas of cattle in my series were situated as follows: Lateral side of the distal third of the mandible; uterus; region of the pancreas; upper third of the neck; distal portion of the penis, and the left vesicogenital pouch. Those of the dog, of which there were three, affected the region of the larynx, the scrotum, and the skin of the lateral surface of the elbow joint (Fig. 26). The two obtained from the mule

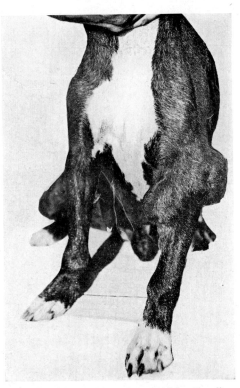

Fig. 26.—Multiple fibrosarcomas of the tissues overlying the elbow joint of a dog.

affected the head. One tumor extended from the right facial crest to the external canthus of the eye, and the other was just above the eye. The one from the horse affected the lower posterior border of the concha, and one from a sheep involved the anterior surface of the scapula. One of the two tumors that were obtained from chickens involved the muscles and tendons of the anterior side of the right fibula, with tumorous foci in the muscles of the left thigh, the gizzard, and the lung. The other affected the entire left portion of the keel bone of a six-month-old white Leghorn cockerel (Fig. 27).

The possible influence of color, breed, sex, and species on the occurrence of fibrosarcoma is not apparent. Age likewise is not a factor. The cases reported, as well as those in my collection, have been of animals the ages of which varied from a few months to several years; the majority occurred, perhaps, in adult life.

Effects.—Fibrosarcomas influence the well-being of the host by their size and position, and as a consequence they may interfere seriously with the proper functioning of some vital part. The infiltrative manner of growth results in progressive destruction of all tissues encountered

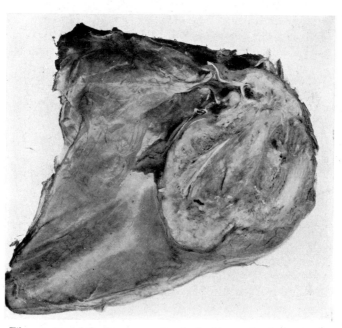

Fig. 27.—Fibrosarcoma of the tissues covering the keel bone of a chicken. Involvement was bilateral and metastasis had occurred to the lungs.

by the proliferating cells. Growths of the exterior of the body usually become traumatized, thus permitting subsequent invasion by pyogenic bacteria. The effect of such a condition on the host is problematic.

Internal growths often cause digestive or respiratory disturbances, depending on the exact position of the growth. Inappetence and chronic indigestion may be observed if the fibrosarcoma is in the abdominal cavity. Yet, as is the case with many other even extremely large abdominal tumors, the animal frequently fails to give the slightest symptom of abnormality, and the tumor is discovered only at necropsy. There is certainly nothing characteristic about internal neoplasms of this variety that would enable one to venture anything more than a clinical diagnosis of tumor, and the likelihood of being correct even then would be largely a matter of chance.

Since fibrosarcomas are malignant they are always dangerous. Even after such of these tumors as are operable have been carefully removed recurrence is common, and if the case is permitted to run its course the usual effects of malignancy can be predicted.

Metastasis and malignancy.—Generally speaking, fibrosarcoma of animals, although capable of being infiltrative and destructive, does not exhibit a degree of malignancy comparable to many other malignant neoplasms. These growths frequently recur rapidly and grow with considerable vigor after successive removals, yet the majority remain more or less localized. Distant metastasis is uncommon. In only two of the fifteen cases of fibrosarcoma in which I made an examination was there demonstrable metastasis. When one considers the malignant histologic appearance of most of these tumors, it is difficult to explain why more of them fail to metastasize.

Gross characteristics.—Fibrosarcomas are irregular nodular masses, occasionally more or less circumscribed, and the pedunculated varieties are usually encapsulated. The capsules of those in the abdominal cavity may be formed by a deflection of the peritoneum which appears as a smooth, glistening, flesh-colored membrane. Those found externally are often just under the skin, and as a consequence the surface is usually covered by hair. They often ulcerate and give off a foul-smelling discharge. The growth is grayish-white or flesh color, and may have a mottled appearance. It is usually firm, but occasionally it is soft, and there is more or less fluid within cyst-like cavities. The blood supply is usually abundant, and if the surface is subjected to frequent injury, hemorrhage is not uncommon, and the dried blood forms a brownish-black crust over the surface which sometimes leads the clinician to suspect pigmented tumor. In size the growths vary from nodules 1 cm. or more in diameter, up to large, fleshy masses weighing many kilograms. The average growth weighs from a few grams to less than 1 kg.

Microscopic appearance.—A fibrosarcoma consists of practically the same elements as a fibroma with the majority of the cells more or less embryonic (Figs. 28 and 29). Fibroblasts are present in abundance, and possess large, well-stained nuclei, with considerable chromatin material in the form of granules diffusely scattered throughout the nuclear substance. The individual fibroblasts appear in an irregular arrangement, and in a given section one may observe cells disposed at every conceiv-

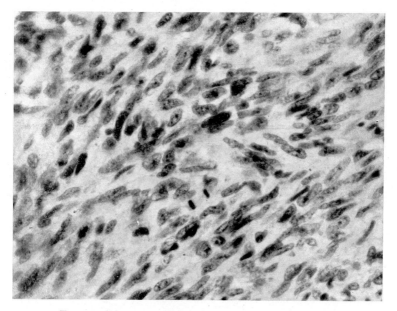

FIG. 28.—Fibrosarcoma from the scapula of a sheep (× 525).

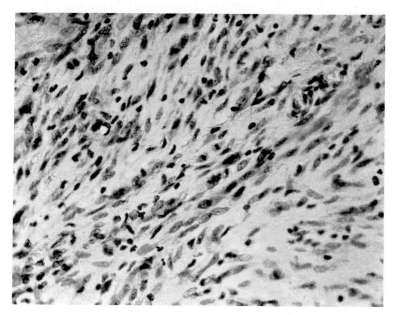

FIG. 29.—Fibrosarcoma from the scrotum of an eight-year-old dog (× 300).

able angle (Fig. 30). As further evidence of the immature nature of the type cell, mitotic figures are present, and in particularly rapidly growing tumors many interesting phases of mitosis may be observed in the same field. Collagen is present in varying amounts; it is more abundant in the slow-growing tumors than in those which grow rapidly. In fact, many fields of vigorously growing tumors of this type do not contain demonstrable collagen fibrils. When present, the collagen frequently presents a tangled, twisted appearance. Definite stroma may be missing, and, in the more slowly growing fibrosarcomas, it may be difficult to determine. However, in some, definite strands of stroma, resembling septums, may be present. The blood vessels appear in elements of the stroma, or, as often happens, in the midst of the parenchyma of the

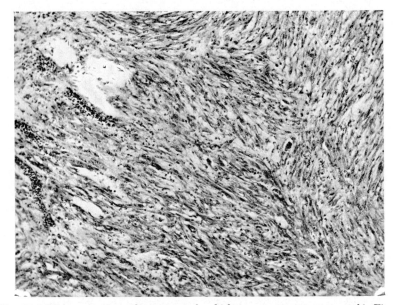

Fig. 30.—Fibrosarcoma over the sternum of a chicken; same case as represented in Figure 27 (× 120).

tumor. In some instances they are large and immature, whereas others are smaller, with the structure of the walls similar to that of adult vessels. Large accumulations of eosinophiles and lymphocytes may occur, and if the mass is infected, polymorphonuclear leukocytes are numerous.

Clinical considerations.—The possibility of fibrosarcoma should be considered in the presence of any fibrous tumor that does not develop in a wound, or as the result of definite trauma, and which shows a tendency to recur after its removal. The multiple character of the tumor, or the appearance of secondary nodules is also suggestive, but one should, when possible, resort to examination of microscopic sections before arriving at a definite diagnosis. Microscopically the immature fibroblasts, with their aggressive infiltrative tendencies, assist in reaching proper conclusions.

Keloids may be mistaken for fibrosarcomas, and one must be alert for any evidence of granulation tissue in growths from the region of wounds (page 87).

Fibrosarcomas in operable situations often can be removed surgically. Although the growth frequently recurs with surprising rapidity, if the operation is done in the early stage of the disease and a considerable amount of the adjacent tissue is removed, definite retardation of the process may be expected.

Before surgical interference with these tumors is attempted the diagnosis should be made certain by biopsy. If microscopic study of the tissue sustains the clinical study, removal of the growth should be attempted with knowledge that recurrence is probable. However, operation often will prolong the life and usefulness of an animal that might otherwise have to be killed for humane or economic reasons.

BIBLIOGRAPHY

1. Cadiot: Quoted by Kitt.
2. Casper, M.: Geschwülste bei Tieren. Ergebn. d. all. Path. u. path. Anat., **11**: 1068–1122, 1907.
3. Crocker, W. J.: Three thousand autopsies. Cornell Vet., **9**: 142–161 (Jan.), 1919.
4. Fölger, A. F.: Geschwülste bei Tieren. Ergebn. d. all. Path. u. path. Anat., **18**: 372–676, 1917.
5. Fox, Herbert: Disease in captive wild mammals and birds: incidence, description, comparison. Philadelphia, J. B. Lippincott Co., 1923, 665 pp.
6 Fröhner: Quoted by Casper.
7. Fuchs, M.: Quoted by Fölger.
8. Fumagalli: Quoted by Casper.
9. Galli, R.: Fibroma of the testicle in domestic animals. Abstract: Am. Vet. Med. Assn., **55**: 89, 1919.
10. Kinsley, A. T.: A text-book of veterinary pathology. Ed. 3. Chicago, A. Eger, 1917, p. 315.
11. Kitt, Theodor: Text book of comparative general pathology. Chicago, Chicago Medical Book Co., 1906, 471 pp.
12. Law, James: Textbook of veterinary medicine. Ed. 3. Ithaca, New York, 1910–1912, **2**: p. 372.
13. Mallory, F. B. and Wright, J. H.: Pathological technique. Ed. 8. Philadelphia, W. B. Saunders Co., 1924, p. 120.
14. Mann, F. C.: Attempts to obtain a transplantable tumor in the higher species of animals. Jour. Cancer Res., **4**: 331–347 (Oct.), 1919.
15. Noack: Quoted by Fölger.
16. Parker: Quoted by Fölger.
17. Petit, G.: Quoted by Casper.
18. Ribbert, Hugo: Transplantation eines Fibroms beim Hunde. Zentralbl. f. allg. Path. u. path. Anat., **21**: 625–628, 1910.
19. Thompson: Quoted by Casper.

CHAPTER V

MYXOBLASTOMA

DEFINITION

Myxoblastomas are composed of connective tissue, consisting of specialized fibroblastic cells which produce mucin in addition to fibroglia, collagen, and elastic fibrils. A benign tumor which comes under this heading is the myxoma. Myxosarcomas are malignant, and there are other terms which will be mentioned in the paragraphs on microscopic description. It is convenient, however, to consider the entire class, without such attention to subdivision, under the heading of myxoblastomas.

HISTOGENESIS

Primary myxoblastomas are not commonly observed in lower animals. However, extensive portions of myxomatous tissue are not infrequently seen in certain adult connective tissue tumors, such as fibromas, lipomas and chondromas, and the clinical terms myxofibroma, myxolipoma, and myxochondroma are appropriately used for such growths. Ewing called attention to the fact that in the early, undifferentiated state, connective tissue has a mucous quality. Such tissue is abundantly distributed throughout the subcutaneous regions in the embryo, and Ewing has expressed the belief that many primary mucous tumors of man arise from such deposits. Whether such histogenesis accounts for certain myxoblastomas in lower animals is a matter of conjecture. The fact, however, that most of the primary myxomatous tumors of animals which have been described have not involved the subcutaneous regions, would seem to require a different explanation for their origin. Of these, the characteristics of a myxoblastoma probably have been acquired in the majority of instances by the metaplastic transformation of fibrous connective tissue elements. In other words, the type cell of most myxoblastomas is a modified fibroblast that has assumed the capacity of producing mucin in addition to the usual products of this cell. The histogenesis and structure of primary myxoblastoma is so closely related to fibroblastoma that aside from the gross characteristics little more description is necessary than that which was given for fibroblastomas.

INCIDENCE

The available statistics on the incidence of myxoblastoma indicate definitely that this form of neoplasm seldom affects domestic animals. Casper quoted Fröhner's observations for a period of eight years, during which time 643 dogs were operated on for tumor and myxomas were not found. Casper also mentioned that among 335 tumors removed from horses in the Prussian army in a period of seven years primary myxoma was not encountered, although one myxofibroma was seen. Johne's statistics, compiled from material collected during twenty-five years at the Pathological Institute of the Dresden High School, showed the following:

Among 250 tumors of horses there was one myxoma; among 417 tumors of cattle there were three myxomas; among 209 tumors of dogs there were three myxomas, and among ninety-two tumors of hogs there were no myxomas. Only a portion of the tumors in Johne's series were primary myxomas. Many were mixed varieties such as myxofibroma and myxochrondroma.

Among 510 tumors in my collection there were only six myxomatous tumors. In 214 tumors of cattle one was a myxofibroma and one a primary myxoma. Among seventy-eight tumors of the dog one myxofibroma was found and among forty tumors of the horse one myxosarcoma was found. One myxosarcoma was also secured in a total of seventy-six neoplasms of swine. The only tumor from the cat was a fibromyxoma.

From these data it is evident that myxoblastoma constitutes a group of tumors of relatively little significance so far as the general animal population is concerned. Their occurrence, although serious enough so far as the affected individual is concerned, is so uncommon that one must consider them as neoplasms of minor significance.

OCCURRENCE AND POINTS OF ORIGIN

The subcutis, submucous, and subserous regions are the points of predilection for the occurrence of myxoblastoma. Most of the reported cases have been those of horses, and although a few cases have been described in which the disease affected cattle and dogs, few examples of the tumor in other species have been reported.

Horse.—Many of the reported myxoblastomas of the horse have been malignant, and a large number has involved the tissues of the head. Calamida observed a horse which died in convulsions, and at necropsy a tumor weighing 35 gm. was found in the left lateral ventricle of the brain and one weighing 5 gm. was found in the right lateral ventricle. The growths were diagnosed microscopically as myxosarcomas. A myxosarcoma of the sphenoid sinus of a horse was reported by Brazzola. Bernardini removed at operation a myxosarcoma which involved the frontal sinus, the maxillary sinus on the left side, and the upper portion of the nasal cavity, destroying the adjacent bone. Middlehurst observed a myxosarcoma of a horse, which affected the posterior portion of the tongue on the left side, and the soft palate, and extended to the lower jaw. Fölger quoted Achilles as having described two cases of myxosarcoma of the intestine of horses. One occurred near the end of the cecum and weighed 870 gm. with some evidence of metastasis to a nearby lymph node. The second tumor reported by Achilles also involved the cecum; it was situated in the serosa of the middle portion of this structure. A myxofibroma which was attached to the mucosa of the rectum by a pedicle 3 cm. long was described by Cadéac. The growth interfered with defecation and was removed. Multiple myxosarcomas were observed by Angelo in a horse which suffered with dyspnea. Necropsy revealed a large number of yellowish-white nodules distributed throughout both lungs. The extent of the involvement can be appreciated by the fact that the lungs were four times heavier than normal. Although the bronchial and mediastinal lymph nodes were affected, metastasis to the abdomen had not occurred.

The myxosarcoma of the horse in my series occurred on the gums of the maxilla, near the lateral incisor teeth of a suckling colt. It was removed surgically, but there was recurrence within a few weeks.

Bovine.—The literature contains records of few cases of myxoblastoma of cattle, which attests to the rarity of the growth in this species. A myxosarcoma of the rumen in the vicinity of the esophageal groove was observed by Ball, and Fölger mentioned a case described by von Gellmann in which the tumor occupied the wall of the left ventricle of the heart. Kitt contended that these tumors are frequently seen on and in the heart of cattle, where they arise from the remains of fetal mucous tissue in the subpericardial and subendocardial regions. Gehrig described a pedunculated myxoma that practically filled the right ventricle of the heart of a cow. One of the two specimens I secured from cattle was a myxofibroma attached to the lining of the rectum near the anus. The mass weighed 960 gm. The other, which was designated myxoma, consisted of a multiple, polypus-like structure resembling a cluster of grapes which occurred in the mucous lining of the esophagus about 15 cm. from the larynx. A similar growth was also present in the esophagus, approximately 15 cm. from the rumen.

Dog.—A myxosarcoma in the region of the front shoulder of a dog was reported by Murray, and Bodon described a somewhat unusual case of myxosarcoma of this animal, in which there was more or less general involvement. The parts affected included the lungs, bronchial and mediastinal lymph nodes, heart, pancreas, kidney, and omentum. A large myxosarcoma of the ovary was reported by Hebrant and Antoine. Little gave an account of a myxosarcoma which occurred on the superior portion of the outer border of the lower jaw of a four-year-old male hound. Following two unsuccessful attempts to remove the growth by surgical means, its final disappearance was effected after prolonged treatment with radium emanations.

The only myxomatous tumor obtained from the dog in my series was a myxofibroma. The growth, which had occasioned symptoms for one year before the death of the animal, involved the mediastinum of a

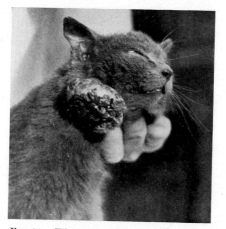

Fig. 31.—Fibromyxoma of the skin of a cat.

six-year-old Spitz. The tumor weighed 1,440 gm. The one tumor of swine in my collection was obtained from the right side of the thoracic cavity of an eight-month-old male hog. The growth was racemose and measured 6 cm. by 15 cm. Adhesions were present which joined the tumor to the lung and to the thoracic wall.

Murray noted an unusual myxosarcoma in which the tumor occupied axillary space of an old male cat. The tumor I obtained from a cat was situated in the skin just below the right ear. It had a short, constricted, neck-like attachment and was pendulous from the skin (Fig. 31). It contained two definite varieties of tissue; one was loose and fibrous, and the other consisted of immature myxomatous elements. The latter, a definite nodular mass, was embedded in the adult connective tissue of the growth. A diagnosis was made of fibromyxoma.

EFFECTS ON THE HOST

The mucin-producing tumors are similar in effect to the fibroblastomas, and the effect on the host depends largely on the size and situation of the growth, and on the secondary changes to which it may be subjected. If it is external, the effect on the patient is not serious; if it is internal and adjacent to, or within a vital part, the mechanical interference exerted may be disastrous.

METASTASIS AND MALIGNANCY

Although many myxomatous tumors remain localized, and have none of the features of malignant growths, it is not uncommon to observe rapid recurrence after removal, and microscopically the growth has every appearance of an immature destructive type. Histologically and clinically two varieties of myxoblastoma are recognized. The benign form is designated myxoma, and the form with characteristics of malignancy, myxosarcoma. Distant metastasis as a consequence of these growths is seldom observed.

GROSS CHARACTERISTICS

The size of these tumors, like that of most other tumors, varies within wide limits. Occasionally a tumor attains generous proportions and weighs as much as 3 to 4 kg., but the majority are much smaller. These growths may appear as lobulated grape-like clusters or more frequently as irregularly rounded nodular tumors. Many of them are encapsulated or partially encapsulated, and practically all of them are soft and slimy to the touch and have a peculiar gelatinous consistence which may cause them to be mistaken for fat. They are somewhat translucent and often are yellowish and streaked. Many are grayish-white or almost colorless. A pedicle type of attachment is occasionally observed.

MICROSCOPIC DESCRIPTION

The histologic structure of a myxoblastoma is fairly simple, and consists of spindle-shaped or stellate cells resting in a homogeneous, slightly basophilic mucinous matrix (Fig. 32). Many of the stellate cells give off long cytoplasmic processes, which anastomose in the matrix, and collagen fibrils in varying amounts are present. The relative proportion of cells and matrix is never constant. In the benign or slow-growing type of myxoma the matrix is usually abundant, and the cells are comparatively few, whereas in the rapidly growing myxo-

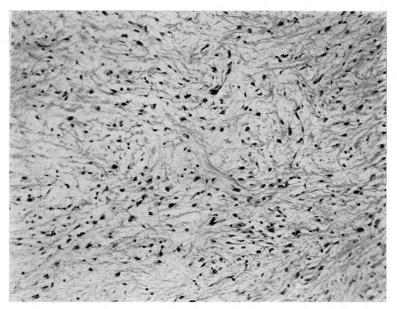

FIG. 32.—Myxoma (× 120).

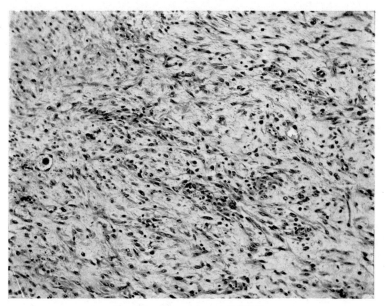

FIG. 33.—Myxosarcoma (× 120).

sarcoma, the mucinous matrix is scant and the cells are numerous (Fig. 33). Ewing has expressed the opinion that the bulk of the matrix depends on the capacity of the mucinous material to absorb water. How-

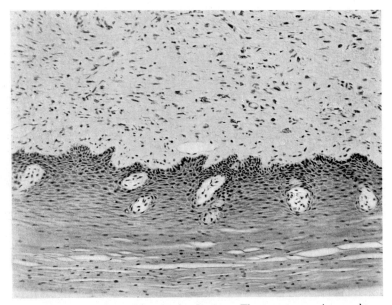

FIG. 34.—Myxoma of the esophagus of a bovine. The tumor occupies a submucous position (× 120).

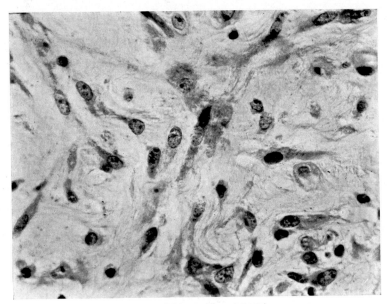

FIG. 35.—Myxosarcoma (× 525).

ever, the rate of growth must have some influence on the quantity of the matrix, since the more immature, rapidly growing cells produce less mucin than the more adult or differentiated cells (Fig. 34).

In the rapidly growing tumors, the myxosarcomas, mitotic figures usually can be demonstrated, and their presence, together with the clinical features of recurrence, infiltration, or metastasis indicates a sarcomatous type of growth (Fig. 35).

If the myxomatous changes have occurred secondarily in primary neoplasms consisting of fibrous connective tissue, cartilage, fat, or bone, remains of the initial tumor elements can usually be found. In such a case, the secondary character of the mucoid material can be indicated by combining the prefix "myxo" with the term ordinarily used for the process constituting the primary tumor; for example, "myxofibroma" and "myxochrondroma."

DIAGNOSTIC CHARACTERISTICS

As I have mentioned, myxoblastomas are often secondary in other primary tumors of connective tissue, and, if they are external, they may be confused with soft fibromas or lipomas. Grossly, however, there are a few features that will assist in determining the true nature of these tumors. Their slimy, gelatinous consistence, and their grayish or yellow-streaked color are valuable aids. Microscopically the star-shaped or stellate cells and the finely granular, fibrillated, or homogeneous matrix are fairly characteristic. Specific stains to aid in the recognition of mucin are often of much assistance in identifying these tumors and should always be used when doubt exists as to their true character.

CLINICAL CONSIDERATIONS

Since many of the myxoblastomas occur internally, their inaccessability makes surgical procedures for their removal difficult if not impossible. Those that are situated on the exterior of the body usually can be removed, although the incomplete encapsulation of many of the growths makes it difficult to remove them completely and recurrence of the growth is frequently observed. Little's experience with radium should encourage the further use of this form of treatment by those who possess the necessary equipment.

BIBLIOGRAPHY

1. Achilles, A.: Quoted by Fölger.
2. Angelo, F.: Quoted by Fölger.
3. Ball, V.: Néoplasmes gastriques. Jour. de méd. Vét. et Zootech., s. 5, 10: 709–716, 1906.
4. Bernardini: Quoted by Fölger.
5. Bodon, M.: Quoted by Fölger.
6. Brazzola, G.: Quoted by Fölger.

7. Cadéac, C.: Sur les retrécisséments et les tumeurs de rectum. Jour. de méd. Vét. et Zootech., s. 5, **12**: 513–517, 1908.

8. Calamida: Quoted by Fölger.

9. Casper, M.: Geschwülste bei Tieren. Ergebn. d. all. Path. u. path. Anat., **11**: 1068–1122, 1907.

10. Ewing, James: Neoplastic diseases. Ed. 3. Philadelphia, W. B. Saunders Co., 1928, p. 183.

11. Fölger, A. F.: Geschwülste bei Tieren. Ergebn. d. all. Path. u. path. Anat., **18**: 372–676, 1917.

12. Gehrig, P.: Quoted by Fölger.

13. Hebrant and Antoine: Large ovarian myxo-sarcoma in a slut. Abstract: Am. Vet. Rev., **45**: 100, 1914.

14. Johne: Quoted by Casper.

15. Kitt, Theodor: Textbook of comparative general pathology. Chicago, Chicago Medical Book Co., 1906, p. 350.

16. Little, G. W.: Some studies in the behavior of malignant growths in dogs and horses. Jour. Am. Vet. Med. Assn., **71**: 171–188 (May), 1927.

17. Middlehurst: Malignant tumour in the tongue of a horse. Vet. Jour., **10**: 296, 1904.

18. Murray, J. A.: Malignant new growths from domesticated animals. Third scientific report of the Imperial Cancer Research Fund, London, 1908, pp. 43–44.

CHAPTER VI

CHONDROBLASTOMA

DEFINITION

Chondroblastoma consists principally of cartilage, the cells of which are derived from undifferentiated mesenchymal elements. The benign form is known as chondroma, and if the tumor grows rapidly and metastasizes it is designated chondrosarcoma. All, of course, are basically chondroblastomas, and as such will be considered, without any consistent effort to separate the two subclasses.

HISTOGENESIS

In considering the developmental process of the cartilage cell it is important to keep in mind its relationship to the fundamental connective tissue cell known as the fibroblast. Under a variety of conditions the fibroblast is capable of certain specialization, as a consequence of which it is able to produce additional substances, to assume altered morphology, and otherwise to change its appearance and functional capacity until it becomes differentiated into a cell which has little if any resemblance to its parent. Thus, cartilage cells ordinarily have their origin from the fibroblastic elements which make up the fibrous membrane known as the perichondrium. By a gradual process of transition, fibroblasts of this structure eventually become transformed into cartilage cells. The fibroblasts of the periosteum may also give rise to cartilage cells, and the occasional occurrence of cartilage in situations devoid of perichondrium or periosteum constitutes presumptive evidence that under certain conditions the cartilage cell may be derived from any tissue in which fibroblasts occur.

Specialized fibroblasts which differentiate into cartilage cells are characterized by the production of a homogeneous ground substance known as chondromucin in addition to collagen and elastic fibrils which are the usual products of these cells. Three varieties of cartilage are recognized, dependent on the predominance of certain products produced by the respective cells. Hyaline cartilage is characterized by the presence of an excessive amount of chondromucin, whereas, if the intercellular substance contains large numbers of elastic fibers, the tissue is designated elastic cartilage. Fibrous cartilage is characterized by the large amount of intercellular collagen fibers.

The adult cartilage cell represents the end product of a gradual process of transformation and as such is not concerned in the production of other cartilage cells. These always arise by differentiation from certain fibroblasts which have the latent capacity to produce chondromucin.

The majority of chondroblastomas develop principally in situations which normally contain cartilage, although they may occur in regions where cartilage is ordinarily absent. For the latter, a histogenesis based on the occurrence of fetal or embryonal displacement of chondrogenic tissue frequently has been advanced. In view, however, of the relationship of chondrogenesis to the fibroblast it seems more logical to assume that the appearance of a cartilaginous tumor in regions where cartilage or bone does not normally occur is, in most instances, the result of metaplasia, by virtue of which any fibroblasts may differentiate into a cartilage cell. The possibility of the occasional occurrence of a chondroblastoma from misplaced chondrogenic rudiments is, however, tenable.

INCIDENCE

Chondroblastoma is one of the rarer neoplasms of the lower animals, although Ewing has expressed the opinion that this tumor is more common in animals than in man. My experience agrees with that of Casper in that with the exception of chondroblastomas which affect the mammary gland of the dog, the tumors are extremely uncommon.

Johne's statistics on the occurrence of cartilaginous tumors are quoted by Casper. At the Pathological Institute of the Dresden Veterinary High School during a period of twenty-five years the tumors were observed as follows:

Among 250 tumors of horses there was one chondroma; among 417 tumors of cattle chondroma was not found; among ninety-two tumors of swine chondroma was not found, and among 209 tumors of dogs there were three chondromas.

Fröhner failed to observe chondroblastoma among 150 tumors of horses, and except for those which involved the mammary gland, he failed to encounter a single specimen among 643 tumors of dogs. Casper stated that among 335 tumors obtained from horses of the Prussian army there were only two chondromas (0.6 per cent).

Among the seventy-eight tumors in my series obtained from dogs there was only one tumor which contained cartilage, a chondrosarcoma.

Among forty tumors of sheep there was one chondroma. Chondroblastoma was not encountered among 214 tumors of cattle, seventy-six tumors of swine, forty tumors of horses, and fifty-three tumors of chickens.

OCCURRENCE AND POINTS OF ORIGIN

Since the greatest number of chondromas arises from regions where cartilage normally occurs, it is to be expected that most of them should develop in association with the skeleton or the cartilage of the respiratory tract.

Horse.—In this animal tumors containing cartilage occasionally arise from the bony structure of the thoracic wall, and since it has been noted that severe trauma to the ribs has been followed by the development of such a tumor, a possible cause for certain chondromas has been advanced. However, one must be cautious in attaching undue significance to trauma in the subsequent development of neoplasm.

The relatively few cases of chondroblastoma reported in the literature are worthy of mention. Chondroma of the wall of the thorax of the horse was reported by Leisering and by Bruckmüller, and Casper quoted Gurlt as having observed a similar tumor that involved the maxilla. Fölger mentioned that Eeckhout described a fibrous, cartilaginous tumor involving the right arytenoid cartilage of the larynx. A large chondrosarcoma of the left lung of a horse was found by Dürbeck, and Kitt is mentioned by Casper as having observed a large, cauliflower-shaped chondroma which originated from the wall of the right bronchus of a horse; the growth penetrated into the lumen of the bronchus, and additional tumorous foci were distributed in the substance of the lungs.

A most remarkable instance of the occurrence of chondroma was reported by Renner. The condition affected a colt which had been born totally blind. Examination revealed the presence of small chondromas in the vitreous humor of both eyes. The masses were encapsulated and attached to the choroid by multiple nonpigmented strands of connective tissue.

Tumors containing cartilage have been reported occasionally as occurring in the intestines. A case of this kind was reported by Joest, who found a small, nodular mass in the wall of the ileum, about 10 cm. from the ileocecal opening in a gelding aged between eighteen and twenty years. A similar tumor of the cecum was described by Schelameur. The occurrence of chondroma of the testis of the horse also has been demonstrated.[3, 27]

Bovine.—Relatively few cases of chondroblastoma of cattle have been reported. Moussu observed a large, osseous chondroma of the turbinated bones of a three-year-old animal. The growth filled the nasal cavity and extended into the nasopharynx. A chondrosarcoma was found by Menicagli in an eight-year-old cow that had been dyspneic for two months. The tumor was close to the lower angle of the right nasal opening and was adherent to the cartilaginous nasal septum. The growth, which was hard but not painful, was removed surgically. Morot is quoted by Casper as having observed a chondroma weighing 4.5 kg.; it was attached to the second and third cervical vertebræ on the left side of the neck of a cow aged fifteen years.

Casper noted in the literature that many chondromas had been described as originating from the cartilage of the bronchi of cattle. A large growth, which involved several ribs of a cow, was reported by Petit and Germain.[30] The mass, which had a nodular, rounded surface, measured 20 by 30 cm., and weighed 8 kg.; its inner surface was covered with pleura, and although there were multiple lesions in the pleura the lung was not affected.

Chondromas arising from the scapula of cattle have been reported by Ball and by Nencioni. Dammann described a cystic chondroma of the bones of the elbow joint. The tumor affected the medullary portion of the humerus and apparently had its origin in the epiphysis of the radius. A chondroma of the humerus, which weighed about 9 kg., was reported by Eisenmenger, and a chondroma which contained some bone was observed by Siedamgrotzky at the fetlock joint of a cow. An enormous chondrosarcoma weighing 28 kg. was observed in the subcutis of the left flank by Janson. The tumor metastasized in the lungs. Kitt mentioned the occurrence of a chondroma in the wall of the rumen of a calf and Fölger quoted Bomhard as having found a tumor containing cartilage in the urethra of a young animal.

Dog.—Cartilaginous tumors of the lower animals occur most frequently in the mammary glands of dogs. Since cartilage is not a normal constituent of this organ, the occurrence of the tumor must be dependent on one of two circumstances; the cartilage cells are either derived from embryonal fetal deposits of chondrogenic tissue, or they arise through a metaplastic transformation from fibroblasts. The fact that all transitions from fibrous connective tissue to cartilage can be observed in many of these tumors favors the latter hypothesis for the development of the majority of chondroblastomas of the mammary gland. The process appears to begin in the interstitial tissues of the milk ducts and alveoli and whereas fibrous or hyaline cartilage is the predominating tissue in most tumors, ossification is sometimes in evidence, particularly in the central portions of cartilaginous masses. In tumors which have existed for a considerable time, and in which degeneration is in progress, calcification may occur. On the basis of the pathologic changes that may ensue, Cornil classified the cartilaginous tumors of the mammary gland as pure chondroma, ossified chondroma, and calcified chondroma.

One must also recognize that the multipotency of the fibroblast from which these tumors arise is such that several varieties of tissues may sometimes occur as a result of fibroblastic activity. Although the initial and predominating proliferation of cells is such as to characterize the growth as a cartilaginous tumor it is not uncommon to find also fibrous, mucous, or even osseous tissue. Various names are sometimes used to designate tumors that contain such tissues in different combinations. Myxochondroma, fibrochondroma, and myxofibrochondroma are common names in the literature, descriptive of these growths. If portions of the epithelial structures are isolated by encroachment of the tumor, cystic cavitations may result. The cystic character of such a tumor is often implied by a combination of terms such as cystochondroma, cystomyxochondroma, and cystofibrochondroma.

Besides the cartilaginous tumors of the mammary gland of the dog, many of which have been described in the literature, chondroblastoma has sometimes been observed in other anatomic situations.

Fölger stated that Joest found a hard, cartilaginous tumor of a dog aged eight years that had destroyed much of the osseous tissues of the frontal region and in which there were spicules of bone. Zahn reported a large osteoid chondroma involving the larynx and the trachea, the exact genesis of which was not determined. Siedamgrotzky found an osteoid chondroma in the thyroid gland. Multiple cartilaginous tumors were found in the thoracic cavity of a dog by Hilden who considered that the growth had originated from the cartilage of the ribs. A similar tumor was observed by Joest in a dog aged four years which had suffered a fracture of the seventh rib. The growth, which was nodular, measured 19 by 11 cm. and extended from the second to the eleventh rib on the left side. Murray reported a chondrosarcoma of the axillary space of a dog, and Cadéac reported a large chondroma of the humerus of a dog aged ten years. The tumor, which also involved the scapula, weighed 4.7 kg. and was considered to be a pure chondroma, since bone was not demonstrable. A malignant form of chondroma that originated on the small toe of the right front foot of a dog was reported by Ball. The primary growth was hard and ulcerated and measured 4 by 5 cm. At necropsy secondary foci were revealed in the lungs and kidneys. The pancreas was also involved. Casper quoted the case of Janson in which a chondroma was found in the spinal canal of a young dachshund; the posterior portions of the animal's body suddenly had become paralyzed. The tumor was situated at the juncture of the fourth and fifth lumbar vertebræ. A somewhat unusual case of chondrosarcoma of the dog was that described by Petit. At necropsy he found a cartilaginous tumor about 7 cm. in diameter in the small intestine of a dog aged eleven years. Metastasis to the lungs had occurred and they contained enormous numbers of nodules of variable size. The intestinal growth consisted

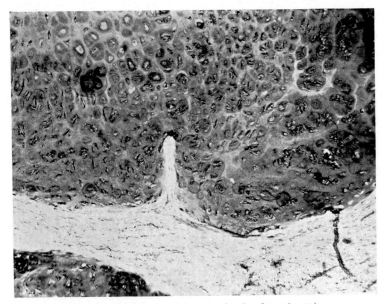

Fig. 36.—Chondroma of the scapula of a sheep (× 85).

entirely of cartilage cells and their precursors. The tumors of the lung had undergone variable degrees of ossification. Casper quoted Mocard and Cadéac as having observed primary chondromas of the bronchi in dogs.

I observed a chondroma which involved the right superior gums and dental spaces of a collie aged nine years.

Other species.—Judging from the reports obtained from the literature, chondroblastoma does not commonly affect domestic animals other than horses, cattle, and dogs. Wooldridge observed a very large cartilage tumor of a cat which contained some spicules of bone. The tumor arose from the right humerus and involved the scapula; it weighed approximately 1.9 kg. A large tumor involving the anterior edge of the concha of a goat aged six years was seen by Nemesek, and a chondroma of the maxilla of a goat was seen by Gurlt. Chondromas of the region of the shoulder in sheep were seen by Gurlt and Röll, and a specimen in my collection involved the right scapula and the surrounding muscle and connective tissue of a sheep aged five years (Fig. 36). The tumor, in which there was some necrosis, weighed 960 gm. In Kitt's textbook of comparative general pathology is a striking illustration of a fibro-chondroma affecting the ovary of a sheep. Kinsley mentioned a chondroma weighing 12 kg. that was obtained from a sheep's sternum.

In Fox's series of nearly fifty neoplasms of captive wild mammals a cartilaginous tumor appeared but once, an osteochondroma of the nose of a caracul.

Kaupp reported a large cartilaginous tumor from the tibia of a hen. The tumor measured 7 by 10 by 11 cm. and was not encapsulated. It consisted principally of cartilaginous tissue in various stages of development, the central portion of which was undergoing ossification. Smaller tumors were also present on the right and left walls of the thorax, and were probably of the same character as the tibial growth. Kinsley mentioned the finding of a chondrosarcoma of the sternum of a chicken. A chondroma of the tarsal region of a parrot was described by Petit and Germain.[29] The mass was egg shaped and covered with skin.

EFFECTS ON THE HOST

Chondroblastomas usually exert their effect by interfering with the proper functioning of a part. Occasionally a tumor may metastasize to distant parts. However, most growths remain localized, and the harmful effect they may exert is dependent largely on their situation and size. Those of the mammary gland of dogs preclude the further functional activity of the parts affected, and those involving or adjacent to the respiratory apparatus may cause severe dyspnea. Those of the skeletal system may induce paralysis if nerves are encroached on, and if joints are involved, lameness occurs.

METASTASIS AND MALIGNANCY

If metastasis occurs it is usually by way of the blood stream and the cells concerned in the initiation of secondary foci are the immature chondrogenic elements, and not the mature cartilage cells of the parent growth. The same variations, which not uncommonly are seen in the structure of the primary tumor may be seen in the metastatic growths, and various combinations of different tissues may occur.

GROSS CHARACTERISTICS

Cartilaginous tumors vary grossly, depending on the amount and quality of the secondary changes which have occurred and the different types of tissues constituting the growth. The majority of these tumors are encapsulated and have a nodular, lobulated, or rounded contour. They are rather firm except when combined with other tissues or when retrogressive changes are present; then they may be softer. Those which consist predominantly of hyaline cartilage are opaque, and milky white to bluish gray. Those of the mammary gland are not uncommonly multiple and are lumpy and sharply limited; occasionally they attain considerable size. Cysts are often encountered which contain a soft, red or brown, slimy, mucus-like material, or a yellowish gelatinous fluid. Fibrous connective tissue in variable amounts is a constituent of many chondroblastomas, serving as a capsular investment, or extending into the substance of the growth. Like most other tumors they vary widely in size, depending on rate of growth and duration. Many of the tumors reported have weighed from one to several kilograms; Kitt gives the upper limit of weight as 28 kg.

MICROSCOPIC CHARACTERISTICS

In a typical chondroblastoma cartilage cells are often in groups of two or more, lying in a homogeneous, somewhat basophilic matrix of chondromucin. The matrix varies in amount; it is most abundant when the hyaline variety of cartilage is present, and is less abundant when the cartilage is of the fibrous or elastic type. In the majority of instances, however, the cartilage is of hyaline nature (Fig. 37). Strands of fibrous connective tissue of variable width frequently separate the cartilaginous tissue into irregular lobular-like areas. This feature is more pronounced in a slowly growing chondroma. In rapidly growing tumors the greatest variability in the appearance of the type cell may be recognized. All gradations, from the most immature to the fully adult cartilage cell are readily demonstrable. The undifferentiated forms which are found in the peripheral region of the respective cartilaginous units are spindle shaped, whereas they become large and polymorphous as the zone of fully differentiated cartilage cells is approached. Between these extremes all gradations occur (Fig. 38). In chondrosarcoma, the rapidity of the growth is evidenced by the num-

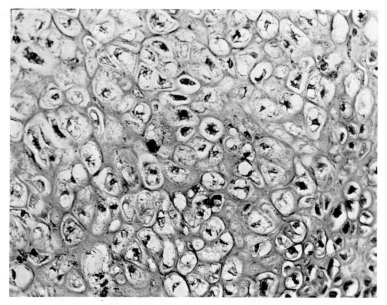

Fig. 37.—Chondroma of the gums of a dog's mouth (× 285).

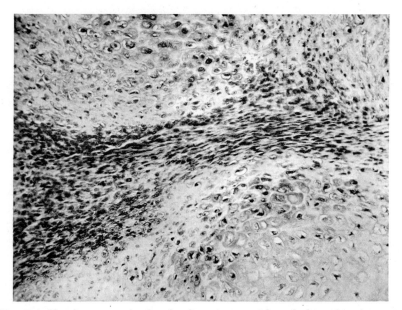

Fig. 38.—Chondrosarcoma showing chondrogenic zone with gradual transition into more adult type of cartilage cells (× 150).

ber of mitotic figures present in the less differentiated portions of the peripheral zones of the various groups of cartilage. Since the cartilage

8

cell represents the end product of cellular differentiation, the mitotic figures are limited to the less mature chondrogenic elements. The blood vessels are confined to the connective tissue which separates the various collections of cartilage cells and are rather few in the slow growing benign forms of the tumor. As a result of inadequacy of the blood supply, large portions may undergo necrosis or calcification. Cystic collections of gelatinous, mucoid material are sometimes seen.

In the rapidly growing tumor the proximity of the immature, vigorously proliferating chondrogenic cells to the poorly formed blood channels constitute a favorable circumstance for vascular invasions and subsequent metastasis.

CLINICAL CONSIDERATIONS

The relative infrequency of the occurrence of cartilaginous tumors makes chondroblastomas as a group of little clinical significance. If their situation makes them operable, removal is worthy of trial. Recurrence will depend on the degree of maturity of the chondrogenic tissue and the thoroughness with which it is removed. If metastasis is evident, operative interference with the primary tumor is futile.

BIBLIOGRAPHY

1. Ball: Chondrome de l'humérus. Jour. de méd. Vét. et Zootech., 140, 1903.

2. Ball, V.: Chondroma of the fingers. Abstract: Am. Vet. Rev., **45:** 242–243 (May), 1914.

3. Bruckmüller: Quoted by Casper.

4. Cadéac: Chondrome du coude. Jour. de méd. Vét. et Zootech., **59:** 72, 1908.

5. Casper, M.: Geschwülste bei Tieren. Ergebn. d. all. Path. u. path. Anat., **11:** 1068–1122, 1907.

6. Cornil: Quoted by Fölger.

7. Dammann: Quoted by Casper.

8. Dürbeck: Quoted by Fölger.

9. Eisenmenger: Chondrome de l'humérus chez une vache. Rev. gen. de méd. vét., **13:** 378, 1909.

10. Ewing, James: Neoplastic diseases. Ed. 3. Philadelphia, W. B. Saunders Co., 1928, p. 202.

11. Fölger, A. F.: Geschwülste bei Tieren. Ergebn. d. all. Path. u. path. Anat., **18:** 372–676, 1917.

12. Fox, Herbert: Disease in captive wild mammals and birds, incidence, description, comparison. Philadelphia, J. B. Lippincott Co., 1923, p. 478.

13. Fröhner, E.: Statistische und casuistische Mittheilungen über das Vorkommen und die chirurgische Behandlung der Geschwülste beim Hunde. Monatschr. f. prakt. Thierh., **6:** 1–19, 1894–1895.

14. Gurlt, E.: Quoted by Casper.

15. Hilden: Quoted by Fölger.

16. Janson: Über zwei Fälle von Enchondrom. Arch. f. Tierh., **7:** 207, 1881.

17. Joest: Quoted by Fölger.

18. Kaupp, B. F.: Sarco-chondro-osteomata of a hen. Jour. Am. Vet. Med. Assn., **55:** 424–427 (July), 1919.

19. Kinsley, A. T.: A text-book of veterinary pathology. Ed. 3. Chicago, A. Eger, 1917, p. 285.

20. Kitt, Theodor: Text-book of comparative general pathology. Chicago, Chicago Medical Book Co., 1906, p. 353.

21. Leisering: Quoted by Casper.

22. Menicagli, Luidi: Chondro-sarcomatous growth. Abstract: Am. Vet. Med. Assn., 49: 114, 1916.

23. Moussu, G.: Des tumeurs des cavités nasales chez les animaux de l'espèce bovine. Rec. de méd. vét., 83: 610, 1906.

24. Murray, J. A.: The zoological distribution of cancer. Third scientific report on investigations of the Imperial Cancer Research Fund, London, 1908, pp. 41-60.

25. Nemesek: Quoted by Casper.

26. Nencioni: Quoted by Casper.

27. Pascale: Quoted by Fölger.

28. Petit, G.: Relation d'un cas de chondrosarcome intestinal généralisé un poumon, chez un chien; considérations sur le mécanisme probable de généralisation des chondromes. Bul. de la Soc. centr. de méd Vét., 59: 283-286, 1905.

29. Petit, G. and Germain, R.: Chondrome à cellules ramifes, de la region tarsienne chez un perroquet. Bul. de la Soc. centr. de méd. Vét., 63: 344, 1909.

30. Petit, G. and Germain, R.: Large ossified costal chondroma generalized to the pleura in a cow. Abstract: Am. Vet. Rev., 42: 349 (Dec.), 1912.

31. Renner: Quoted by Casper.

32. Röll: Quoted by Casper.

33. Schelameur: Chondrome de la crosse du coecum. Jour. de méd. Vét. et Zootech., 41: 342, 1900.

34. Siedamgrotzky: Quoted by Casper.

35. Wooldridge, C. H.: An enormous chondroma of the right fore limb of a cat. Abstract: Am. Vet. Rev., 41: 476 (July), 1912.

36. Zahn, F. W.: Beiträge zur Geschwulstlehre. Deutsch. Ztschr. f. Chir., 23: 297-314, 1886.

CHAPTER VII

OSTEOBLASTOMA

DEFINITION AND GENERAL CONSIDERATION

Osteoblastomas are derived from the progenitors of cells which when fully differentiated become osteoblasts. The benign form is known as osteoma and the malignant variety as osteogenic sarcoma. The succeeding paragraphs will consist of general comment on the whole class of osteoblastoma, rather than on the subclasses separately. Little is known of this phase of oncology as it relates to the lower animals. True osteogenic neoplasms are not often encountered, and opportunity for their study is extremely meager. Seemingly, these tumors vary widely in their clinical and pathologic aspects, and if a comprehensive understanding of them is to be gained it would be essential to examine a large number of specimens. Unfortunately no such examination has been made, and much of the information available has been obtained from occasional reports of cases.

The subject of bone tumors is confused by the difficulty of separating the genuine osteoblastomas from the not uncommon osseous processes that are often associated with inflammatory and degenerative changes. Inflammatory proliferations, particularly of the epiphysis, may result in bony outgrowths on account of the deposition of lime salts in the osseomucin which has been produced by the connective tissue cells concerned in the excessive reparative process. Such hard, jagged, multiple, nodular masses of the surfaces of bones are sometimes extensive and are referred to as examples of exostosis. Ossification of muscles, fascia, and aponeurosis following more or less chronic injuries not infrequently occurs among cattle and horses, but these changes are best considered as part of the phenomenon of repair of tissue and outside the realm of neoplasia. However, it is sometimes extremely difficult, if not impossible, to determine the exact character of certain of these conditions.

Among the lower animals a true bony tumor may occasionally arise in the soft tissues, separate from the skeleton. These tumors, which may arise in the heart, the subcutis, the peritoneum, and the lung, are the result of metaplastic transformation of the multipotent connective tissue fibroblasts, as a consequence of which they assume the rôle of osteoblasts, or bone-forming cells. The acquired functional capacity of the cells permits production of osseomucin in which lime salts are deposited. Ewing stated that the several factors which seem to influence the acquisition of osteoblastic properties by fibroblasts are: (1) Proximity to bone; (2) the presence of calcific deposits; (3) active productive inflammation, and (4) special predisposition to calcification and ossification associated with disturbance of calcium metabolism. Ossification of fibroblastoma, myxoblastoma, and chondroblastoma not uncommonly occurs, and the tumors often become a complex combination of tissues, so that it may be difficult to determine the character of the tissue concerned in the initial proliferation.

As examples of heteroplastic ossification are the new bone formations which are sometimes found in the walls of the right side of the hearts of horses and cattle. Fölger noted that the condition exhibits a predilection for the tissues of the right side and that it never occurs on the left. Joest observed a large bony tumor in the lateral wall of the right auricle of a cow, which was considered to be due to metaplasia of connective tissue as a consequence of an inflammatory process. Joest also described extensive ossification in both posterior lobes of the lungs of a cow, the bony changes having followed interstitial pneumonia. Kitt[31] quoted Even and Cope as having found cattle in Argentina in which the connective tissue of the lungs was so calcified and ossified that the affected parts resembled an encrusted sponge. Bruckmüller found completely developed bone tissue in irregular masses, distributed in the lungs of an old dog, and Coremans found a spongy osteoma, about 8 cm. in diameter, in the lungs of a bovine. Beel came to the conclusion that the peritoneum in domestic animals, particularly in the hog, is likely to undergo ossification and that traumatic influences perhaps have some part in the process. Ossification of the peritoneum of cattle, swine, and dogs was described by Gurlt.

Virchow found osteomas of the vitreous humor of horses to be common. They develop from connective-tissue elements and assume the form of friable plates or spongy, bony masses. Bony new growths of the testis of a stallion were described by Gurlt, and several instances of ossification of the fibrous covering of the testis of horses were recorded by Bruckmüller. An ossifying sarcoma of the scrotal region of a nine-year-old castrated bovine was described by Daille and Sabatte. Metastasis had occurred to the lumbar lymph nodes, the lungs, the bronchial and mediastinal lymph nodes and to the pleura. A case of multiple osteomas of the lung of a bear was reported by Bollinger.

HISTOGENESIS

The origin of the type cell of bone tumors is not unlike that of cells concerned in the development of normal bone. The histogenesis, which is rather complex, has been summarized briefly by Mallory as follows: "Under normal conditions bone cells arise from fibroblasts either directly or through an intermediate form of it called the osteoblast. The fibroblasts which produce bone cells are known as periosteal and endosteal cells. They produce fibroglia, collagen, and elastic fibrils. In addition they are capable of secreting a dense homogeneous intercellular substance called osseomucin which binds the fibrils together rendering them more or less invisible and attracts lime salts. While this substance is being deposited the fibroblast contracts and alters its shape. The cell finally comes to occupy a cavity called a lacuna surrounded by the homogeneous substances in which the lime salts are deposited. From the cell cytoplasmic processes and perhaps fibroglia fibrils extend in all directions through canaliculi to connect with other cells. Bone cells are formed in this way in the skull, and so forth. In other places the fibroblasts change first into polymorphous osteoblasts often with fine granules in their cytoplasm."

It is generally considered that bone cells do not originate from cartilage. The ossification of cartilaginous structures is brought about by the proliferative activity of osteoblasts which arise from the osteogenic tissues. These invade the cartilage and gradually replace it by formation of bone. The fully differentiated bone cell, like the cartilage cell, is an end product and is not capable of giving rise to other bone cells by mitosis.

ETIOLOGY

The possible part of trauma in the etiology of bone tumors has been suggested by several case reports in which the tumor became apparent following a disturbance of this kind. The relationship, however significant, is devoid of proof, although in discussing the possible influences of trauma on the occurrence of osteogenic sarcoma of human beings, Kolodny stated: "It is believed that sarcoma of bone is frequently a result of a loss of growth restraint following an accidental or occupational trauma to a previously normal bone or a surgical trauma to an existing benign tumor growth." Kolodny also emphasized the significance of certain predisposing factors in the development of neoplasia. Although trauma may result in a definite urge of the injured tissues to initiate regeneration and repair, trauma hardly can be responsible for the loss of restraint of growth which characterizes the biology of the tumor cell. This is apparently due to some obscure, intangible factor designated perhaps unsatisfactorily by the word "predisposition."

The data pertaining to the incidence of tumors arising from bone are few. Reliable statistics are not available from American sources.

Casper reported that osteoma was not found among 335 tumors observed in horses belonging to the Prussian army, and none was found among 643 tumors of dogs examined by Fröhner[18]; however Fröhner[19] reported finding two osteomas among 150 tumors in a series of 5,000 horses. The incidence of osteomas among the material seen during twenty-five years in the Pathological Institute of the Dresden Veterinary High School is given by Johne as follows:

Among 250 tumors of horses there were two osteomas (0.5 per cent); among 416 tumors of cattle there were two osteomas (0.25 per cent); among ninety-two tumors of swine there were no osteomas, and among 209 tumors of dogs there was one osteoma (0.25 per cent). These statistics on the incidence of osteoblastoma are apparently limited to osteoma, which is the benign form of the disease. Definite data on the incidence of osteogenic sarcoma, as it affects animals, are not to be had. However, if one may judge from the cases reported in the literature, malignant tumors of bone are much more common in lower animals than benign tumors. The lack of a uniform nomenclature for the malignant varieties of bone tumor makes satisfactory classification of many of the reported cases impossible. For this reason the use of an inclusive term such as "osteogenic sarcoma" is desirable in referring to the sarcomatous growths which arise from the progenitors of cells which ordinarily become transformed into osteoblasts. To create different names to provide for the minor and often secondary features of certain of these tumors only adds confusion to a group of neoplasms which are often of a complex character.

OCCURRENCE AND POINTS OF ORIGIN

Most osteoblastomas occur in relation to bone; usually they arise from the bones of the head and of the extremities. Many of those in the head originate from the sphenoid and the ethmoid bones, where they may attain considerable size and replace adjacent normal structures of bone. According to Kitt, those which start from the ethmoid bone may penetrate into the cranial cavity and compress the brain. They are often malignant. Many cases have been reported in which osteomas have been found free in the respective cavities of the head, separation from the walls of a cavity occurring as a consequence of pressure atrophy or necrosis. Cases have been observed in which bony growths were expelled from the nasal passage.

The following are examples selected from the literature of the distribution of osteoblastomas of domestic animals.

Horse.—If one may judge from the reported cases the majority of bone tumors affecting horses arise from the tissues of the head;* many of the tumors described exhibited malignant tendencies although distant metastasis seemed to be uncommon.

Fölger quoted Coquot as having operated in a case in which a sarcomatous bony tumor affected the turbinated bones and part of the ethmoid bone on the right side of a three-year-old horse. Hendrix found a massive growth of similar nature on the dorsum of the nose of a horse. The growth was 34 cm. in circumference and 18 cm. long. Ripke removed an osteoma from the alveolar border of the maxilla, and Schimmel reported what he considered to be an osteofibroma which arose from the alveolar border of the mandible of a two-month-old colt.

Hendrix and Swaenepoel observed a malignant osteoma which apparently had its origin from the alveolar border of the maxilla. The growth had invaded and destroyed the palate, and the vomer had likewise disappeared. The ethmoid bone and the meninges of the brain were also involved. As a result of the tumor in the orbital spaces exophthalmos was present. Ehers is quoted by Fölger as having observed a case similar to this.

A tumor of the frontal sinus of a horse, designated as osteofibrosarcoma, was described by Schade. The growth had penetrated into the cranial cavity and destroyed the right olfactory lobe of the brain. A sarcomatous bony growth that had penetrated the ethmoid bone was found by Hartmann in the upper half of the right nasal cavity of a thirteen-year-old horse, and a case is recorded by Duschanek of an osteoma in a one-year-old horse which completely filled the frontal sinus, both maxillary sinuses, and the upper part of the nasal cavity. Although the tumors in Duschanek's case were of ivory-like consistence, the multiplicity of the lesions would suggest osteogenic sarcoma. Kinsley stated that osteoma is a common tumor of mules, occurring as projecting, pedunculated masses attached to the inferior maxilla.

* The bony, horn-like projections that sometimes occur under the skin of the frontal bones of horses are probably not true neoplasms but are the result of fetal mishap in the development of the bones of the head.

The reported instances of tumors derived from bone as they affect horses indicate that in this species the tumors occur most frequently in the following situations: The alveolar border of the mandible and maxilla, the upper nasal cavity, and the respective sinuses of the head. Apparently the bones of the body, or those of the extremities of horses, are seldom concerned in the genesis of osteoblastoma.

Bovine.—Tumors originating from bone seem to arise more commonly from the tissues of the head than from other tissues. Kitt[32] considered malignant tumors of the ethmoid bone and frontal bone to be common in these animals and cases of this kind were described by Leibenger. A hard osteoma of the nasal cavity, which had originated from the alveolar border of the maxilla, was described by Joest. Poletajew reported a rapidly developing osteoma weighing 786 gm. from the ramus of the mandible. Metzger, as quoted by Fölger, observed what was considered to be an osteosarcoma of the maxillary sinus, and an illustration depicting an osteoma of the horn of a cow appeared in Kitt's textbook of comparative general pathology. Multiple osteosarcomas of a cow were reported by Schimmelpfenning. The tumors were in the form of small nodules on the fifth cervical vertebra, on several of the dorsal vertebræ, and on almost all of the ribs. Petit[38] saw a huge bony sarcoma weighing 17 kg. which involved the last four ribs on the left side.

I have not observed true bone tumors affecting the extremities of cattle; apparently they are among the rarer forms of the disease. The only case of osteoblastoma which I observed in a series of 225 neoplasms obtained from bovine sources was a tumor, weighing approximately 19 kg., on the scapula of an old Jersey cow. The prescapular and prepectoral lymph nodes were involved metastatically, and there were also many tumorous nodules throughout the lungs. The parent tumor of the scapula was bone-like in every respect although the lesions of the lymph nodes and the lungs, while firm, were composed largely of undifferentiated tissue with little ossification. Histologically the tumor was considered to be an osteogenic sarcoma.

Dog.—The head of the dog, like that of the horse and the cow, has been the origin of many of the bone tumors which have been reported as occurring in this animal. A moderate number of osteoblastic tumors involving the extremities of the dog have been reported. In fact, available data indicate that the bones of the extremities of dogs are much more prone to neoplasia than the extremities of other species. Also the majority of the osteogenic tumors of the dog seem to be malignant. Benign osteoma rarely occurs.

Fölger mentioned Joest as having described an osteosarcoma which almost destroyed the squamous portion of the temporal bone of a female hunting dog. The growth had obliterated the articular fossa of the temporomaxillary articulation and had invaded the cranial cavity. Petit[40, 41] found an osseous sarcoma in the middle of the forehead in a six-year-old dog, which exhibited evidence of subnormal mentality. The tumor was connected with a similar large growth within the cranial cavity, which had seriously compromised the brain tissue, without, however, penetrating the dura mater. A so-called telangiectatic osteosarcoma of the left maxilla of a dog was reported by Petit and Almy. Petit[37] described an ossifying telangiectatic sarcoma that occurred on

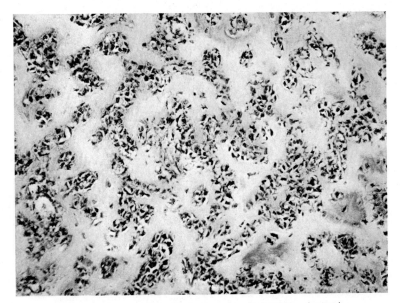

Fig. 39.—Osteoma from the laryngeal region of a dog ($\times$ 160).

the left side of the frontal region of a great Dane. The growth, which extended into the left nasal fossa, was infiltrative and destructive.

Among my collection of eighty-one tumors of the dog only two were osteoblastomas. One was an osteoma that originated from one of the bones of the larynx of a three-year-old fox terrier. It was bony, hard, and involved the laryngeal structure so intimately as to make it difficult to distinguish normal anatomic landmarks (Fig. 39). Adenocarcinoma of the thyroid gland and metastasis to the lungs and the liver were also present. The other tumor was an osteogenic sarcoma that involved the distal portion of the left ulnar of a two-year-old male English setter (Fig. 40). After a period of about six months the tumor had destroyed the epiphysis of the ulnar and the adjacent portion of the radius, and had extended into the upper portions of the carpal bones. Although metastasis was not revealed in roentgenograms of the thorax at the time the affected leg was amputated metastasis to the lungs was eventually demonstrated.

An osteogenic sarcoma of a seven-year-old St. Bernard dog, designated giant-cell sarcoma of the periosteal type, was studied by Mc-Whorter and Whipple. The growth, which was a fusiform mass situated largely in the distal portion of the diaphysis of the right radius, measured

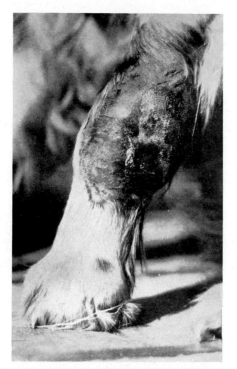

Fig. 40.—Osteogenic sarcoma of the ulnar of a dog.

27.5 cm. in diameter. It developed rapidly, but metastasis was not observed. An osteosarcoma originating from periosteal tissues of the diaphysis of the femur of a dog was observed by Petit,[39] and an enormous osteosarcoma of the left femur, weighing 5,800 gm. was described by Hogard; this animal was a six-year-old Newfoundland dog. The tumor, which evidently arose from the periosteum, involved the distal epiphysis and the adjoining half of the diaphysis. Fölger quoted Leblanc as having described an osteosarcoma of the proximal end of the femur of a six-year-old bitch. The tumor had infiltrated the adjacent musculature and produced small metastatic nodules in the lungs, although the regional lymph nodes were not involved. Joest reported a rapidly developing osteogenic sarcoma that occurred at the distal end of the forearm of a two-year-old dog. Among the necropsy data concerning a total of 1,548 dogs, Crocker listed an osteosarcoma of the left femur. An osteogenic sarcoma of a six-year-old great Dane was reported by Stewart. The tumor was of about five months' duration when the animal was killed, and the roentgenograms revealed a highly osteoplastic neoplasm involving the distal fourth of the right radius.

An osseous sarcoma that involved the thoracic wall of a two-year-old dog was reported by Petit.[38] The growth was telangiectatic and extended from the ninth to the twelfth ribs. The diaphragm was also affected, and metastasis was noted in the omentum, spleen, and liver. The liver weighed 3,700 gm. The lungs, pleura, and heart were not involved.

Other species.—Bone tumors have occasionally been observed in a few of the other domesticated mammals, and a few instances have been recorded in which wild mammals were affected.

An osteosarcoma of a sheep, which involved the left maxilla and extended to the palate, was observed by Horne, and a similar tumor of this species, affecting the mandible, was mentioned by Bashford and Murray. In a total of 401 cats examined at necropsy Crocker noted one osteosarcoma of the left femur. Cadéac described an osteosarcoma of the maxilla of a one-year-old cat, and an osteosarcoma of a deer was reported by Teetz. The mass, which originated from the spinal column of the scapula weighed approximately 3.3 kg. and had a circumference of 73 cm. Among Fox's series of neoplasms of captive wild mammals and fowls is listed on osteoma of the sternum of a Beechy's spermophile (Citellus grammurus beecheyi) and an osteofibroma of the jaw of an Isabelline gazelle (Gazella isabella).

Ratcliffe* described a malignant osteogenic tumor that appeared in or near the epiphysis of the ulna of a Chacma baboon (Papio porcarius). Metastasis eventually occurred to the lungs, walls of the right ventricle, and the right gluteus muscles.

EFFECTS ON THE HOST

Since the majority of bone tumors of animals arise in the tissues of the head, serious consequences are not uncommon. A benign osteoma

---

* Although Ratcliffe designated the neoplasm a giant-cell tumor, the process had many of the characteristics of an osteogenic sarcoma with the giant cells of secondary importance.

is usually disfiguring and may prove harmful on account of the situation, but the tendency of a large number of osteogenic tumors to exhibit the characteristics of malignancy constitutes a menace to the life of every individual who harbors such a tumor. Although distant metastasis is less common than from many other malignant tumors, the local destructiveness occasioned by these infiltrating growths is sufficient to consider the appearance of one of them a matter of major importance. If the tumors are situated in the oral cavity their presence may interfere with the proper taking of food and those that involve the air passages frequently cause dyspnea. Tumors of the long bones may infiltrate joints, and lameness may result. Instances have been observed of fractures of bones that have been weakened by invasion of the friable tumorous tissue, and such an accident may seriously imperil the life of the animal on account of the ensuing hemorrhage.

METASTASIS AND MALIGNANCY

Slow-growing, noninfiltrating, benign osteomas remain as localized nodular masses which may persist for years, with no inclination to become malignant. The malignant varieties, on the other hand, are malignant from the time of their inception. They exhibit different rates of growth, but in many of the cases reported they attained generous proportions and death followed within a few months to several months.

As I have mentioned, most osteogenic sarcomas exert their malignant propensities by their local invasive destructiveness, although occasionally a tumor may be capable of widespread metastasis. The proximity of many of the tumor cells to the blood vascular system, and capacity to infiltrate tissues of this kind, probably accounts for the metastatic dissemination of these tumors by way of the blood stream. It is not surprising, therefore, that occasionally a case is observed in which the lungs are studded with enormous numbers of secondary tumors. Instances in which metastatic tumors have been found in the liver, spleen, and kidneys are rare.

GROSS CHARACTERISTICS

Bone tumors vary widely in their gross appearance; the difference is due to the rate of growth, the anatomic situation, and the histologic character of the elements constituting the tumor. The slowly growing, benign forms are usually of a firm to stone hard consistence, although more or less soft masses of tissue, with numerous bony spicules may occasionally be found. The latter are somewhat spongy, and are most frequently seen in situations where bone does not occur normally. The amount of bone present, and the intimate relationship of the mass to the bone structure from which it originated, is frequently such as to require the use of a cleaver or a saw to separate the growth from the body. In the primary lesions of osteogenic sarcoma considerable bone tissue may occur whereas the metastatic foci frequently contain little of this substance, and are frequently irregular, compact, or hemorrhagic masses of tissue without resemblance to bone. Although osteoblastomas are irregular, somewhat nodular, and occasionally pedunculated, their physical characteristics are subject to so much variation as to make it

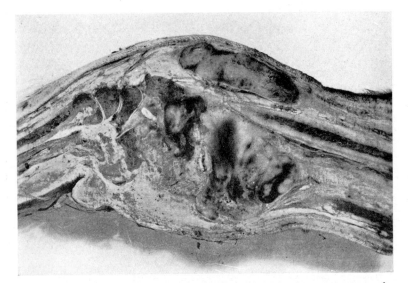

FIG. 41.—Sectional view of osteogenic sarcoma of the ulnar of a dog; same case as shown in Figure 40.

impossible to determine what should be considered typical. The majority of such tumors reported have been intimately associated with the tissues from which they originated (Fig. 41). A capsule usually covers the protecting surfaces, although one may expect the rapidly growing malignant forms occasionally to permeate the initial membranous investment and to infiltrate the surrounding soft tissues. If a soft tumor is near the surface and subject to trauma, ulceration associated with infection, and suppuration may occur.

The hard, benign osteoma is white to yellowish white, whereas the malignant, rapidly growing osteogenic sarcoma is likely to appear grayish or flesh colored.

MICROSCOPIC CHARACTERISTICS

The tumors vary as much in their microscopic appearance as they do grossly, largely because of the rate of growth and the degree of differentiation attained by the respective elements of the tumor. Since differentiation is a variable factor one may expect to see different stages in the transition of the osteogenic cell from the primitive to the most adult state in the same tumor (Fig. 42). These changes are to be seen in the malignant rather than in the benign forms of the disease. In the latter the growth progresses so slowly as to obscure the different stages in the developmental process.

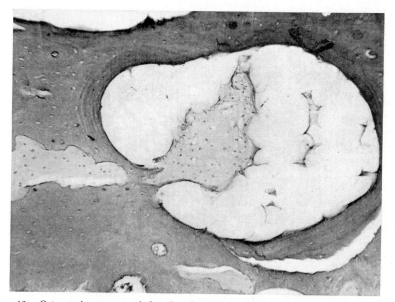

FIG. 42.—Osteogenic sarcoma of the ribs of a sheep. Adult tissue predominates in this field in which there are also a few islands of cartilage ($\times$ 120).

In structure, osteoma simulates bone. The resemblance, however, is seldom complete, and much of the finer histologic detail of normal bone is lacking. In the compact, benign forms which have been decalcified, one usually sees a diffusely disposed acidophilic matrix of osseomucin interrupted at irregular intervals by collections of osteoblasts, many of which may be atrophic (Fig. 39). Lamellæ may be distinguishable, and channels comparable to haversian canals are sometimes seen. In the soft or spongy bone tumors, numerous large and irregular spaces are present, and the bone, which appears as anastomosing trabeculæ, is correspondingly reduced in amount.

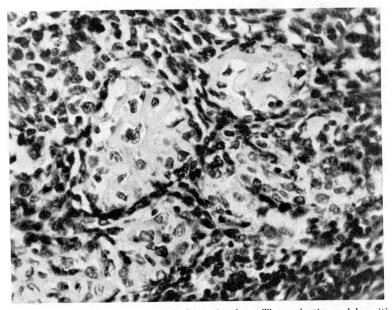

FIG. 43.—Metastatic osteogenic sarcoma; lung of a dog. The production and deposition of osseomucin has occurred although mineral salts are not demonstrable (× 440).

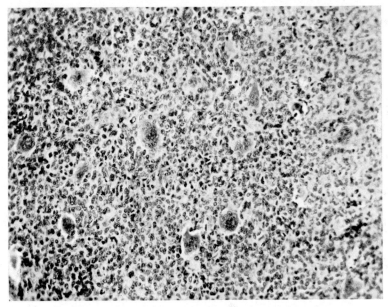

FIG. 44.—Osteogenic sarcoma of ulnar of a dog (× 225).

The microscopic structure of osteogenic sarcoma is usually that of a very cellular, infiltrative type of growth, in which destruction of normal

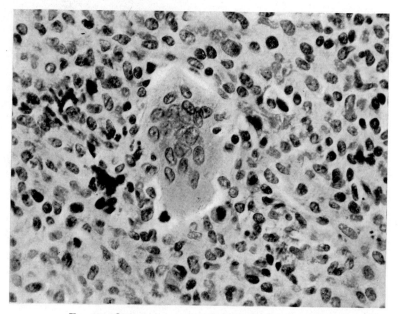

FIG. 45.—Osteogenic sarcoma of ulnar of a dog (× 660).

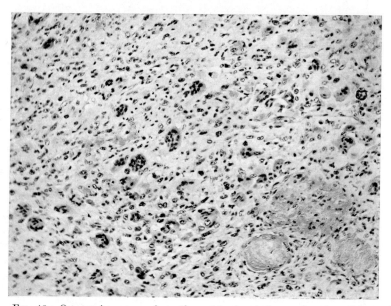

FIG. 46.—Osteogenic sarcoma from the wrist of a baboon; the photomicrograph (× 120) was prepared from a slide obtained through the courtesy of Dr. Herbert L. Ratcliffe of Philadelphia.

elements is usually evident. The morphology of the cells concerned in the structure of the tumor is not constant. The cells may be spindle,

9

ovoid, or polyhedral, and cells usually appear in compact, diffuse collections, and occasionally giant cells may be seen in the midst of the vigorously proliferating neoplastic elements (Figs. 43, 44, and 45). The giant cells are probably formed by the fusion of endothelial leukocytes (Figs. 46 and 47), and function in a manner comparable to osteoclasts by digesting and removing débris resulting from retrogressive influences to which the tumor cells may be subjected.[36] Mitotic figures are very often numerous, and a great many different phases of this phenomenon may be seen in the same microscopic field. Although some of the cells usually express sufficient differentiation to lay down osseomucin,

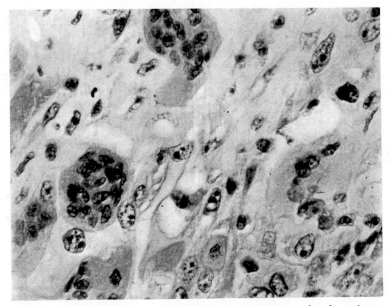

Fig. 47.—Giant cells of an osteogenic sarcoma of a baboon; the photomicrograph (× 525) was prepared from a slide obtained through the courtesy of Dr. Herbert L. Ratcliffe.

which subsequently may become bony trabeculæ, large groups of cells may occur in which bone or its precursor, osseomucin, is not apparent.

A considerable number of the reported cases of osteogenic sarcoma in animals has been described as being of a telangiectatic character. Ewing has observed that such tumors in man are characterized by overdevelopment of the blood spaces, with interstitial hemorrhages. The essential features of such a tumor are the blood sinuses, of variable size, which are "lined by hyperchromatic spindle and polyhedral cells."[15]

Rarely a tumor associated with bone may possess, as a striking characteristic, large numbers of giant cells of variable shapes and characteristics. These large, cytoplasmic masses, containing numerous nuclei, constitute such a prominent feature of these growths that they are usually referred to as giant-cell sarcomas or giant-cell tumors. The exact nature of the growths has been the subject of much controversy in which there is as yet no unanimity. Certain observers insist that these are the product of inflammation and repair, whereas others contend that they represent a definite neoplastic entity.[33]

Data on the occurrence of giant-cell tumors of domestic animals are rather meager, which would indicate that such growths must be among the rarer forms of animal tumors.

A few cases of a variety of giant-cell tumor of animals known as epulis, which springs from the alveolar processes of the jaw, have been reported. Meyer is quoted by Fölger as having observed such a tumor in the left maxilla of a hog. Boucek[5] reported two cases in which similar growths occurred in dogs. A giant-cell sarcoma arising from the posterior portion of the palate of a twelve-year-old dog was described by Douville, and Crocker listed a giant-cell sarcoma of the left scapula of a dog which was found at necropsy of 1,548 dogs. Crocker also mentioned that among 401 cats examined at necropsy there was a giant-cell sarcoma of the left foreleg.

A very unusual instance of giant-cell sarcoma of the wall of the left ventricle of the heart of a bovine was described by Gehrig. Whether the tumor was a primary growth, or metastatic, could not be determined. A giant-cell sarcoma of the nasal septum of a horse was noted by Boucek,[6] and a rapidly growing giant-cell sarcoma with hyaline degeneration was mentioned by Roth as occurring in the subparotid region of a horse.

Baker reported multiple giant-cell bone tumors of a Plymouth rock hen. At necropsy a new growth of soft, jelly-like consistence was found within the substance of the proximal portion of the metatarsus. The growth was limited by the cartilaginous tissue of the surface of the joint. A similar, but somewhat firmer tumor also was present at the proximal end of the tibia. Baker commented on the similarity between the giant-cell tumors in the case he studied, and in those encountered in man.

CLINICAL CONSIDERATIONS

In the diagnosis of bone tumors, particularly those of benign character, it may be exceedingly difficult to distinguish between bony outgrowths of inflammatory inception and true bone tumors. In this connection it is helpful to keep in mind that osteoma of the extremities of animals is a rather rare condition and that the majority of the bony protuberances of these parts are of inflammatory origin.

In the diagnosing of bone tumor of the smaller animals, use can be made of the roentgen ray by those having access to the necessary equipment. By this means presence of disease within bony cavities might be demonstrated, where otherwise it would escape detection (Fig. 48).

The malignant forms of the disease usually progress rapidly, and the tumors attain generous proportions within a relatively short time. The growth may occasion a definite bulging of the affected part, and if the bones of the extremities are involved, the tumor eventually causes such deterioration of the normal tissues that fracture of the diseased part

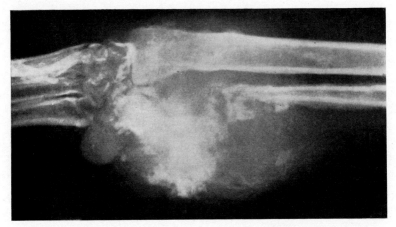

Fig. 48.—Roentgenogram of osteogenic sarcoma of the ulnar of a dog.

may ensue as a consequence of ordinary function. Such a happening is calamitous, since satisfactory relief cannot be accorded the unfortunate animal, and for humane reasons it should be killed.

Malignant osteogenic tumors may cause considerable pain, and progressive loss of weight. If the tumor is on one of the extremities, the pain seems to be lessened when the animal is in a recumbent position; in one of my cases, the dog preferred to lie on his back with the affected leg elevated.

The intimate association of the growth with the tissues from which it originated, and the anatomic inaccessability of many of the growths, particularly those of the head, are serious obstacles in the way of surgical treatment of tumors of this kind. If the lower extremities of the smaller animals are affected, amputation in the early stages of the disease may be tried. Although the tumor may eventually appear in other tissues as a consequence of metastasis before amputation, the relief from pain and the subsequent betterment of the general physical well-being of the animal justifies removal of the affected part. Growths of the epulis type, and others of the oral cavity, that may be pedunculated usually can be removed without difficulty.

Generally speaking, however, operation should be considered a rather futile procedure in combating osteogenic sarcoma as it occurs in the lower animals. The value of the roentgen ray in treatment is problematic. In one of my cases, an osteogenic sarcoma of the ulna in which the neoplastic cells were very immature, an intensive course of roentgen-ray treatments failed to have a restraining influence on the tumor and amputation was finally necessary. However, failure to obtain satisfactory results in this instance does not indicate that the treatment of others would likewise be futile. As material becomes available this problem should be investigated further.

BIBLIOGRAPHY

1. Baker, S. L.: Giant-cell tumours of bone in a fowl. Jour. Path. and Bacteriol., **31**: 657–658, 1928.

2. Bashford, E. J. and Murray, J. A.: Comparative cytological characteristics of malignant new growths. Scientific reports on the investigations of Cancer Research Fund, London, 1904, pp. 16–36.

3. Beel: Quoted by Fölger.

4. Bollinger: Quoted by Casper.

5. Boucek, Z.: Mitteilungen über 35 histologisch Tiergeschwülste. Arch. f. wiss. u. prakt. Tierh., **32**: 585, 1906.

6. Boucek, Z.: Quoted by Fölger.

7. Bruckmüller: Quoted by Casper.

8. Cadéac: Sarcome ossifiant de la bouche du chat. Jour. de méd. vét., **50**: 405, 1899.

9. Casper, M.: Geschwülste bei Tieren. Ergebn. d. all. Path. u. path. Anat., **11**: 1068–1122, 1907.

10. Coremans: Quoted by Casper.

11. Crocker, W. J.: Three thousand autopsies. Cornell Vet., **9**: 142–161 (Jan.), 1919.

12. Daille, A. and Sabatte, J.: Osteosarcome de la region testiculaire, avec generalisation, chez in beouf bistourne. Rév. vét., **33**: 65, 269, 1908.

13. Douville: Tumeurs malignes chez la chien. Sarcome a myéloplaxes de la voute palatine. Bul. de la Soc. centr. de méd. vét., **66**: 451, 1912.

14. Duschanek: Osteo in den Kopfhohlen des Pferdes. Tierarzt. Zentralbl., **26**: 533, 1903.

15. Ewing, James: Neoplastic disease. Ed. 3. Philadelphia, W. B. Saunders Co., 1928, pp. 218–292.

16. Fölger, A. F.: Geschwülste bei Tieren. Ergebn. d. all. Path. u. path. Anat., **18**: 373–676, 1917.

17. Fox, Herbert: Disease in captive wild mammals and birds, incidence, description, comparison. Philadelphia, J. B. Lippincott Co., 1923, 665 pp.

18. Fröhner, E.: Statistische und casuistische Mittheilungen über das Vorkomen und die chirurgische Behandlung der Geschwülste beim Hunde. Monatschr. f. prakt. Tierh., **6**: 1–19, 1894–1895.

19. Fröhner, E.: Hundert weitere Geschwülste bei Pferden. Monatsch. f. prakt. Tierh., **13**: 35, 1902.

20. Gehrig, P.: Quoted by Fölger.

21. Gurlt: Quoted by Casper.

22. Hartmann: Quoted by Fölger.

23. Hendrix, F.: Osteosarcome der chanfrein chez un poulain. Ann. de med. Vet., **61**: 648, 1912.

24. Hendrix and Swaenepoel: Quelques considerations sur les osteosarcomes du maxillaire superieur chez le cheval. Ann. de med. Vet., **53**: 433, 1904.

25. Hogard: Quoted by Fölger.

26. Horne: Quoted by Fölger.

27. Joest: Quoted by Fölger.

28. Johne: Quoted by Casper.

29. Kinsley, A. T.: A text-book of veterinary pathology. Ed. 3. Chicago, A. Eger, 1917, p. 290.

30. Kitt, Theodor: Text-book of comparative general pathology. Chicago, Chicago Medical Book Co., 1906, p. 355.

31. Kitt: Quoted by Casper.

32. Kitt: Quoted by Fölger.

33. Kolodny, Anatole: Bone sarcoma. The primary malignant tumors of bone and the giant-cell tumor. Surg., Gynec., and Obst., Suppl. 1, **44**: 1–214, 1927.

34. Leibenger: Osteosarkom. Wchnschr. f. Tierh., **42**: 336, 1898.

35. McWhorter, J. E. and Whipple, A. O.: Studies in cancer. George Crocker Special Research Fund, Columbia University Press, 1913, **3**: 117–124.

36. Mallory, F. B.: The principles of pathologic histology. Philadelphia, W. B Saunders Co., 1914, p. 295.

37. Petit, G.: Sarcome ossifiant des cornets et de la face, chez une chienne. Bul. de la soc. Anat. de Paris, s. 6, **2**: 1012–1013, 1900.

38. Petit, G.: Sarcome ostéoïde telangiectasique des côtes chez une vache. Bull. de la Soc. centr. de méd. vétér., **57**: 208, 1903.

39. Petit, G.: Ostéosarcome de l'extrémité inférieure du femur chez un chien. Bull. de la Soc. centr. de méd. vétér., **57**: 222, 1903.

40. Petit, G.: Sarcome ossifiant de la voûte cranienne ayant provoqué l'aplatissement des hémisphères cérébraux avec atrophie cérébelleuse consécutives, chez un chien. Bull. et mém. Soc. anat. de Paris, s. 6, **8**: 43–46, 1906.

41. Petit, G.: Compression et atrophie cérébrales par une tumeur de la voute du crâne, chez un chien. Bull. soc. centr. de méd. vét., **59**: 312, 1907.

42. Petit, G. and Almy: Sarcome ostéoïde, de la mâchoire supérieure chez le chien. Bull. de la soc. centr. de méd. vét., **15**: 469, 1901.

43. Poletajew, L.: Quoted by Fölger.

44. Ratcliffe, H. L.: Tumors in captive primates with a description of a giant-cell tumor in a Chacma baboon, *Papio porcarius.* Jour. Cancer Res., **14**: 453–460 (Aug.), 1930.

45. Ripke: Quoted by Fölger.

46. Roth, J.: Quoted by Fölger.

47. Schade: Quoted by Fölger.

48. Schimmel, W. C.: Quoted by Fölger.

49. Schimmelpfenning: Quoted by Fölger.

50. Stewart, W. H.: Periosteal sarcoma in a dog. Am. Jour. Roentgenol. and Radium Therap., **5**: 192 (April), 1918.

51. Teetz: Osteosarkom beim Reh. Berlin Tierarz. Wchnschr., 579, 1889.

52. Virchow, Rudolph: Die krankhaften Geschwülste. Berlin, A. Hirschwald, **2**: 1864–1865, p. 100.

CHAPTER VIII

LIPOBLASTOMA

DEFINITION

Lipoblastoma is a new growth consisting principally of fat cells and their supportive elements. Since lipoma is the only pure lipoblastoma to be considered, terminology requires little attention. Fibrolipoma, which, as its name suggests, is a mixture of fat and fibrous tissue, will be mentioned only.

HISTOGENESIS

Fat cells are derived, by a process of developmental changes, from certain elements of the embryonal mesenchyme. In their immature state, the cells may assume a polyhedral contour, contain an acidophilic cytoplasm without demonstrable fat, and in general resemble certain epithelial cells. Fat in the form of fine droplets eventually appears in the cytoplasm, and as the droplets increase in number they tend to coalesce and thus form large fat globules. As these continue to increase in size and number the entire interior of the cytoplasmic structure eventually becomes filled with fat, and the nucleus may be crowded to the periphery of the cell. The fat cell varies in its appearance, depending on its state of maturity, and the recognition of these variations in structure is essential to the interpretation of the histologic features of certain lipoblastomas that may be encountered.

Concerning the etiology of fat tumors in man, Ewing wrote: "A congenital tissue predisposition seems to be an essential factor in the origin of most lipomas." Whether predisposing influences are significant in the occurrence of these tumors of lower animals is a matter of conjecture. Although the fact has not been established it would seem reasonable to assume that the same etiologic influences are probably responsible for the inception of these tumors regardless of the species in which they occur.

INCIDENCE

Although fat tumors are by no means among the commoner neoplasms, they seem to be somewhat more common than the meager statistics indicate. In the neoplastic material observed at the Pathological Institute of the Dresden Veterinary High School during a period of twenty-five years, Johne noted only seventeen lipomas among 968 tumors of lower animals. The incidence of lipoma among the respective species was as follows:

Among 250 tumors of horses, six were lipomas; among 417 tumors of cattle, eight were lipomas; among 209 tumors of dogs, two were lipomas, and among ninety-two tumors of swine, one was a lipoma.

Casper mentioned that only three lipomas were observed among 335 tumors of horses in the Prussian army during seven years, and Fröhner[14] noted four fat tumors among 150 neoplasms secured from 5,000 horses observed at a veterinary clinic during a similar period. Fröhner also obtained thirty-nine lipomas from a total of 643 dogs operated on for neoplasia. The lipomas in my collection were obtained from the different species as follows: Among seventy-eight tumors of dogs two were lipomas, one lipoma was found among each of the following three groups, forty tumors of horses, 214 of cattle, and seventy-seven of swine.

OCCURRENCE AND POINTS OF ORIGIN

Lipomas occur with greatest frequency in regions where considerable adipose tissue normally exists, such as the connective tissues of the subcutaneous, intramuscular, submucous, and subperitoneal regions. Rarely they may arise from almost any place where fat tissue is normally present, as well as in situations normally free of fat cells, but possessing them because of some prenatal developmental mishap. Although the points of predilection vary somewhat with the different species the greater number of fat tumors which have been described have occurred in the subcutis of the extremities, and in the subserosa of the abdominal cavity.

Horse.—The literature contains a few references to lipoma originating from the membrana nictitans, and bilateral involvement of this kind was reported in a four-year-old stallion by Williams.[5] Lipoma of this structure was also observed by Schimmel and by Puschmann.

Casper quoted Joest as describing a somewhat unusual case of multiple lipoma in which seventy to eighty tumors had developed within a few weeks. The growths were situated on the head, neck, shoulder, withers, and abdomen. Tumorous nodules were also present between the muscles, especially in the cervical region. Casper mentioned the report by Schneidemühl of an instance of multiple lipomas of an emaciated horse. The tumors were in the subcutis, over the thorax and abdomen. They had developed within a year and were beginning to undergo calcification. Multiple lipomas in the subcutis posterior to the right scapula and in the lumbar region of a six-year-old stallion were described by Sawwaitow. A large growth was situated between the kidney and the liver and one was found in a testis.

Several cases of lipoma of the subcutis have been reported in which the tumor was freely movable over a considerable area. In the case observed by Bartke, a flattened lipoma on the left side of the back could be moved from the withers to the sacral region.

A huge lipoma in the region of the right flank of a horse was described by Hendrickx. The tumor measured 92 by 42 by 45 cm. and weighed 42 kg.; it had been present for six years. Casper stated that Essen had removed a lipoma weighing 4 kg. from the left half of a mare's udder, and Gooch noted a lipoma of the testis of a small four-year-old horse. Möller observed a large lipoma weighing 26.5 kg. in the subcutaneous tissues near the distal portion of the biceps femoris muscle, and Kinsley mentioned a diffuse lipoma of generous proportions in the subcutaneous tissues of the left hind leg of a two-year-old horse. It would appear from the illustration in Kinsley's case that the growth extended from the stiffle to below the hock, and that the affected leg seemed to be at least twice the circumference of the opposite leg which was not affected. Kitt noted the frequent occurrence of lipomas of considerable size in the subcutaneous tissues in the region of the knee of horses. Lipomas of horses usually occur in the abdominal cavity, where they commonly arise from the omentum or the mesentery. These growths are usually single although they may be multiple. They are sometimes pedunculated, and this may be responsible for serious twists or entanglements of the intestines that usually terminate in the death of the animal. Many cases of this kind have been mentioned by various observers.

Fölger considered that lipomas of the stomach and walls of the intestine occur infrequently; he quoted the case reported by Achilles in which there was a ring-shaped tumor of the wall of the intestine situated 2.5 cm. posterior to the stomach. Hurpez observed a lipoma that involved both the colon and the cecum, and Brose removed a lipoma about 12 cm. in diameter from the rectum of a horse. Casper mentioned an irregularly shaped lipoma, weighing 2.25 kg., that occurred in the right ventricle of the heart of a fourteen-year-old horse.

The one lipoma of the horse in my collection was obtained from a three and a half-year old Percheron. The history of the case is of some interest. When the animal was about a year old an abscess occurred in the tissues over the hip joint. This was drained and the wound apparently healed. Sometime later the horse received a kick in the region where the abscess had formed, and a fat tumor subsequently appeared in this area, which eventually attained a diameter of 40 cm. The growth was extirpated and had not recurred when the last observation was made eighteen months following removal.

Bovine.—Lipomas do not appear to occur in cattle as frequently as in horses. Furthermore, in cattle they seem to arise less commonly in the subcutaneous tissues; in the majority of reported cases the growths were situated in the interior of the body. In by far the greater number of reported cases the lipoma originated in the abdominal cavity (Fig. 49).

A lipoma weighing approximately 4.7 kg. was removed surgically from the left foreleg of a cow by Dey, and a lipoma of a calf was ob-

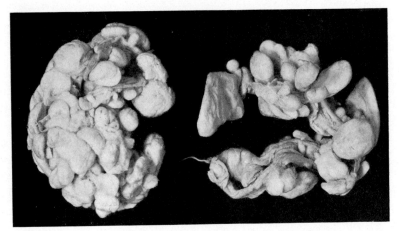

Fig. 49.—Multiple lipoma of the parietal peritoneum of a cow.

served in the same situation by Vielhauer. The growth surrounded the muscles completely, causing their atrophy. A lipoma was also present under the left scapula; this had penetrated into the intercostal spaces, and fatty masses had developed on the inner surface of the wall of the thorax.

Trotter observed in the left flank of an ox multiple nodules of variable sizes that had some resemblance to tuberculous nodules or to carcinoma. Microscopically the tumors were found to be lipomas. A pedunculated lipoma of the rumen of a cow, situated 3 cm. from the opening of the esophagus, was reported by Schweinhuber, and Kühnau observed in a three-year-old cow, affected with generalized tuberculosis, numerous fat tumors involving the omentum and both the visceral and parietal peritoneum. Casper quoted Verner as having recorded a strangulating lipoma of the abdomen of an ox, and Steuding reported a lipoma weighing 3.3 kg. in the region of the kidney of a three-week-old calf.

A lipoma of the mesentery of a calf was described by Giannini, and Lessa is credited by Casper as having demonstrated a pedunculated lipoma about 5 cm. in diameter in the rectum of a cow 6 cm. anterior to the anus. Joest described a lipoma weighing 8.7 kg. in the pelvic region of a cow. The tumor had interfered with parturition, as a consequence of which death had occurred. McFadyean described a lipoma, about 8 cm. in diameter, of the frontal bones of a calf nine months old. The growth, which appeared to have had its inception during fetal life, had interfered with the development and ossification of the cranial vault, and there was a large irregular opening in the lower part of the forehead representing a defect in the frontal bones. This space was occupied by the tumor.

A rare instance of the occurrence of lipoma was reported by Kühnau. The tumor, which measured 4 cm. in diameter, originated in the left hemisphere of the brain, in front of a vascular loop lying in the pia mater, in the region of the corpus callosum. The growth encroached on the brain tissue, and finally penetrated the frontal bone. Kühnau believed the tumor to be congenital. Ebinger is quoted by Casper as having found an extradural lipoma that compressed the spinal cord in the lumbar portion of the vertebral canal of a nine-year-old cow, and a somewhat similar tumor of the region of the sacrum of a cow was reported by Pfister. Kitt mentioned that Lund had recorded a huge lipoma of the submucosa of the uterus of a cow. The mass had the remarkable weight of 75 kg.

I have in my collection a specimen obtained from the abdominal cavity of a twelve-year-old grade cow. The entire visceral and parietal peritoneum was studded with small, grape-like clusters of light yellow fat tumors. Lesions of actinomycosis were present in the submaxillary and retropharyngeal lymph nodes.

Dog.—The sites of predilection of lipoma in dogs seem to be in the subcutaneous tissues of the inner surface of the thigh, the region of the shoulder, over the abdomen, and near the anus. They do, however, occur occasionally within the abdomen, and are commonly observed in well-nourished old dogs.

From the cases reported in the literature one may obtain a general idea concerning the distribution of fat tumors as they affect dogs. Fröhner[13] observed lipoma originating from the membrana nictitans of dogs, and in several instances he removed fat tumors from the anal region. Douville described a subcutaneous lipoma weighing approximately 1.9 kg. from a six-year-old female fox terrier. The growth, which was painless, extended from the lumbar region to the base of the tail and partially involved the upper part of the thigh. The animal died following operative removal of the growth. Douville described several other cases of lipoma of dogs. One tumor, weighing 4.5 kg., could not be removed because of the intimate involvement of the muscles of the thigh, and another tumor weighing 900 gm., was found in the region of the flank. Heney and Wooldridge removed a lipoma from the perineum of an old female dachshund. The occurrence of lipoma in the mammary gland of obese female dogs was described, according to Casper, by Stockfleth and Bang. Corst and Thomas reported on an invasive type of fat tumor of the mammary gland of a bitch which they designated "liposarcoma," and Petit and Peyron encountered in a female dog an invading liposarcoma of the mammary gland, which also possessed a mixed tumor consisting of epithelial elements, cysts, and cartilage. A pedunculated lipoma, which hung from the umbilicus of a dog, was described by Lawrence. The mass almost reached the ground when the animal was in a standing position.

Relatively few internal lipomas of the dog have been reported. Petit observed a large irregularly lobulated angiolipoma on the pelvic wall, and Williams[43] reported a pedunculated lipoma arising from the mesentery of a terrier. Some idea of the size of the tumor in this case may be obtained from the fact that the weight of the mass was equal to a fourth of the weight of the affected animal. Casper mentioned the reports of Trasbot of the finding of two large lipomas in the liver of a dog, and Bruckmüller found small lipomas of the kidney. Lipoma of the spleen was observed by Stephan in a fourteen-year-old terrier, and Semmer is quoted by Casper as having seen multiple small lipomas in the lungs of an old dog.

I have observed a lipoma weighing 85 gm. that developed under the skin over the hip joint of a three-year-old dog. The growth appeared following trauma to the affected region, and whereas a definite etiologic significance could not be ascribed to the trauma in this instance its possible influence was nevertheless suggested. A somewhat unusual example of lipoma occurred in a twelve-year-old female poodle. The animal's abdomen was noticeably pendulous and on palpation a rather large, firm, irregularly spherical mass could be demonstrated in the midabdominal region. Necropsy disclosed a smoothly lobulated, somewhat spherical mass weighing approximately 2 kg. and measuring 15 cm. at its greatest dimension (Fig. 50). The tumor was covered with a sheet of omental tissue, and was attached to the middorsal region by a short pedicle-like structure. The growth, which was covered with a capsule, consisted of two major portions, one of which resembled collapsed pulmonary tissue. When cut across, the growth presented a fatty or greasy appearance, and by appropriate stains its lipoblastic character was demonstrated. The liver contained several small fat foci, but the possible relationship of these to the growth was not established. The other organs were normal. This particular specimen was of considerable interest because of the extreme variation in the morphology of the type cell. All gradations, from the most immature to the adult types, were readily demonstrable.

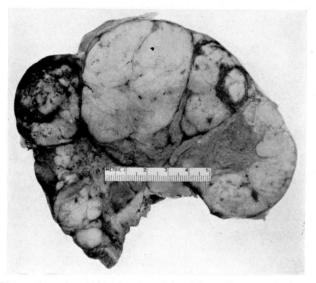

Fig. 50.—Lipoma from the middorsal region of the abdominal cavity of a dog. Sectional view.

Other species.—A huge lipoma weighing approximately 20 kg. which originated from the mesentery of a mule was reported by Stewart. On the surface of the liver were several small fat tumors. A subendocardial lipoma of the right ventricle of the heart of a two-year-old sheep was found by Messner, and Piper observed in the liver of a two-year-old wether numerous small, definitely limited, grayish-white nodules which were considered, microscopically, to be lipomas.

I recently obtained an intracranial lipoma that was found by a butcher engaged in the removal of the brains of hogs in a large midwestern slaughtering establishment. The tumor which was firm and the color of hog fat, was said to have been half the size of the brain.

The circumstances under which the growth was found precluded detailed data concerning it. Frozen sections of the tumor, stained with scarlet red, revealed a structure made up principally of fat-engorged cells.

Fox did not observe a lipoma in an extensive experience with captive wild mammals. Eight lipomas, however, were observed in captive wild birds. With two exceptions, these were disposed under the skin of the thorax and abdomen. One lipoma occurred under the scalp, and one occurred as a pelvic mass surrounding the cloaca of a hawk.

EFFECTS ON THE HOST

The deleterious effects of lipoma are largely of a mechanical nature. The tumors may become so large as to impede the natural movements of the animal. Those in the abdominal cavity often are attached by a pedicle and may become twisted around a loop of intestine with the usual results of intestinal strangulation. Again, these pendulous tumors may become separated from their attachments, and remain free among the abdominal viscera. When they occur within the orbit, or associated with the conjunctival mucosa, considerable interference with vision often results. Those that are congenital are often dangerous due to the pressure exerted on a vital part.

METASTASIS AND MALIGNANCY

The clinical observation of these tumors as they affect animals yields little data that would suggest metastasis, and although they may cause serious disturbances because of their size and situation, they are not ordinarily considered malignant in the usual sense of this term. Although, in an occasional case, multiple tumors may be present in situations suggestive of metastatic dissemination, proof that metastasis actually has occurred is difficult to establish. However, the embryonal appearance of many of the cells in certain of these tumors strongly suggests malign possibilities. Mitosis often can be demonstrated, and relationship of the neoplastic cells to the generous blood supply are circumstances favoring metastasis. The majority of fat tumors must be considered as belonging among the benign growths, but it cannot be denied that an occasional lipoblastoma, possessing the usual attributes of potential malignancy may occur. If malignancy can be demonstrated, such a tumor might properly be considered liposarcoma. Lipomas usually grow slowly and increase in most instances by expansion. Occasionally a diffuse type of growth may be encountered. Recurrence after removal is not infrequent, and is probably due to incomplete removal of the tumors at the initial operation.

GROSS CHARACTERISTICS

In size and shape these tumors, like most other tumors, are subject to more or less variation. Although remarkably large lipomas have been observed, they seldom attain a weight of more than 3 to 5 kg., and most of them weigh much less. They are usually rounded and multilobulated, although diffusely disposed masses of adipose tissue may occur which are difficult to describe.

The subperitoneal lipomas of the abdominal cavity may appear as small multiple tag-like masses or grape-like clusters of fat tissues, whereas those of the mesentery are elongated and pedunculated. Not uncommonly lipomas may be found free within the abdominal cavity following separation from their attachments.

Although most lipomas are firm, they are usually more or less elastic. They have a decided fatty appearance and impart a greasy film to the blade when cut with a knife. The color varies somewhat with the species. Lipomas of hogs are whitish, not unlike the color of lard, those of cattle are commonly whitish yellow, resembling suet, those of horses are often dirty yellow, and those of dogs are usually dirty white.

Lipomas that originate in the subcutis are seldom encapsulated, although those within the abdominal cavity frequently are. Even without a capsule most lipomas are circumscribed in shape; the exceptions are those that grow diffusely.

Secondary changes that may occur in lipoblastoma include necrosis, as a consequence of which the tumor may become dry and almost chalk-like or firmly calcified. Mucinous degenerations resulting in the formation of cysts may also occur. Occasionally there may be considerable laking of blood, or hemorrhage, and tumors situated externally often become ulcerated, the result of trauma.

If the tumor contains an excessive amount of fibrous connective tissue, it is often referred to clinically as "fibrolipoma."

MICROSCOPIC DESCRIPTION

The ordinary adult type of lipoma has a relatively simple structure. It usually consists of closely arranged fat cells, somewhat larger than normal, cells which are polyhedral and loaded to capacity with one large fat globule or several smaller ones. The nucleus is displaced by the excessive fat and may be obliterated. Interspersed irregularly among the

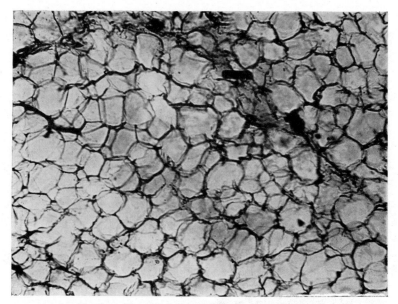

FIG. 51.—Lipoma of the subcutis of a horse ($\times$ 150).

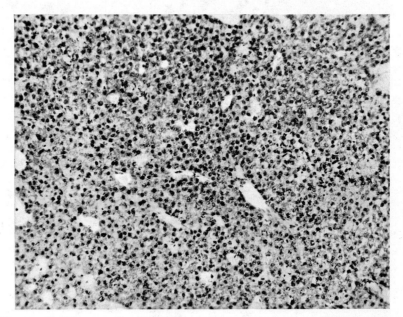

FIG. 52.—Lipoblastoma of a dog. Diffuse collection of immature undifferentiated lipo-blasts ($\times$ 120).

fat cells are various strands of fibrous connective tissue, which support the blood vessels of the tumor (Fig. 51).

Lipomas of the immature type frequently are more or less complex structurally, due to potential variability in the morphologic characteristics of the lipoblast. In the embryonic type of fat tumor these cells, which may be disposed in diffuse sheets, have a general resemblance to certain epithelial elements and may be likened to those of the parenchyma of the liver or those of the adrenal cortex (Fig. 52). They possess a rather prominent nucleus, somewhat eccentrically situated, which contains a particulate chromatin substance and a finely granular, acidophilic cytoplasm. A nucleolus usually can be seen, although this feature is best demonstrated in frozen sections that have been lightly

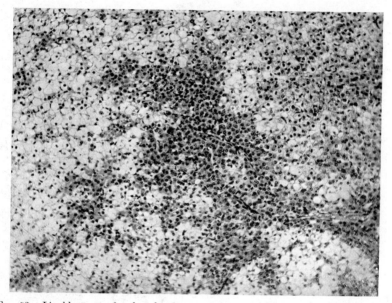

FIG. 53.—Lipoblastoma of a dog showing many immature fat-free lipoblasts (× 115).

stained with hematoxylin. Mitotic division of the cells can be seen occasionally. The continuity of the cellular accumulations may be broken by irregular spaces filled with blood and only a minimal amount of fibrous stroma is discernible. By appropriate stains, large numbers of the immature fat cells may be seen to be entirely devoid of demonstrable fat; in others, a few small globules may be present (Fig. 53). In other parts of the same tumor one may expect to find large regions in which the fat cells assume a distinct adult character and all the characteristics of a fully mature lipoma (Fig. 54).

In order to obtain a comprehensive idea of fat neoplasms one should always resort to study of sections that have been treated with one of the

10

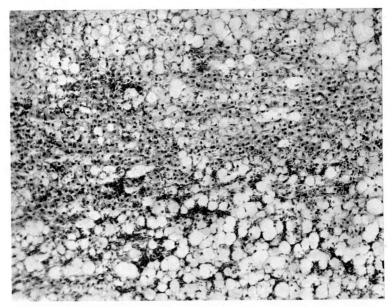

Fig. 54.—Lipoblastoma of a dog; lipoblasts in various stages of differentiation (× 120).

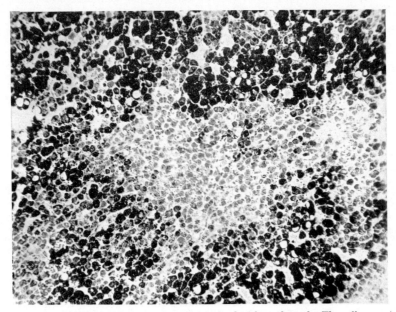

Fig. 55.—Lipoblastoma of a dog; preparation stained with scarlet red. The cells containing fat appear black in the photomicrograph (× 120).

specific fat stains. Scarlet red, osmic acid, or sudan III, are all serviceable for this purpose. Fat tumors, however, should not be preserved in alcohol or in any agent that is a fat solvent. Frozen sections prepared from formalin-fixed tissue, and stained with scarlet red, usually provide satisfactory preparations (Fig. 55). Although it is ordinarily not necessary to resort to special methods in order to recognize fat tumors, the finer histologic details of many of them can best be appreciated in preparations which have been handled so as to retain their cellular integrity.

CLINICAL CONSIDERATIONS

The gross anatomic characteristics of the majority of lipomas, particularly those of the adult type, usually are sufficient to enable them to be recognized without resorting to the microscope. Their color, that of normal adipose tissue, and their fatty constituents suggest at once their true character. In case of doubt, frozen sections stained with one of the specific fat stains reveal the exact nature of the growth. The reactions are characteristic.

Usually only lipomas that are situated subcutaneously are amenable to treatment. Those within the abdomen are seldom, if ever, discovered in life, and the difficulties in the way of successful operative procedures in the abdominal cavity, of the larger mammals, preclude the possibility of resorting to them, even though the actual separation of the tumor from the body might of itself be a simple matter.

The part played by pedunculated lipomas in causing intestinal strangulation has been mentioned. It usually terminates fatally. The symptoms are sudden of onset, and death usually occurs within a day. At necropsy a loop of intestine is found entangled with the pedicle of a tumor having its origin usually in the mesentery. Death results from rupture of the intestine, general sepsis or intoxication.

Surgical removal of subcutaneous lipomas is worthy of trial. If the mass is not excessively large, and had not extensively infiltrated the surrounding interstitial tissues, it can usually be extirpated without difficulty. However, Douville emphasized the danger of operative removal of diffuse interstitial lipomas because of the likelihood of death due to what he considered traumatic shock. Many of the tumors possess a generous blood supply, and control of hemorrhage is frequently difficult.

If all parts of the tumor have been removed, it will not recur; if remnants remain, reappearance may be expected. The rate of growth of most lipomas is so slow that recurrence may not become apparent until lapse of considerable time.

BIBLIOGRAPHY

1. Achilles, A.: Quoted by Fölger.

2. Bartke: Ueber Wandergeschwulste bei Pferden. Deutsch. tierärztl. Wchnschr., 357, 1898.

3. Brose, O.: Ein Fall von Mastdarmtumor. Ztschr. f. Veterinark., 6: 379, 1894.

4. Bruckmüller: Quoted by Kitt.

5. Casper, M.: Geschwülste bei Tieren. Ergebn. d. all. Path. u. path. Anat., 11: 1068–1122, 1907.

6. Corst and Thomas: [Liposarcoma in mammary gland of a dog.] Bull. de l'Assn. franç. p. l'étude du cancer, 16: 142–152, 1927. Abstr. in: Cancer Rev., 2: 403 (Nov.), 1927.

7. Dey, D.: A fibro-lipoma on the forearm of a cow. Vet. Jour., 64: 85, 1910.

8. Douville: Lipomes chez le chien. Rec. de méd. vét., 84: 361, 1907.

9. Douville: Lipomes chez le chien. Rec. de méd. vét., 84: 566, 1912.

10. Ewing, James: Neoplastic diseases. Ed. 3. Philadelphia, W. B. Saunders Co., 1928, p. 196.

11. Fölger, A. F.: Geschwülste bei Tieren. Ergebn. d. all. Path. u. path. Anat., 18: 372–676, 1917.

12. Fox, Herbert: Disease in captive wild mammals and birds: incidence, description, comparison. Philadelphia, J. B. Lippincott Co., 1923, p. 473.

13. Fröhner, E.: Ueber das Vorkommen der Geschwülste bei Hunden. Monatschr. f. Tierheilk., 6: 124, 1895.

14. Fröhner, E.: Quoted by Casper.

15. Giannini: Quoted by Casper.

16. Gooch, F. L.: Tumour of a cryptorchid testicle. Vet. Jour., 62: 138, 1906.

17. Heney and Wooldridge: Lipom of the perineum and fibroma of the mammary gland of a bitch. Vet. Jour., 63: 465, 1907.

18. Hendrickx: Lipome énorme chez un cheval. Ann. de méd. vét. (Dec.), 1899.

19. Hurpez: Lipomes ayant envahi tout l'epipoon. Rec. d'hyg. et de méd. vétér., s. 8, 3: 327, 1906.

20. Joest: Grosses Lipom im Beckenbindegewebe des Rindes. Dresden, Dresdener Hochschulber, 1907, p. 121.

21. Johne: Quoted by Casper.

22. Kinsley, A. T.: A text-book of veterinary pathology. Ed. 3. Chicago, A. Eger, 1917, p. 287.

23. Kitt, Theodor: Text-book of comparative general pathology. Chicago, Chicago Medical Book Co., 1906, p. 348.

24. Kühnau: Quoted by Casper.

25. Lawrence, H. L.: A lipoma in a dog. Case report. Cornell Vet., 2: 84, 1912.

26. McFadyean, J.: A remarkable case of congenital lipoma in a calf. Jour. Comp. Path. and Therap., 14: 291–293, 1901.

27. Messner: Lipom im Herzen eines Schafes. Ztschr. f. Fleisch. und Milchhyg., 7: 239, 1897.

28. Möller, H.: Quoted by Casper.

29. Petit: Angio-lipome chez une chienne. Rec. de méd. vét., 235, 1903.

30. Petit and Peyron: Two mammary tumors in a bitch. Bull. de l'Assn. franç. p. l'étude du cancer, 16: 510–515, 1929.

31. Pfister: Quoted by Casper.

32. Piper: Lipome in der Schafleber. Ztschr. f. Fleisch. u. Milchhyg., 13: 89 1903.

33. Puschmann, O.: Quoted by Fölger.

34. Sawwaitow: Quoted by Casper.

35. Schimmel, W. C.: Quoted by Fölger.

36. Schweinhuber: Lipom an der Schlundeinpflanzung beim Rind. Wchnschr. f. Thierheilk. u. Viehzucht., **4**: 463, 1902.

37. Stephan, L.: Quoted by Fölger.

38. Steuding: Lipom beim Kalbe. Ztschr. f. Fleisch. u. Milchhyg., **8**: 14, 1898.

39. Stewart, H. A.: Diffuse lipomatosis in a mule. Abstract: Am. Vet. Rev., **42**: 455 (Jan.), 1913.

40. Trotter, A. M.: Multiple lipomata of peritoneum of the ox. Jour. Comp. Path. and Therap., **22** : 353, 1909.

41. Vielhauer, K.: Quoted by Fölger.

42. Williams: Quoted by Casper.

43. Williams: Veterinarian, **70**: 361, 1897.

CHAPTER IX

LEIOMYOBLASTOMA

To myoblastomas, as a group, belong the new growths composed of muscle tissue. Growths made up of smooth muscle cells are known as leiomyoblastomas. These include leiomyomas, which are benign, and leiomyosarcomas, which are malignant, but since the latter are rare, most of the space will be devoted to leiomyoma.

DEFINITION AND IDENTITY

Leiomyoma is of mesenchymal origin, and is made up of smooth muscle cells and associated elements. The type cell is characterized by longitudinally disposed, homogeneous, thread-like fibrils within its cytoplasm known as myofibrils. These fine fibrillary structures ordinarily are not demonstrable by the usual hematoxylin-eosin stain. Their demonstration is dependent on fixing perfectly fresh tissue in Zenker's solution and staining it with Mallory's phosphotungstic acid hematoxylin.

INCIDENCE

Leiomyoma, although not common, is by no means rare. Statistics on the incidence of its occurrence are very meager but the numerous cases reported in the literature indicate that it is fairly common among practically all species of common domestic animals. Data compiled by Johne at the Pathological Institute of the Dresden Veterinary High School gives the incidence of leiomyoma as follows:

Among 250 tumors of horses, there were four leiomyomas; among 417 tumors of cattle, there were thirteen leiomyomas; among 209 tumors of dogs, there were four leiomyomas, and among ninety-two tumors of swine, there were seven leiomyomas.

In a series of 533 tumors in my collection there were twenty-three leiomyomas. These were distributed as follows:

Among 227 cattle, there were ten leiomyomas; among eighty-two dogs, there were six leiomyomas; among forty sheep, there were two leiomyomas; among fifty-five chickens, there were five leiomyomas, and among forty-two horses and eighty-seven swine, leiomyomas were not found.

Failure to find leiomyomas in swine may have been due to the fact that they are usually slaughtered at a relatively early age, and perhaps the small number of tumors of the horse accounts for my inability to secure a leiomyoma. The literature contains many references to leiomyomas of horses, although Crocker did not mention having seen any at necropsy of 768 horses.

OCCURRENCE AND ORIGIN*

Tumors made up of smooth muscle usually arise in the interior of the body, where most of the structures which contain a predominance of smooth muscle are found. There are but few elements on the surface of the body essential to the development of leiomyoma, and consequently such tumors seldom occur. The uterus, vagina, stomach, intestine, esophagus, and urinary bladder are common sites for the occurrence of leiomyomas. They may also occur in association with the blood vessels, the cervix, the prostate gland, the gallbladder, and the spleen.

The twenty-three tumors of smooth muscle in my collection were distributed among the respective organs and tissues as follows: Eight in the uterus, three in the spleen, two in the bladder, two in the cecum, two in the small intestine, one tumor in the cervix, one in the oviduct, and two tumors in the broad ligament; the site of two was not determined.

Horse.—The majority of leiomyomas that have been found in horses have originated from tissues along the alimentary tract. Röder, however, observed a somewhat unusual, diffusely growing leiomyoma of the right lower eyelid of a horse, and Kitt is quoted by Casper as having described a similar growth in the region of the carpal joint; this tumor weighed 250 gm. and was thought to have originated from the smooth muscle fibers which are said to occur in this region.†

Leiomyoma of the esophagus is more common in horses than in other animals and is usually situated in the thoracic portion of the canal. Leiomyoma of the horse's stomach has been described by Johne, Rabe, Lothes, Maguire, and others. Cocu observed a leiomyoma of the stom-

---

* The use of the term "spindle-cell sarcoma" in older literature makes it impossible to recognize with certainty many tumors reported; they may have been malignant tumors of smooth muscle.

† Dr. James Farquharson, anatomist, Division of Veterinary Medicine of the Colorado Agricultural College does not agree with Kitt's statement concerning the occurrence of smooth muscle fibers in the region of the carpal joint. In a personal communication, Dr. Farquharson denies the existence of smooth muscle in this region except for that contained within the walls of blood vessels. Kitt's tumor originated perhaps from the latter.

ach in a thirteen-year-old Percheron gelding that died suddenly as a consequence of rupture of the stomach at the middle of the great curvature. The gastric wall was greatly thickened by the tumorous process, and the pyloric opening was so small that it would admit only one finger. What was perhaps a smooth muscle tumor, but which was designated "spindle-cell sarcoma," was reported by Holle. The growth was within the stomach and was 25 cm. long and 23 cm. wide. There was also a large mass free within the stomach and a smaller one in the duodenum. Ball reported a spindle-cell sarcoma in the greater curvature of the stomach of a mare; from the description it is likely that the growth was composed of smooth muscle. Messner described as spindle-cell sarcoma a somewhat unusual tumor in the stomach of a twelve-year-old gelding that was probably also a variety of leiomyoma. The tumor was in the subserosa of the greater curvature, and was connected by a neck of tissue to a much longer mass, covered with mucous membrane, in the submucosa. A leiomyoma that was attached to the stomach by a broad pedicle was seen by Petit,[48] and two leiomyomas, in which the stomach was involved, were reported by Ball. The one that arose from the left half of the stomach projected into the lumen; the other was an ovoid, pedunculated tumor 15 cm. long and 10 cm. wide, embedded in the muscularis of the organ and covered with peritoneum.

Tumors arising from the musculature of the intestines of the horse have been noted by several observers. In most of the reported cases the tumors involved the duodenum or the jejunum. Görig[24] reported finding a tumor about 5 cm. in diameter in a twelve-year-old horse, which originated in the muscularis of the duodenum a considerable distance from the pylorus. Cadéac noted a large leiomyoma of the same region that surrounded the intestine and caused a narrowing of the lumen; Freude found in a horse that died following an attack of colic a leiomyoma, about 4 cm. in diameter, which had arisen in the muscular layer of the jejunum and caused diminution of the intestinal lumen. Achilles found a dome-like, edematous leiomyoma 14 cm. long and 8 cm. wide, weighing 960 gm. in the middle portion of the jejunum of a horse.

I found only one case of leiomyoma of the uterus of the mare described in the literature.[57] The tumor was 28 cm. long and 13 cm. wide and weighed approximately 5.2 kg. Its presence was not suspected until it was forced out through the vulva by the strenuous exertions of the animal. The tumor was removed surgically but death soon occurred from hemorrhage of the uterine artery which had been ruptured by traction of the expelled growth.

Casper stated that a leiomyoma of the urinary bladder of a horse was observed by Johne and that Siedamgrotzky had described a leiomyoma of the testes of an old horse; this growth was situated on the outer surface of the testes in the space between the two glands, and was intimately associated with the tunica albuginea. Besides the main tumor, a number of smaller tumors were present. The growths probably arose from the unstriped muscle that is normally present in the tunica albuginea.

Bovine.—Most leiomyomas of cattle arise from the smooth musculature of the genital tract. As a rule, they contain a large amount of fibrous connective tissue and are often referred to clinically as "fibromyomas" or "fibroids."

The uterus of cattle seems to possess a particular predilection for myomatous tumors. Six of the ten specimens in my series of leiomyomas obtained from cattle were derived from this organ, and in most of the cases reported in the literature the uterus was involved. The tumors may originate anywhere along the uterine musculature, and some enormous specimens have been reported. Although these tumors usually occur singly, Spreule is quoted by Casper as having found at necropsy fifteen large tumors and many smaller ones in the uterus of a cow; their total weight was 80 kg. In one case the interior of the uterus was studded with large numbers of nodular growths from 3 to 20 cm. in diameter. Such tumors are not consistent in anatomic position, shape, or form. A leiomyoma weighing 4,840 gm. was observed in the cervix of a cow by Amaducci, and in the material I have studied was a small but definite area of myomatous neoplasia in the cervical tissue of a seven-year-old Hereford cow. The vagina may occasionally give rise to leiomyomas; cases of this kind have been reported by Albrecht, Johne, Kohlhepp, and Barbier. Görig[23] found in the vagina of a slaughtered cow five leiomyomas; the largest was about 14 cm. in diameter (Fig. 56).

Smooth muscle tumors of the digestive tract also have been observed in cattle. Bohm found a leiomyoma of the rumen, about 15 cm. from the esophageal opening, and in its vicinity was a smaller tumor. Moussu found a leiomyoma 10 c.c. long involving the small intestine of a cow that had suffered recurrent attacks of indigestion. Similar tumors of the intestine of cattle have been observed by Joest[30] and by Johne. One of the leiomyomas in my series occurred near the juncture of the small and the large intestines. The growth was nodular, about 4 cm. in diameter, and firmly embedded in the wall of the intestine. The exposed portion was covered with peritoneum. A pedunculated leiomyoma about 6 cm. in diameter was reported by Görig, arising from the mucosa of the rectum.

Voirin described a leiomyoma about 12 cm. in diameter that involved the dorsal wall of the urinary bladder of a five-year-old bovine, and Goldman described the unusual occurrence of a smooth muscle tumor of the gallbladder. The surface of the much enlarged gallbladder appeared rough as a consequence of the presence of multiple, closely disposed nodules of variable size, and the wall of the bladder was about 5 cm. thick. Practically the entire surface of the mucosa was extensively involved by calcified, villus-like projections, made up of swollen connective tissue, and invested with normal columnar epithelium.

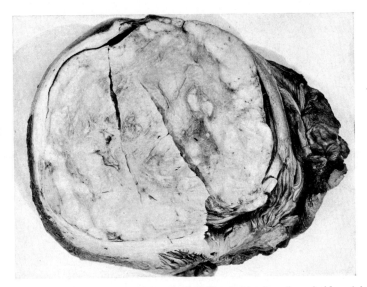

Fig. 56.—Leiomyoma occupying the vaginal vault of a bovine; it probably originated from the cervix.

Joest is credited by Casper as having found two leiomyomas of the aorta of a cow, but details were not given. A tumor designated "adenoleiomyoma" was reported by Craig and Doyle. It was observed at necropsy in an emaciated seven-year-old cow; many firm, nodular masses throughout the liver, omentum, and peritoneum were found. The tumors were composed of irregular, alveolar-like spaces lined with epithelium, with a predominance of unstriped muscle occupying the portions between the adenomatous structures. Its origin was not determined. One of the cases of leiomyoblastoma of the bovine which I studied was somewhat unusual in that the tumor probably originated from the smooth muscle of the splenic capsule (Fig. 57). The spleen and the liver were extensively involved by metastasis.[17]

Dog.—Tumors of the dog, consisting of smooth muscle, are widely distributed. Data are not sufficient to enable one to determine the exact sites, or organs in which there is a tendency for the development of new growths of this kind.

A leiomyoma containing foci of necrosis was described by Mettam as occurring in the posterior portion of the esophagus, near the opening into the stomach, of a twelve to thirteen-year-old Irish setter. Paukul found a soft leiomyoma that projected, dome-like, into the lumen of the jejunum of a young dachshund. The tumor, which was 75 mm. long and 60 mm. wide, had caused narrowing of the intestinal lumen. The two leiomyomas I observed were primary in the musculature of the cecum.

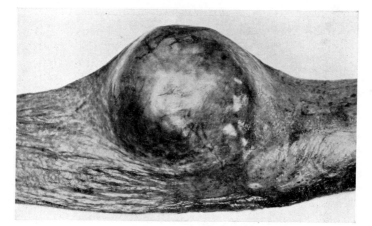

Fig. 57.—Leiomyosarcoma of the spleen of a bovine.

Both of the tumors projected above the external surface of the intestine; the intestinal lumen was not invaded, although in one instance the deeper portions of the mucosa were involved. One of the leiomyomas occurred in a thirteen-year-old male shepherd dog; several forms of primary neoplasm were also found at necropsy.[18] The other leiomyoma in my collection occurred in a two-month-old male Boston terrier. The tumor was pedunculated and weighed approximately 480 gm. Although the exact anatomic situation was not definitely determined, it appeared to be attached to the pancreas.

Fölger quoted Maggi who found at necropsy, in the right cornu of the uterus of a twelve-year-old St. Bernard dog, a tumor which was designated a "lipofibromyoma" because it contained smooth muscle, connective tissue, and fat. The tumor weighed 980 gm. and measured, at its greatest diameter, 40 cm. Hobbs found at necropsy a fibromyoma about 3 cm. in diameter in the uterus of a fourteen-year-old dog that had not been pregnant in the last twelve and a half years of life. In the vulva was a smaller tumor that had recurred a few months after removal. Auger removed a cystic fibromyoma weighing 150 gm. from the cervix of a bird dog. Johne found two leiomyomas in the vagina of dogs. Leisering found a large number of variable sized tumors, designated as fibromyomas, in the vaginal submucosa.

Leiomyoma arising from the smooth muscle of the wall of the urinary bladder of dogs has been reported by several observers, including Johne, Liénaux, and van Tright. Two of the myomatous tumors, obtained from dogs which I examined, originated in this structure. The tumors may be situated under the serosa or in the submucous region. The tumor described by Liénaux weighed 3 kg.; most of them, however, are much smaller.

Fölger noted the report by Tabusso of a somewhat unusual cystic fibromyoma of the prostate gland of a seven-year-old pug dog. The involved structure was 6 cm. long and 4 cm. wide and weighed 58 gm.

Swine.—A few cases of leiomyoma of swine have been reported; the tumors were all in the uterus. Two such tumors were observed by Joest[29]; one weighed 9 kg. and arose in the left cornu of the nongravid uterus of a sow that had farrowed a number of times, the other weighed 8.5 kg. and was found in the left cornu of a sow that was pregnant. The uterus in the latter case contained four macerated fetuses, and purulent metritis was present. Four leiomyomas of the uterus of swine were reported by Johne; one that extended into the lateral ligament was noted by Bohm; one was found in the uterus of a sow by Beiss, and weighed, together with the uterus, 36 kg., and one was found by Zietzschmann in each cornu of the uterus of a hog. In the smaller of these two tumors, muscle elements predominated, although a sufficient amount of fibrous connective tissue was present to justify a designation of "fibroleiomyoma" for the larger of the two.

Fowls.—Leiomyoma undoubtedly occurs more frequently in the common fowl than the number of reported cases would indicate. A leiomyoma of the mesentery of a hen was described by Tyzzer and Ordway. It was firm and round, was covered by peritoneum, and measured 7 by 5 by 5 cm. A smaller tumor, measuring 2 by 1.5 cm. was present between the larger tumor and the intestine. A leiomyoma of the muscular stomach or gizzard was reported by Ehrenreich and Michaelis.

The mass, which was described as being about 3 cm. in diameter, was covered by peritoneum and extended diffusely into the adjacent musculature of the gizzard. Leiomyomas were also observed in chickens by Joest and Ernesti. In one instance two firm nodules, about 1.5 cm. in diameter, originated from the outer muscular layer of the small intestine 4 cm. anterior to the large bowel. The second tumor, which weighed 35 gm., apparently involved one of the ligaments of the oviduct. Joest and Ernesti also described a tumor designated as "adenomyoma" in the wall of the rectum or large intestine about 5 cm. anterior to the cloaca. Besides the smooth muscle, the mass contained gland or tubular-like structures.

Of the fifty-five neoplasms in my collection that were obtained from chickens, five, approximately 9 per cent, were leiomyomas. Two of the tumors were situated in the dorsal ligament of the oviduct, and one involved the substance of the oviduct proper; in one case irregular, elongated nodules were distributed along the musculature of the intestines, and in one the heart, lungs, spleen, and wall of the abdomen of a seven-month-old barred rock hen were involved. The origin of the primary tumor in this instance was not determined.

Other species.—Smooth muscle tumors occasionally have been observed in cats. Petit[47] found a leiomyoma in the uterus of this animal, and Richard found a cystic fibromyoma of the left cornu of the uterus of a nine-year-old cat. The mass in the latter instance was 6 cm. long and 15 cm. wide.

I have observed two leiomyomas that were obtained from old female sheep. In both instances the tumors occurred in the uterus and were found at necropsy following slaughter of the animals for food. One of the tumors weighed 15 gm. and the other 2.4 kg.

A leiomyoma 9 cm. long and 4 cm. thick, involving the small intestine of a mule, was reported by Blanc and a similar tumor of the esophagus of a mule was observed by Lucet; this tumor was 17 cm. in diameter and occupied the thoracic portion of the esophagus for a distance of 25 cm. Two leiomyomas of the ileum, approximately 50 c.c. anterior to the ileocecal valve, were found by Kinsley in a seven-year-old mule that had suffered intermittently with indigestion. The tumors were about 8 cm. in diameter and had practically occluded the intestinal lumen.

A fibroleiomyoma was found by Malvicini in a lioness. It weighed 880 gm. and was situated in the lateral ligament in the space between the ovary and cornu of the uterus. Joest[30] observed 100 tumors of variable sizes in the submucosa of the uterus of a fifty-year-old elephant. The growths were diagnosed microscopically as leiomyomas. Johne is quoted by Casper as having seen a leiomyoma of the intestine of an elephant, and Fox observed a leiomyoma of the uterine cornu and fimbria in an Indian elephant.

The finding of three leiomyomas of the uterus of a muskrat was reported by Hilgendorf and Paulicki. The largest tumor was about 1.5 cm. in diameter; the lumen of the affected organ was filled by the growths.

EFFECTS ON THE HOST

Ordinarily, tumors consisting of smooth muscle grow slowly and seldom cause symptoms until they are large enough to interfere with the proper functioning of the part involved. The fact that the majority of leiomyomas occur in hollow organs such as the stomach, intestines, and uterus enhances the probability that these tumors will eventually cause mischief. However, the direction which the growth takes is of much importance in determining the subsequent effect the tumor may have on the proper functioning of the involved part. Those that grow outward from the wall of the structure from which they arise may attain great size and not interfere to any appreciable degree with the well-being of the affected animal. If the tumor encroaches on the lumen of a hollow organ such as the intestine or the uterus, the function of the affected part may be seriously impaired. If the alimentary tract is involved, persistent indigestion is likely to ensue, and the tumor may eventually be the indirect cause of death. Pregnancy may be complicated if the body of the uterus is affected, or if the tumors are multiple and in both cornua. Williams and Williams mentioned a fibromyoma in one cornu of the uterus of a cow that became pregnant several times in the opposite cornu. The animal eventually became sterile, perhaps due to the increased size of the tumor, which had reached a diameter of from 26 to 30 cm. The presence of such tumors within the uterus, the cervix, or the vaginal passage may be the cause of maternal dystocia which may or may not be difficult to treat, depending on the anatomic situation of the tumor, and its size.

The presence of unusually large tumors within the abdominal cavity undoubtedly affects the well-being of the animal, even though the physiology of the involved part is not noticeably disturbed. It seems reasonable to assume that the constant traction and pressure caused by a tumor weighing from a few to many kilograms would influence the animal's health, and give rise to symptoms that might be somewhat obscure but nevertheless real.

METASTASIS AND MALIGNANCY

Malignant leiomyomas or leiomyosarcomas are characterized by their highly cellular structure and an infiltrative and destructive type of growth. Widespread metastasis may occasionally be observed, but as a rule malignancy is suggested by evidence of rapid growth and by the tendency of the neoplastic elements to infiltrate and replace the adjacent normal tissue (Fig. 58). In this malignant type of leiomyoma the cells of the tumor are immature, and mitosis is readily demonstrable (Fig. 59).

It should be kept in mind that leiomyomas are sometimes multiple primarily, therefore the presence of several such growths is not neces-

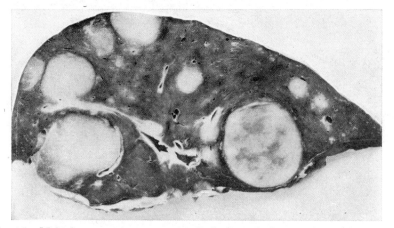

Fig. 58.—Multiple metastatic tumor masses in the liver of a bovine; the primary growth was in the spleen. Same case as shown in Figure 57.

sarily evidence of metastasis or of malignancy. This is particularly true if the tumors are situated within the same general region, as for example, along the intestine or within the uterus. On the other hand, if a leiomyoma is situated in a part normally rich in smooth muscle, and one or more tumors are present in a distant and unrelated organ, the first tumor should be considered clinically malignant, and to have resulted in metastasis.

Among the malignant leiomyomas in my series of neoplasms were the following: (1) Primary tumor in the splenic capsule of a cow with multiple and extensive metastasis in the liver; (2) malignant leiomyoma of the uterus of two cows, in one of which the tumor metastasized to the lungs and associated lymph nodes and in the other of which nodules were found in the liver; (3) malignant leiomyoma of the cecum of a dog that had every appearance of a malignant neoplasm but metastasis had not occurred, and (4) numerous leiomyomas distributed in the spleen, liver, and kidneys of a seven-year-old male collie. The primary growth in this case measured 12 by 7 by 6 cm., and was situated in the ventral portion of the spleen.

In the material I studied, metastasis seemed to have occurred in every instance by way of the blood stream; it was not uncommon to find blood vessels, even of large size, entirely occluded by plugs of vigorously growing neoplastic cells.

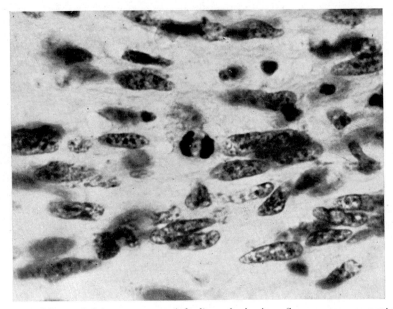

Fig. 59.—Metastatic leiomyosarcoma of the liver of a bovine. Same case as represented in Figure 58 (× 675).

From what is known concerning smooth muscle tumors it would seem proper to conclude that they seldom exhibit a tendency to become malignant, and even those that locally have every characteristic of malignancy are slow to metastasize to distant parts. An occasional specimen, however, is capable of extensive and widespread metastasis.

GROSS CHARACTERISTICS

The size and shape of leiomyoblastomas like that of most tumors are subject to considerable variation. Although most of them weigh from a few grams to a few kilograms, depending on the species affected, extremely large specimens are occasionally observed. Bidault described a fibromyoma, 32 cm. in diameter and weighing 30.5 kg., of the uterus of an old cow. I observed portions of a leiomyoma, approximately 90 cm. in diameter, of the uterus of a cow.   These two specimens no doubt represent the upper limit of size attained by these tumors, and most of them are much smaller. A pedunculated form of attachment is sometimes observed, although usually the tumors are attached by a rather broad base, or over a considerable portion of their structures, by tissues derived from the organ from which they arose. Usually they are smooth and round although they may be elongated, oval, or irregularly spherical. The benign forms are usually encapsulated; the capsule is removed with difficulty.   Most of the tumors are resilient and of firm consistence, but occasionally a soft or flabby specimen may be seen.

When cut across, the exposed tissue presents a shiny appearance, flesh-pink to grayish-white.   The structure is irregular and lobulated, and the respective units of leiomyomatous tissue are separated from each other by bands of fibrous connective tissue of variable thickness. Leiomyomas of this character are frequently encountered in the uterus and are often designated clinically "fibromyomas" or "fibroids." However, it should be recognized that the fibrous connective tissue plays a secondary part in the structure of these tumors.   Although fibrous connective tissue may sometimes equal or exceed in amount the myomatous elements present, particularly in cases of long standing, nevertheless, the neoplastic process involves fundamentally the smooth muscle cells, which are the elements concerned in the inception of these tumors.

The surface exposed on section commonly reveals conglomerate masses of twisted interlacing fibers, interspersed at irregular intervals by strands of connective tissue. The elongated, myomatous elements seem to run in every conceivable direction, although this feature is best demonstrated in histologic sections. In the slowly growing tumors well-formed blood vessels usually insure an ample supply of blood, although in unusually large specimens extensive areas of necrosis indicate that the blood supply is at times inadequate.   Besides the necrosis, other retrogressions that may occur, particularly in tumors of unusual size, are calcification, edema, and cystic degeneration.

MICROSCOPIC DESCRIPTION

The microscopic appearance of smooth muscle tumors varies somewhat with the rate of growth. Those that progress slowly and retain their benign character have a somewhat different appearance than those which grow rapidly and exhibit other evidences of malignancy.

11

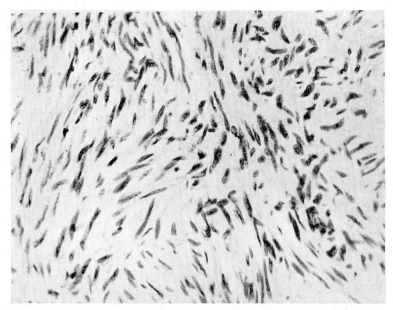

Fig. 60.—Leiomyoma of the urinary bladder of a dog (× 285).

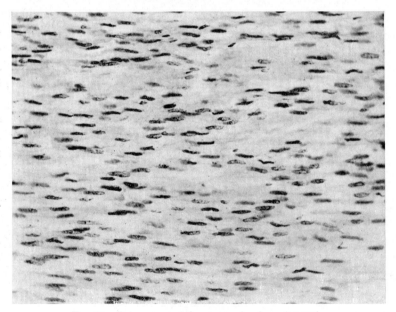

Fig. 61.—Leiomyoma of the uterus of a sheep (× 285).

The cells of a slowly growing, benign leiomyoma are usually organized into units or bundles which are disposed at every conceivable angle (Fig. 60). Variable proportions of strands of fibrous connective tissue appear promiscuously, and serve as a stroma for the blood vessels, which may be abundant and well formed. The smooth muscle cells are usually elongated, spindle-shaped forms arranged in a parallel fashion, but plump, ovoid cells may predominate. It is usually difficult or impossible to discern the respective cellular outlines, although the nuclei are sharply defined (Fig. 61). The nuclei are ovoid to rod shaped, and numerous chromatin granules give the nucleus a coarse, roughened appearance (Fig. 62). In sections that have been properly prepared, myoglia fibrils which appear as longitudinal striations in the cuticle of the cytoplasm may be demonstrated.[41] A few fibroblasts usually

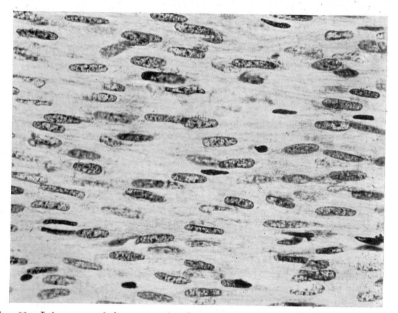

FIG. 62.—Leiomyoma of the uterus of a sheep. Same case as represented in Figure 61 (× 525).

occur among the muscle cells. These produce collagen in variable amounts, which tends to bind the various constituents of the growth into a firm, resilient whole. Sections stained by the method of van Gieson reveal distinctly the wavy connective tissue fibrils (Fig. 63).

In the malignant forms of leiomyoma the smooth muscle cells exhibit characteristics of immaturity which are particularly noticeable in the nuclei. The cells are more abundant than in the slowly growing benign type, and the nuclei are larger and contain an abundance of granular chromatin (Figs. 64 and 65). An eccentrically situated nucleolus may be observed in some of the nuclei, and mitotic division is fre-

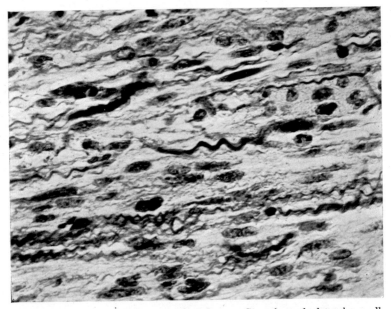

FIG. 63.—Leiomyosarcoma. Section stained by van Gieson's method to show collagen fibrils (× 500).

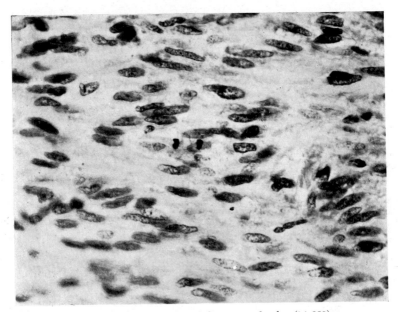

FIG. 64.—Leiomyosarcoma of the cecum of a dog (× 660).

quently a striking feature in many malignant leiomyomas. Many of the blood channels consist of nothing more than a layer of endothelium resting on the surrounding neoplastic elements.

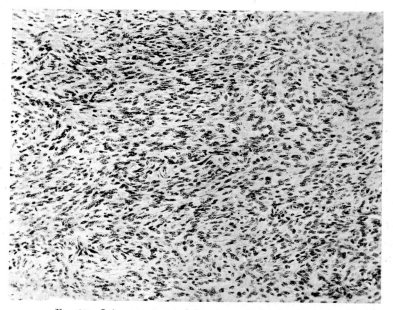

Fig. 65.—Leiomyosarcoma of the uterus of a bovine (× 120).

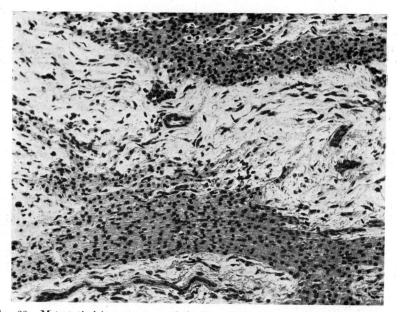

Fig. 66.—Metastatic leiomyosarcoma of the liver of a bovine showing infiltrative character of the growth (× 175).

The invasive tendencies of the malignant forms of leiomyoma are usually apparent. The vigorous proliferating cells extend in every direction, as a consequence of which they replace less resistant normal constituents (Fig. 66).

It may sometimes be difficult to determine microscopically whether one is confronted with a smooth muscle tumor or with fibroblastoma, and special stains, such as van Gieson's, are often helpful in determining the true character of the tumor in question. Material that has been fixed in Zenker's solution may be stained by phosphotungstic acid hematoxylin as recommended by Mallory and Wright for the purpose of demonstrating myoglia, which are specific for tumors of this kind. If uncertainty exists concerning the myomatous character of the growth the anatomic situation from which the tumor originated must be considered carefully in reaching a decision. Most leiomyomas arise from structures such as the uterus, stomach, and intestine, which normally contain much smooth muscle. Nonepithelial tumors of these parts are likely to consist of myomatous elements.

CLINICAL CONSIDERATIONS

Since leiomyomas usually arise from structures in the interior of the body, opportunities for their surgical removal are not common. Their presence in the organs of predilection is usually difficult to diagnose, particularly in the larger animals, and the instances when a tumor of this kind may be extirpated successfully are few. Unless malignancy is manifest, the presence of a leiomyoma of the uterus or intestine is hardly likely to give rise to symptoms that would disclose its presence.

Leiomyoma in the esophagus, stomach, or intestines is likely to cause intermittent indigestion, varying in severity, and similar tumors of the uterus may be responsible for an animal's inability to breed. If the uterus of cattle or horses is involved, the tumors often can be discovered by palpation through the rectum. In most instances, however, leiomyomas, even of large proportions, fail to exhibit diagnostic symptoms, and the growths are found only at necropsy.

If tumor is discovered in the smaller animals, such as cats and dogs, those of the uterus may be removed. If the growth is limited to the uterus their removal is not particularly formidable.

In a few instances the presence of a leiomyoma within the genital passage has occasioned a foul-smelling bloody discharge that was instrumental in drawing attention to the presence of the growth. However, such discharge might indicate several diseases of the genital apparatus.

BIBLIOGRAPHY

1. Achilles, A.: Quoted by Fölger.

2. Albrecht, M.: Über ein Myofibrom in der Scheide eines Rindes. Wchnschr. Tierh., 265, 1896.

3. Amaducci, P.: Fibro-mioma dell'utero, operazione. Clin. vet., **29**: 562–564, 1906.

4. Auger: Tumeur du col. utérin chez une chienne. Jour. de méd. Vét., **61**: 449, 1910.

5. Ball, V.: Néoplasmes gastriques. Jour. de méd. Vét. et Zootech., s. 5, **10**: 709–716, 1906.

6. Barbier: Quoted by Casper.

7. Beiss: Leiomyom des Uterus eines Schweines. Ztschr. f. Fleisch. u. Milchhyg., **8**: 139, 1898.

8. Bidault: Fibro-myome de l'utérus chez une vache. Rec. de méd. Vét., **89**: 487–489, 1912.

9. Blanc: Tumeur de l'iléon représentant le diverticule de Meckel. Jour. de méd. Vét., 712, 1896.

10. Bohm, E.: Quoted by Fölger.

11. Cadéac, C.: Rev. vet., 6, 1885.

12. Casper, M.: Geschwülste bei Tieren. Ergebn. d. all. Path. u. path. Anat., **11**: 1068–1122, 1907.

13. Cocu: Diffuse leiomyoma of the stomach and rupture of the organ. Jour. Am. Vet. Med. Assn., **52**: 210 (Nov.), 1917.

14. Craig, R. A. and Doyle, L. P.: Adenoleiomyomata in a cow. Jour. Am. Vet. Med. Assn., **63**: 482–484 (July), 1923.

15. Crocker, W. J.: Three thousand autopsies. Cornell Vet., **9**: 142–161 (Jan.), 1919.

16. Ehrenreich, M. and Michaelis, L.: Ueber Tumoren bei Hühnern. Ztschr. f. Krebsforsch., **4**: 586–591, 1906.

17. Feldman, W. H.: Leiomyosarcoma of the spleen in a bovine. Am. Jour. Path., **4**: 139–144 (March), 1928.

18. Feldman, W. H.: Multiple primary neoplasms in lower animals: Report of a case. Am. Jour. Path., **4**: 497–506 (Sept.), 1928.

19. Fölger, A. F.: Geschwülste bei Tieren. Ergebn. d. all. Path. u. path. Anat., **18**: 372–676, 1917.

20. Fox, Herbert: Disease in captive wild mammals and birds, incidence, description, comparison. Philadelphia, J. B. Lippincott Co., 1923, p. 479.

21. Freude: Kolik infolge Myoms im Leedarm. Ztschr. f. Veter., **18**: 384, 1906.

22. Goldmann: Leiomyom der Gallenblase des Rindes. Sächs. Ber., **45**: 245, 1900.

23. Görig: Multiple Leiomyome in der Scheide einer Kuh. Deutsch. tierärztl. Wchsnschr., 29, 1896.

24. Görig: Zum Vorkommen von Darmtumoren. Deutsch. tierärztl. Wchnschr., 29, 1896.

25. Hilgendorf, F. and Paulicki, A.: Mehrfache Myome in dem Uterus einer Biberratte (Myopotamus corpus). Virchow's Arch. f. path. Anat. u. Physiol., **49**: 295–296 (Jan. 18), 1870.

26. Hobbs, F. C.: An interesting case of uterine tumor. Vet. Jour., **62**: 205–206, 1906.

27. Holle: Quoted by Fölger.

28. Johne: Quoted by Casper.

29. Joest, E.: Zwei Fälle von Leiomyom am Uterus des Schweines. Dresdener Hochschulber, Dresden, 1912, p. 154.

30. Joest, E.: Quoted by Casper and by Fölger.

31. Joest, E. and Ernesti, S.: Untersuchungen über spontane Geschwülste bei Vöglen mit besonderer Berücksichtigung des Hauschuhns. Ztschr. f. Krebsforsch., **15:** 1–75, 1915–1916.

32. Kinsley, A. T.: Fatal colic, a result of obstruction with a leiomyoma. Am. Vet. Rev., **35:** 574–576 (Aug.), 1909.

33. Kitt, A.: Quoted by Casper.

34. Kohlhepp: Quoted by Casper.

35. Leisering: Quoted by Casper.

36. Liénaux, E.: Myome de la vessel chez un chien. Ann. de méd. Vét., **43:** 662, 1894.

37. Lothes: Myoma laevicellulare an der Cardia des Pferdemagens. Ber. thierärztl. Wchnschr., **6:** 185, 1890.

38. Lucet, A.: Myome à fibres lisses de l'oesophage. Rec. de méd. Vét., 741, 1894.

39. Maggi, U.: Quoted by Fölger.

40. Maguire: Veterinarian, **67:** 609, 1894.

41. Mallory, F. B. and Wright, J. H.: Pathological technique. Ed. 8, Philadelphia, W. B. Saunders Co., 1924, pp. 125 and 149.

42. Malvicini, A.: Un cas de fibroleiomyome de l'uterus d'une lione. Jour. de méd. Vét., **62:** 193, 1911.

43. Messner, E.: Sarkome des Magens bei einem Pferde. Deutsch. tierärztl. Wchnschr., **17:** 19, 1909.

44. Mettam, A. E.: A leiomyoma of the terminal portion of the esophagus in a dog. Vet. Jour., **63:** 269, 1907.

45. Moussu, G.: Occlusion intestinale à répétition. Rec. de méd. Vét., **87:** 697–704, 1910.

46. Paukul, E.: Leiomyom des Jejunums bei einem Hunde. Arch. f. wissensch. u. prakt. Tierh., **33:** 113–119, 1907.

47. Petit, G.: Myomes utérins chez une chatte. Rec. de méd. Vét., 704, 1902.

48. Petit, G.: Léiomyome de l'estomac chez un cheval. Bul. Soc. centr. de méd. Vét., **58:** 452, 1904.

49. Rabe: Quoted by Casper.

50. Richard: Fibro-myome kystique de la corne utérine gauche, chez une chatte laparotomie; hystérectomie abdominale sub-totale; guérison. Bul. de Soc. centr. de méd. Vét., **64:** 163–168, 1910.

51. Röder: Leiomyom am Auge eines Pferdes. Sächs. Ber., **46:** 218, 1901.

52. Schütz: Arch. f. Tierh., **7:** 14, 1881.

53. Siedamgrotzky: Quoted by Casper.

54. von Tright: Quoted by Casper.

55. Tyzzer, E. E. and Ordway, Thomas: Tumors in the common fowl. Jour. Med. Res., **21:** 459–477 (Oct.), 1909.

56. Voirin: Quoted by Casper.

57. Williams, W. L. and Williams, W. W.: The diseases of the genital organs of domestic animals. Ithaca, N. Y., 1921, p. 274.

58. Zietzschmann: Leiomyome im Uterus eines Schweines. Sächs. Ber., **46:** 194, 1901.

CHAPTER X

RHABDOMYOBLASTOMA

DEFINITION AND GENERAL CONSIDERATION

A rhabdomyoblastoma is a tumor composed of muscle cells that have the inherent capacity to produce both longitudinal and cross striations within their cytoplasm. The class includes rhabdomyomas and rhabdomyosarcomas, respectively, as they are benign or malignant, and there are various other growths designated in the literature by combinations of syllables, such as "adenorhabdomyoma"; these are self-explanatory.

Relatively little is known concerning rhabdomyoblastomas as they occur in the lower animals. They are so rarely observed that opportunity for their comprehensive study has not occurred. The literature I examined contained mention of less than twelve cases in which one could be reasonably sure that the tumor in question was a rhabdomyoblastoma. Even in human beings it is rare, although valuable descriptions of it have been contributed by Mallory and by Ewing.

Since many striated muscle tumors arise as a consequence of misplacement of embryonic tissue during fetal development, these tumors may occur in situations normally devoid of striated muscle. Such a tumor is referred to as a "heterologous rhabdomyoma," whereas a striated muscle tumor occurring where striated muscle is normally present is designated a "homologous rhabdomyoma."

INCIDENCE

Casper mentioned a case of rhabdomyoblastoma of a thirteen-year-old horse that was described clinically by Monod and histologically by Coyne and Cavalié. The tumor, which measured 6 by 5 cm., was red brown, had a stalk-like attachment, and in shape somewhat resembled a mushroom. It was situated under the skin between the supraspinatus and the brachiocephalicus muscles. The tissues were arranged in a laminated fashion, radiating toward the periphery.

A very unusual specimen of a striated muscle tumor was observed by Boucek. It was a rounded mass, about 1 cm. in diameter, situated in the midst of the otherwise normal myocardium of a cow. It was composed of bundles of muscle fibers of the skeletal muscle type, connective tissue, and empty, tubular, gland-like cavities lined with cuboidal epithelium. The tumor was considered a heterotopic adenorhabdomyoma and its position was explained on the basis of fetal inclusion.

After the death of a horse from rupture of the stomach, Joest[6] found a firm, nodular tumor weighing 4,500 gm. which surrounded the abdominal aorta for a considerable distance. The mass was connected with the adventitia of the aorta, but the vessel was not compressed. Microscopically, a mixed type of growth was apparent. Although the structure was essentially that of a round-cell sarcoma, there were also traces of both smooth and striated muscle fibers.

Kitt mentioned a rhabdomyoma that was observed by Gratia during the dissection of an old horse. The tumor was fusiform, 8 to 10 cm. in length, in the trunk of the vagus nerve about the middle of the neck. Kitt quoted Kilessnikow as having found a growth designated "rhabdomyosarcoma melanodes" containing pigment cells, in the connective tissue of the tail and perianal region of a twenty-four-year-old stallion. Metastasis had occurred to the liver, spleen, peritoneum, and pleura.

A multiple rhabdomyoblastoma in the neck of a six-months bovine fetus was reported by Prochazka. The tumor consisted of striated muscle fibers in various stages of differentiation.

A remarkable example of a multiple heterologous rhabdomyoma that occurred in the lungs of a four to five-month-old lamb was described by Day. The rarity of this condition justifies quoting from a portion of Day's description of this tumor: ". . . both lungs were found to contain perhaps a thousand or more spherical nodules which ranged in size from 1 mm. to 2 cm. in diameter. A cut surface through the greatest diameter of the caudal lobe of the right lung exposed 185 of these growths which were quite evenly distributed throughout both lungs. Some of the larger growths were situated just beneath the pleura but did not appear to involve this membrane. Generally speaking, the peripheries of the neoplasms were comparatively smooth, yet some of the large ones showed a few bosselations on their surfaces which appeared to be an outgrowth of tumor substance. In a few places there was a coalescence of two or more tumors. . . . The lungs appeared normal in size and the lung tissue which was not involved in the new growths seemed normal in color and texture. All other organs were reported normal by the inspector who conducted the autopsy." Microscopically this tumor consisted essentially of bundles of immature striated muscle cells and scattered among them was a large number of glandular tubules lined with a single layer of cuboidal epithelial cells* (Figs. 67 and 68). Regarding the histogenesis of the tumors Day concluded that they probably originated from misplaced embryonal tissue.

A congenital, multiple rhabdomyoma that involved the heart of a female hog, aged approximately three months was studied by Hieronymi and Kukla. The tumors which were considered the cause of death involved the musculature of one of the ventricles of the heart and the ventricular septum. The nodules, which varied from 1 to 2 cm. in di-

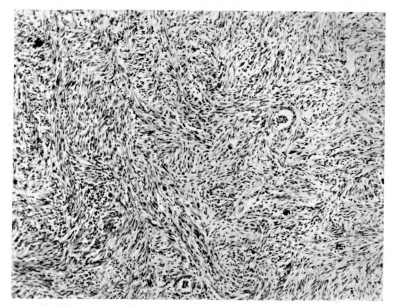

Fig. 67.—Rhabdomyoma of lungs of a sheep; the photomicrograph (× 120) prepared from a slide obtained through the courtesy of Dr. L. Enos Day of Chicago.

ameter, were subendocardial and subepicardial and were not encapsulated. The authors considered that the muscle fibers of the tumors bore a resemblance to the large Purkinje fibers of the bundle of His. A similar tumor was observed by Joest[7] in a slaughtered female hog aged about one and a fourth years. In the myocardium of the outer wall of the left ventricle of the heart, and in the substance of the ventricular septum, were multiple nodules of variable size. Joest considered these to have developed as a consequence of the persistence of embryonal myocardial tissue among fully differentiated myocardial elements. He

* Dr. Day kindly permitted me the privilege of examining histologic sections prepared from this specimen.

was disinclined to accept these tumors as genuine neoplasms on account
of their histogenesis.

Meyer reported the occurrence of multiple rhabdomyoma that
arose from the skeletal musculature of the sternum of a chicken. There
were six tumors varying from 1 to 2 cm. in diameter, which were easily
removed from the surrounding musculature. The tumors consisted
principally of striated muscle fibers which were partially separated
from each other by strands of connective tissue. On account of the mixed
character of the growth Meyer designated the condition "fibromyoma
striocellulare."

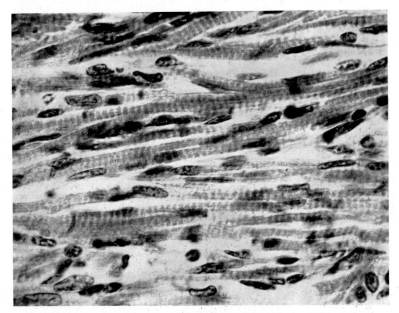

Fig. 68.—Rhabdomyoma of lungs of a sheep; the photomicrograph (× 800) prepared
from a slide obtained through the courtesy of Dr. L. Enos Day.

Only two rhabdomyoblastomas occurred in my series of neoplasms
obtained from animals. One was an infiltrating mass weighing approximately 14 kg. which involved the tissues over the lateral aspect of the
proximal portion of the right humerus of a five-year-old gelding (Fig.
69). The tumor extended anteriorly to the inferior cervical region, pos-
teriorly to the adjacent costal region, and ventrally down the foreleg
for a considerable distance. The growth grew rapidly and it was necessary to kill the animal.

Microscopically this tumor showed all transitions from the very
youngest or immature muscle cells with mitosis to those which were

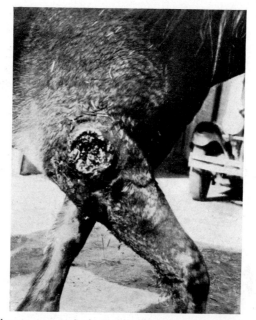

FIG. 69.—Rhabdomyosarcoma of a horse; the photograph obtained through the courtesy of Dr. H. E. Kingman of Fort Collins, Colorado.

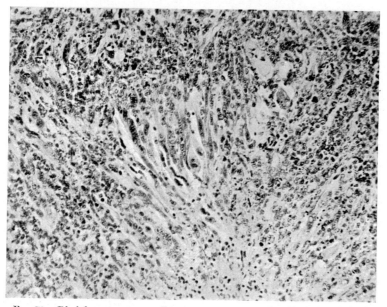

FIG. 70.—Rhabdomyosarcoma. Same case as represented in Figure 69 (× 140).

more mature, and contained transverse striations (Fig. 70). The immature cells, however, predominated, and diligent search was usually necessary in order to find muscle fibers with cross striations. Many of the more mature, elongated muscle fibers possessed more than one nucleus, and it was not uncommon to see as many as six to eight within the same cytoplasmic structure. The tumor was generously supplied with blood channels, some of which were thrombosed. There was also considerable fluid in certain portions of the growth, and the number and character of the leukocytes present suggested infection. Although there is much evidence to indicate that the majority of striated muscle tumors arise from embryonic elements that have been misplaced during fetal development, the specimen just described was probably not of this character.

The second specimen I observed was obtained from the musculature anterior and inferior to the left prescapular lymph node of a one-year-

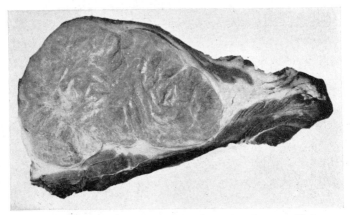

FIG. 71.—Rhabdomyoma of the prescapular region of a year-old sheep.

old sheep. The growth, which was encapsulated, was somewhat dome shaped, and measured 9 cm. in diameter at the base, with a maximal height of 6 cm. (Fig. 71). It was definitely separated from much of the surrounding musculature by a narrow zone of adipose tissue. It was firm, flesh pink, and in a freshly cut surface were seen large numbers of very irregularly disposed strands of tissue. Microscopically the growth consisted of slender, elongated, ribbon-like fibers with a tendency to form irregular bundles disposed in every conceivable direction (Fig. 72). The individual fibers had a marked affinity for the eosin stain, and with subdued light it was not difficult to demonstrate the presence of characteristic cross striations in many of them (Fig. 73). The nuclei were rather prominent. They were slender and elongated, and were usually situated at the periphery of the respective fibers. Mitosis was

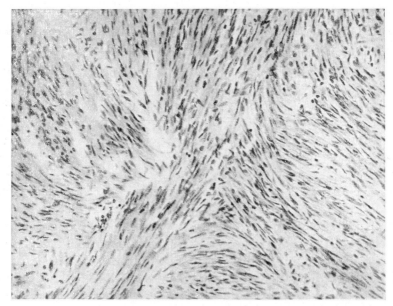

FIG. 72.—Rhabdomyoma of a sheep. Same case as represented in Figure 71 (× 225).

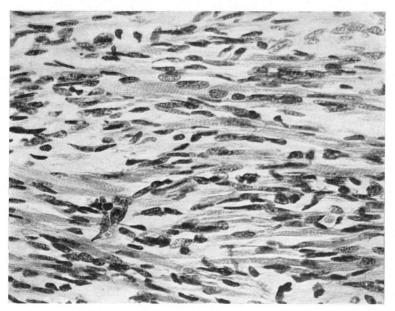

FIG. 73.—Rhabdomyoma of a sheep. Same case as represented in Figure 71 (× 525)

not observed. Blood vessels of different sizes were present, although these structures were not numerous. There was but little fibrous connective tissue except in the capsular structure which consisted of a rather broad band of this substance. Many small lymphocytic cells were to be seen in the zone of contact between the capsule and the neoplastic tissue.

STRUCTURE

Mallory pointed out that the type cell of rhabdomyoma varies in morphology, depending on its histogenesis. Heart muscle cells which arise from the splanchnic mesoderm form compact anastomosing masses in which the limits of the individual fibers cannot be discerned. A tumor originating from such elements consists of myogenic cells, which, to quote Mallory, "are usually very large and may be spherical, elongated or branching and contain one to several nuclei. The cytoplasm of the cells is often coarsely vacuolated, a characteristic which has attracted much attention in the past." Voluntary striated muscle consists of elongated, somewhat cylindric, multinucleated fibers, and a tumor arising from these elements usually consists of thin, ribbon-like immature muscle cells which may be disposed in a parallel fashion to form indefinite bundles, or the fibers may interlace with each other. Variable degrees of maturity may be apparent within a relatively small portion and in general many highly cellular portions often simulate fibrosarcoma. In those portions in which the embryonic type of cell predominates, the cytoplasmic substance is minimal, and most of the cellular bulk is made up of nuclear material. Mitosis is confined to these more immature cells. Cross striations are often difficult to demonstrate, although in the material from Day's case they were to be seen in nearly every fiber.

The paucity of material for study perhaps makes it unwise to attempt to set forth what constitutes the salient features of rhabdomyoblastoma. The embryonic inception of many of these tumors enhances their possibility for variation within wide limits, and each presents a problem in cytology worthy of careful study.

CLINICAL CONSIDERATIONS

Rhabdomyoblastomas are rare, and although they may seriously disturb the well-being of the affected animal because of their situation, as a class they are of more interest to the pathologist than to the clinician.

BIBLIOGRAPHY

1. Boucek, Z.: Mitteilungen über 35 histologisch untersuchte Tiergeschwülste. Arch. f. wissensch. u. prakt. Tierh., **32**: 585–600, 1906.

2. Casper, M.: Geschwülste bei Tieren. Ergebn. d. all. Path. u. path. Anat., **11**: 1068–1122, 1907.

3. Day, L. E.: Rhabdomyoma of the lungs of a sheep. Jour. Am. Vet. Med. Assn., **61:** 436–441 (July), 1922.

4. Ewing, James: Neoplastic diseases. Ed. 3. Philadelphia, W. B. Saunders Co., 1928, pp. 334–339.

5. Hieronymi, E. and Kukla, R.: Ein Beitrag zur Kenntnis der angeborenen Rhabdomyome des Herzens. Virchow's Arch. f. path. Anat. u. Physiol., **232:** 459–479, 1921.

6. Joest, E.: Periaortales Sarko-rhabdo-leiomyom beim Pferd. Bericht über das Veterinärwesen im Königreich Sachsen (1905), **50:** 297–298, 1906.

7. Joest, E.: Quoted by Ackerknecht, Eberhard. Kreislauforgane. In: Joest, Ernest. Handbuch der speziellen pathologischen Anatomie der Haustiere. Ed. 2, Berlin, R. Schoetz, 1925, vol. 4, p. 473.

8. Kitt, Theodor: Text-book of comparative general pathology. Chicago, Chicago Medical Book Co., 1906, p. 354.

9. Mallory, F. B.: The principles of pathologic histology. Philadelphia, W. B. Saunders Co., 1914, pp. 343–347.

10. Meyer: Quoted by Ziegler, M.: Muskeln. In: Joest, Ernest: Handbuch der speziellen pathologischen Anatomie der Haustiere. Ed. 2, Berlin, R. Schoetz, 1929, vol. **5:** p. 489.

11. Prochazka, G.: Rhabdomyoma in a cow foetus. Cas. lék. cesk., **64:** 1476–1481 1925. Abstr. in: Cancer Rev., **3:** 54 (Feb.), 1928.

12

CHAPTER XI

ENDOTHELIOBLASTOMA

DEFINITION AND TERMINOLOGY

Endothelioblastoma is a new growth derived from certain elements of the mesenchyme, the cells of which exhibit a tendency to line blood vessels, lymph vessels, and lymph spaces. Those characterized by the formation of new blood spaces or channels are designated hemangiomas, whereas those in which the spaces or cavities contain a serous lymph-like fluid are referred to as lymphangiomas. The latter is not often observed in animals. Endothelioblastomas are considered collectively by some authors as angiomas, the term indicating a growth composed of newly formed vessels. Mallory designated those in which the cells tend to form blood vessels as hemangio-endothelioblastomas, and those that produce lymph vessels he called lymphangio-endothelioblastomas. Most of this chapter will be devoted to blood vessel tumors. Some of the authors cited have called the tumors they reported hemangiomas or angiomas, whereas in describing my own material I have tended to favor the term "hemangio-endothelioma." Other terms will appear as required. It is generally considered that in man many of the tumors of this group are congenital in origin, and although meager data make it unwise to draw conclusions, it would seem that many of those in animals have a similar origin.*

BLOOD VASCULAR TUMORS

Incidence.—Tumors consisting of elements that normally go to make up blood channels are occasionally encountered in the lower animals, but this variety of neoplasms is by no means common. Casper stated that only one tumor of this kind was found among 335 tumors of horses in the Prussian army observed during a period of seven years. Fröhner[10] found two hemangiomas (0.3 per cent) among 643 tumors of dogs, but failed to find a single specimen among 150 tumors of horses.[11]

---

* A case of multiple endotheliomas of the lungs of a one-day-old colt that was without question of a congenital nature was reported several years ago.[7]

Johne's statistics, obtained from material observed at the Patho-ological Institute at Dresden, show the occurrence of hemangiomas as follows:

Among 250 tumors of horses there were two hemangiomas of the liver and seven of the nose; of 417 tumors of cattle seventy-seven were of the liver and one was of the lung; of ninety-two tumors of swine two were of the liver and one was of the spleen, and among 209 tumors of dogs hemangiomas were not noted. The high incidence of hemangiomas in cattle in this series throws considerable doubt on the true nature of the seventy-seven tumors listed as affecting the liver. The rather frequent occurrence of the pseudoneoplastic condition of the liver of cattle known as telangiectasis would justify one's failure to accept as true hemangiomas all tumors listed in Johne's report.

In my series of 535 new growths obtained from the lower animals there were ten that were designated as hemangiomas. Four of these occurred among 230 tumors obtained from cattle, three among forty-three tumors of horses, two among eighty-one tumors of dogs, and one among forty-one tumors of sheep.

The older literature contains reports of a considerable number of tumors designated hemangiomas and angiomas, and others were referred to as endotheliomas.

Horse.—A diffuse, cavernous angioma that involved the gums and palate of a horse was observed by Grebe. Roder was quoted by Fölger as having found a hemangioma of two to three years' duration on the lower surface of the thorax of a sixteen-year-old horse. An angioma of spongy consistence, that involved the entire thickness of the skin of the upper lip of a horse was described by Rigot, and Gebruth found, in the nictitating membrane of an old horse, two small, flat tumors which he designated as endotheliomas. A tumor of the nictitating membrane of the left eye of a four-year-old horse was also described by Volland. The growth, which was designated as angiosarcoma, was destructive and had spread extensively, involving the antrum of Highmore, and the frontal and sphenoidal sinuses. It was made up of cavities filled with blood and proliferating endothelium.

An instance of multiple angiomas of an old horse was reported by Ravenna.[26] The tumors, which varied in size, were in the heart, lungs, spleen, and kidneys, and consisted essentially of endothelial-lined spaces filled with blood. Casper quoted Françesco as having operated for an ulcerating angioma of the glans penis of a horse; he also cited Bennet's case in which a fibro-angioma about 10 cm. in diameter was situated at the base of the tail of a horse.

A hemangioma involving the endocardium was reported by Montané, and Ercolani is credited by Casper as having found one on the wall of the left ventricle of the heart of a horse.

The material which I obtained from horses included a capillary hemangioma from the midprepectoral region of an eighteen-year-old gelding, and a hemangioma of the left upper eyelid of a horse aged eighteen years; in the latter case, tumors also were present over the temporal fossa, and in the parotid region. There was also present a cystic multilocular tumor, 6 cm. in diameter, near the thoracic aperture, which was filled with blood. The histology of this process wa-indicative of malignancy, although this could not be definitely des

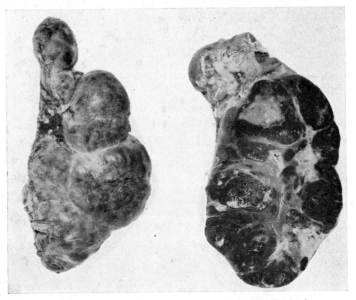

Fig. 74.—Hemangio-endothelioma of the adrenal glands of a horse.

termined. Multiple hemangiomas also were found in various tissues of a twenty-five-year-old mare which had been killed for necropsy. The involved adrenal bodies were filled with blood and were 10 cm. long, 5 to 6 cm. wide, and about 3 cm. thick. The spleen contained numerous, dome-like hemorrhagic cysts from 1 to 3 cm. in diameter. Similar tumor formations were present in the cortical portion of the kidneys, and a few hemorrhagic elevations were found on the surface of the parietal peritoneum. There was no histologic evidence that the process was malignant (Fig. 74).

Bovine.—An angioma of the skin of a cow was described by Trotter,[37] and Stenzel found four angiomas of the udder. One tumor consisted of markedly dilated interalveolar vessels which were greatly in excess of the normal number. From the parent capillaries there was given off a large number of irregularly twisted vessels, which eventually formed anastomoses with others. The vessels were intertwined in a most intricate way. In the three other cases reported by Stenzel angiomas were found to be of a cavernous nature, arising in the interlobular connective tissue. An extensive angioma of the right labia of the vulva of a cow was reported by Leisering, and Eggeling found a pulsating hemangioma about 10 cm. in diameter in the wall of the vagina.

A growth designated as "endothelial sarcoma" was found in the omasum of a thirteen-year-old cow by Ehlers; the process consisted of one large growth about 20 cm. in diameter, and many smaller ones. The laminæ of the organ were destroyed.

Trotter[38] reported the finding of a cavernous hemangioma in the liver of an old cow. The tumor measured approximately 13 by 11 by 8 cm. and was separated from the adjacent hepatic tissue by a fibrous capsule. The tumor consisted of spongy, rather cellular, loose connective tissue which formed blood-filled cavities lined with endothelium. Thrombi were present, many of which were canalized. Boyd, Fitch, Grinnells, and Billings also observed a cavernous hemangioma associated with multiple adenomas of the pancreas in the liver of a ten-year-old cow.

Casper quoted Zschokke as having reported an angioma of the base of the skull of a cow. The presence of the tumor caused strabismus convergens.

My material included multiple hemangio-endotheliomas that occurred in the subcutaneous tissues of a six-year-old cow. The tumors, which were five in number and situated at various places over the body, had been present for about three months. Severe cough developed and the animal rapidly declined and died. Necropsy was not performed. Histologically, the tumor was characterized by a scant amount of connective tissue stroma on which rested one to several layers of endothelial cells, so arranged as to form irregular spaces or cavities. In some of these were red blood corpuscles, and in some organized thrombi.

A similar tumor was obtained from the region of the left iliac lymph node of an eight-year-old cow. Besides the pelvic mass, which weighed 12 kg., there were multiple tumors in the lungs and on the parietal pleura. The pelvic tumor was considered to be hemangio-endothelioma. At necropsy of a seven-year-old Holstein cow, multiple hemangio-endotheliomas were distributed uniformly throughout the lungs. There was also involvement of the parietal pleura, the liver, spleen, kidneys, and adrenal glands. Many lymph nodes, including the bronchial, mediastinal, renal, portal, sublumbar, iliac, supramammary, precrural, and popliteal were involved. Microscopically the tumor consisted of a delicate connective tissue stroma on which rested single layers of endothelial cells. Although many definite blood spaces were to be seen, this degree of differentiation was not attained in much of the material examined.

In another instance, a tumor weighing 120 gm. and approximately 5 cm. long, was found adjacent to the jugular vein in the midcervical region of an old grade cow. The growth was considered to be an endothelioma, although blood spaces or channels were not a part of the structure. The tumor consisted of a more or less diffuse collection of what were considered to be endothelial cells, but conclusive proof of their identity was absent.

Dog.—Two cases of hemangio-endothelioma of the parotid region of dogs were observed by Liénaux. Regenbogen reported four cases of hemangioma of the cavernous type in dogs between the ages of six and ten years. One of the animals was found to have two hemangiomas, one in the subcutaneous tissue near the umbilicus and the other on the ventral surface of the tail, 3 cm. from the anus. In one dog a tumor, about 4 cm. in diameter was firmly attached to the overlying skin, to the right of the median line, near the eleventh or twelfth vertebra. The third case was that of a seven-year-old dog with a hemangioma on the lateral surface of the right antebrachium 7 cm. from the elbow joint. The tumor, which was about 4 cm. in diameter, was firmly attached to the skin. The fourth dog observed had a small hemangioma under the skin of the right side.

Siedamgrotzky described an angioma of the subcutis situated close to the penis in the right inguinal region of a poodle. The tumor, which consisted of a mass of coiled, twisted vessels of variable sizes, appeared as a bluish-black growth under the skin. In the subcutis, near the sacral region of a bird dog, Suffran found a soft, painless tumor 6 by 4 by 1 to 2 cm. The growth was of two months' duration and was composed of alveolar-like spaces which were filled with blood and separated from each other by connective tissue stroma. A capillary hemangioma, which occurred on the ventral surface of the tail, above the anus of a dog, was reported by Leisering. Fölger quoted Galli as describing an endothelioma which he claimed arose from the corpus cavernosum of the penis of a dog. A cavernous hemangioma, about 10 cm. in diameter, which Fölger considered to be a genuine tumor was found by Stephan in the liver of a ten-year-old terrier. In the same animal a carcinoma of the breast with metastasis to the lungs was found.

A somewhat unusual case of malignant endothelioma affecting an old shepherd dog was reported by Kingman and Newsom, who permitted me to examine tissues obtained from the tumor. The history of the case suggested the possible influence of trauma in the inception of this tumor. The dog had the habit of nosing the screen door open, and as he passed through the door, which was equipped with a rather stiff spring, it usually struck him a sharp blow on the right side of the thorax. A large, circumscribed swelling, that was first noticed by the owner four months before the animal died, gradually developed over the right thoracic region. The growth was exceedingly vascular, and when a cannula was thrust into the enlargement a stream of blood escaped, with no diminution in the size of the tumor. The animal was killed for necropsy; the lungs were found to be studded with multiple nodular formations of variable size, and a large mass was found in the posterior mediastinum (Fig. 75). Histologically the tumor was alveolar-like, with the respective compartments lined with endothelial cells. Many of the spaces were filled with red blood corpuscles, although in some portions of the tumor proliferation of the endothelial cells was so profuse as practically to obliterate the cavities.

One of the hemangiomas in my collection occurred in the subcutis over the right posterior part of a mammary gland of an adult female dog. The tumor was nodular, 2 cm. in diameter, and was diagnosed microscopically as cavernous hemangio-endothelioma.

Other species.—Failure to find references in the literature on the occurrence of endothelioblastoma in domesticated mammals other than horses, cattle, and dogs indicates how infrequently these tumors affect other species. Koch, however, reported finding a hemangioma about 2 cm. in diameter in the coccygeal gland of a parrot, and I had occasion to examine a malignant capillary hemangioma from an old ewe. The right kidney and both lungs were extensively involved. The liver revealed vigorous proliferation of the endothelial lining of some of the larger vessels.

Metastasis and malignancy.—Although hemangio-endothelioblastomas, as they occur in animals, are usually localized, occasionally specimens are encountered which appear in widely separated parts of the body. The widespread distribution in many cases is without question a consequence of metastasis, but in some cases the multiplicity of the lesions, and their morphology, strongly suggest primary multiple origin. The tumors usually infiltrate tissues, and distant foci that

appear to have resulted from true metastasis may be in fact proliferative extensions from the parent structure.

The tumors belonging to this group do not ordinarily exhibit marked
malignancy. It is true that an infiltrative type of growth is usually
evident, but it is exceptional for a hemangio-endothelioma to become
severely destructive. The benign tumors exert a locally destructive

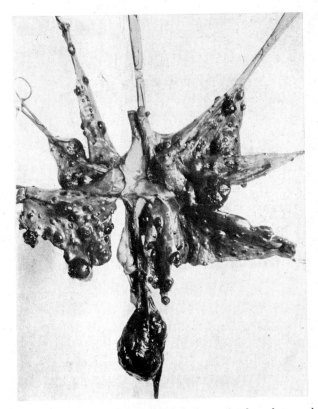

Fig. 75.—Malignant hemangio-endothelioma of the lungs of a dog; photograph prepared
by Dr. Edward Alkire.

influence and may spread extensively by infiltration into the adjacent
tissues and by extending even within the blood channels.

Gross characteristics.—Hemangio-endotheliomas usually are characterized by their color, which varies from dark blood red to purple.
They are of soft consistence, and by pressure the blood can be expressed
from them, to return when the pressure is removed. If a growth is
punctured, much blood is likely to escape. The cavernous varieties are
likely to present a hemorrhagic multilocular aspect, in which well-

organized thrombi may be found. Those of the exterior are covered by the unbroken skin, and have a rather broad base of attachment.

Microscopic description.—It would be extremely difficult, if not impossible, to present under one heading a word picture descriptive of all tumors falling into this group. Generally speaking, however, the majority of hemangio-endotheliomas show a tendency to form multiple, irregular, immature capillaries, spaces, or cavities, varying in size from small alveolar-like openings to large, cavernous compartments which may or may not be filled with blood (Fig. 76). These spaces are lined by one to several layers of endothelial cells. The cells lining many of

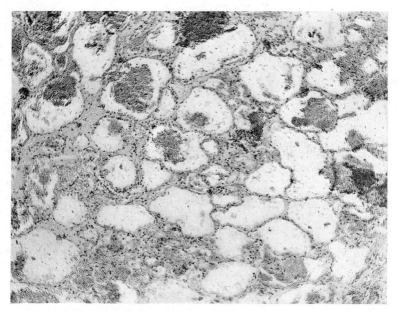

Fig. 76.—Cavernous hemangio-endothelioma of the subcutis of a dog ($\times$ 75).

the cavities may push into the lumens from one side, and by gradual proliferation eventually fill most of the interior, but still retain attachment with the parent cells by a neck, or isthmus. Frequently, solid nests or irregular sheets of cells may present a compact arrangement that simulates certain carcinomatous or sarcomatous structures. This may be due to the vigorous proliferation of the undifferentiated cells which fill the spaces that were formed earlier. In some of the tumors the type cell may occur in small groups or whorl-like clusters, with lumen entirely lacking. The blood in these tumors often undergoes disintegration, due to its being removed from the circulation. Spaces filled with a clear, homogeneous fluid are usually seen, and some of the cavities may be occupied with thrombi showing various degrees of organization (Fig. 77).

The type cell also varies somewhat in appearance. Many cells are oval or polyhedral, depending on whether they occur in a single layer, or in diffuse, nest-like masses with others. Again, they may be flattened and almost spindle-like. In one specimen I examined, the type cell was similar, in many respects, to the ordinary endothelial or mononuclear leukocyte. In compactly arranged portions, many of the cells present a somewhat clear cytoplasm. As a rule, however, the cytoplasm takes a slightly basic stain, and the nuclei, which are fairly large

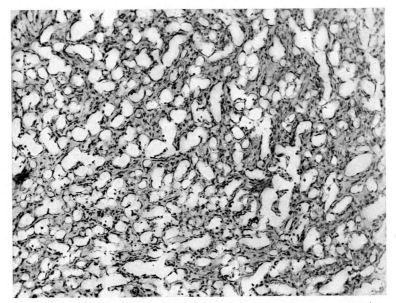

Fig. 77.—Malignant hemangio-endothelioma of the kidney of a sheep (× 120).

or oval, contain considerable chromatin in the form of fine granules. In some material mitotic figures are numerous.

In the recognition of certain hemangio-endotheliomas, particularly in an organ such as the liver, it may be necessary to distinguish between the condition known as capillary telangiectasis and true neoplasm. The former is nothing more than compensatory dilatation and congestion of preëxisting vessels, whereas the latter is characterized by the presence of blood spaces that are newly formed, and which have infiltrated into adjacent tissues.

Endothelioblastomas that are characterized by the formation of multiple capillary-like vessels are conveniently called "capillary he-

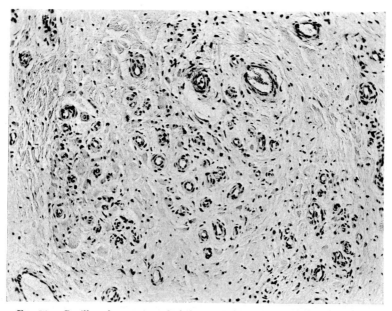

Fig. 78.—Capillary hemangio-endothelioma of the subcutis of a horse (× 120).

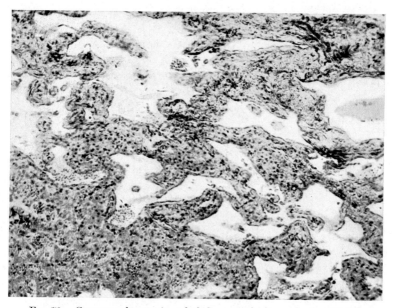

Fig. 79.—Cavernous hemangio-endothelioma of the liver of a dog (× 50).

mangiomas" and if the tumors are composed of dilated, irregular, alveolar spaces of variable dimensions they are termed "cavernous hemangiomas" (Fig. 78, 79 and 80).

Not infrequently one encounters a tumor in which it is difficult to discover criteria sufficient properly to defend a diagnosis of hemangio-endothelioma. Certain tumors that perhaps belong to this group of neoplasms are frequently so devoid of characteristics by which they can be definitely recognized as such, to justify the belief that many lesions designated as hemangio-endotheliomas are considered so erroneously. Although certain forms of hemangio-endothelioma are of simple structure, and possess features that are fairly characteristic, further study will be necessary before all forms of such neoplasms can be correctly designated.

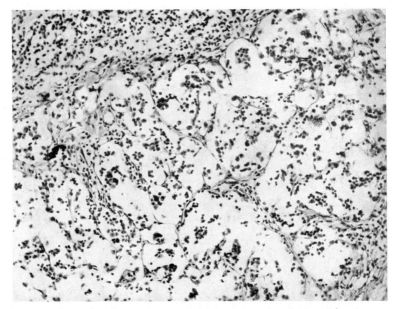

Fig. 80.—Malignant hemangio-endothelioma; bovine (× 150).

Clinical considerations.—Tumors of this group that occur contiguous with the skin are often amenable to operation. The extremely vascular nature of many of them may make it difficult to control hemorrhage if operation is performed carelessly. The infiltrative manner of their growth may prevent complete extirpation, and unless all of the neoplastic process is removed, recurrence is likely.

PSEUDOHEMANGIOMATOUS CONDITIONS

A considerable number of so-called angiomas or hemangiomas of the nasal mucous membranes has been reported. Casper was of the opinion that the condition is relatively common in domestic animals, particularly the horse. The lesions occur as a rule in the upper part of the nasal septum, where they appear as smooth, more or less flattened, red or blue elevations. They are not definitely limited in contour and are particularly prone to bleed if subjected even to slight trauma. This condition probably does not represent a true neoplastic process; it is perhaps due to dilation of the large veins in the submucosa of the nasal mucous membrane.

Telangiectasis is not uncommonly encountered in the liver of cattle, especially old cows, and is designated by different writers as capillary telangiectasis, angiomatosis, cavernous angioma, spotted capillary angiomatosis, and multiple disseminated angioma of the liver; occasionally it has been erroneously grouped with the genuine neoplasms, as noted in the older literature. The disease has been the object of careful investigations by Casper, Stockmann, Stroh, Jaeger, Rühmekorf, Hedrén, and Kettler.

The affected liver appears somewhat enlarged, and single or multiple irregularly shaped, dark red to bluish-black, nonelevated areas can be seen. The color of these areas contrasts markedly with the brownish red of the normal liver. The areas are of a softer consistence than the normal tissue and on section they are generally found to extend throughout the organ, although some are localized. The areas consist of tarlike blood, and extensive thrombosis. Microscopic examination reveals a meshwork of dilated blood-filled cavities surrounded by normal liver tissue. The cavities are interspersed with columns of thin, drawn out remnants of hepatic cells and the blood spaces are lined by endothelium. The cells within an affected area are arranged irregularly, and those near the periphery of the lesion are often more or less retrogressive. Encapsulation does not occur.

Many explanations of the pathogenesis of telangiectasis, as it occurs in the livers of cattle, have been offered. Stroh expressed the belief that the condition results from stasis or congestion caused by compression of the abdominal portion of the posterior vena cava, directly or indirectly the result of pathologically enlarged or misplaced stomachs of herbivorous animals. Stockmann found the condition so frequently associated with hepatic distomiasis that he considered that increase of connective tissue, formed as a consequence of the parasites, caused closure of the blood vessels, with an increase in blood pressure in the noncirrhotic portions. The increased pressure was thought to occasion widening of the capillaries, as a consequence of which the adjacent hepatic cells became atrophic and disappeared. Hedrén concluded that the lesions were of an infectious origin, due to a fungus, which he designated Monilia bovis. Kettler, however, did not accept Hedrén's conclusion and felt that any fungus in telangiectatic lesions was secondary to the inception of the lesions.

The explanation of the process accepted by most pathologists at present is that advanced independently by Rühmekorf and by Jaeger. These investigators found the disease to be essentially telangiectatic degeneration dependent on the focal, fatty retrogression of hepatic cells. The disappearance of hepatic tissue is followed by compensatory dilatation of the blood spaces of the involved part and the formation of new connective tissue. Concerning etiology, Rühmekorf mentioned nutritional disturbances and injury induced by infectious diseases, with individual susceptibility playing a part. Jaeger stated that certain inherent weaknesses of the hepatic cells are contributory factors, and that intoxication or autointoxication may be of significance.

The figures of Rühmekorf, pertaining to the incidence of telangiectasis of the liver of cattle, are of some interest. He examined 3,242 livers and found capillary telangiectasis present in 312 (9.62 per cent). The disease occurred among the various cattle as follows:

In 1,500 livers of cows, telangiectasis was found in 199 (13.27 per cent); in 1,000 livers of steers, telangiectasis was found in 102 (10.2 per cent); in 600 livers of bulls, telangiectasis was found in eight (1.33 per cent), and in 142 livers of heifers, telangiectasis was found in three (2.11 per cent).

Ravenna[27] described the occurrence of telangiectasis of the liver of a mule, and Fölger found the condition in the adrenal glands of forty horses in an examination of 300. The disease was confined to animals aged eight years or more. Fölger thought the changes could be explained etiologically on the basis advanced by Jaeger for telangiectasis of the bovine liver.

Fabris reported finding a hemorrhagic tumor about 4 cm. in diameter in the liver of a young hutch rabbit. Histologic examination of the affected portions disclosed general dilation of the capillaries. The condition might properly be considered telangiectasis.

LYMPH VASCULAR TUMORS

Tumors composed of the essential elements of lymph vessels (lymph-angio-endothelioblastomas) are extremely rare in lower animals. In my collection of approximately 550 tumors, there was none.

Incidence.—Multiple lymphangioma of the visceral and parietal pleura and of the pericardium of a twenty-year-old horse was reported by Markus. The growths consisted of numerous flat, irregular proliferations, varying in size from 1 mm. to 3 cm. Some were attached by a broad base and others were pedunculated. In many of the growths at the distal extremity were translucent, dilated vesicles, about 1 cm. in diameter, which contained clear, serous fluid. The regional lymph nodes and the other organs were not affected. The process was considered to be a lymphangioma on account of the presence of endothelial-lined spaces that contained a serous, lymph-like fluid, and a few small lymphocytes.

Casper mentioned the report of Schindelka in which was described what may have been lymphangioma of a five-year-old cat. In the region adjacent to the teats, and surrounding them were tumors varying in size from 1 to 4 cm. in diameter. The growths were pendulous, yellowish red, and appeared like small bags half full of fluid. When punctured, a yellow, serous fluid escaped. Although the tumors were not examined microscopically, the process was designated "lymphangioma cavernosum."

Medwedew reported a case of lymphangioma of a dog. The growth extended forward under the skin from a few centimeters below the anal opening, and was 10 to 12 cm. wide and 27 cm. long. Fölger mentioned two cases of lymphangioma of horses reported by Nocard. One of the tumors involved the prepuce and the other was in the inguinal region, in the vicinity of the saphenous vein.

Bernardini[1] observed a lymphangioma in the subcutis over the right hip joint of a seven-year-old horse. Following an unsuccessful attempt to remove the tumor by surgical means, a lymph-like fluid flowed continuously from the wound. At necropsy, in the affected region there was found an alveolar, spongy, flesh-colored tissue containing much lymph-like fluid that had replaced the subcutaneous and intermuscular connective tissue and extended into the musculature. Microscopically, a network of connective tissue trabeculæ was found enclosing cavities lined with endothelium. A second, similar tumor was reported later by the same author.[2] This tumor appeared in the submaxillary region of a six-year-old gelding. The growth was about 10 cm. in diameter and had progressed rapidly, so that within six months it extended over most of the region involved. A lymph-like fluid issued through an opening in the overlying skin. A mass weighing 500 gm. was removed surgically, but later recurrence was noted.

The rarity of lymphangio-endothelioma among animals has precluded the examination of sufficient material to make it possible to outline the salient morphologic features of these tumors. When present in human beings they are characterized by proliferation of communicating channels or spaces lined with endothelium and containing a serous, lymph-like fluid.

The dilatation of preëxistent lymph vessels by excessive amounts of lymph sometimes occurs, and is known as lymphangiectasis. Such a lesion should not be confused with neoplasm.

BIBLIOGRAPHY

1. Bernardini, D.: L'infangioma cavernoso sotto cutaneo in un cavallo. Clin. vet., 29: 437–450, 1906.

2. Bernardini, D.: Su di un secondo caso di l'infangioma cavernoso collocutaneo nel cavallo. Clin. vet. (Sez. prat.), 32: 484, 1909.

3. Boyd, W. L., Fitch, C. P., Grinnells, C. D. and Billings, W. A.: Cavernous hemangioma of the liver together with multiple adenoma of the pancreas. Cornell Vet., 9: 169–170, 1919.

4. Casper, M.: Geschwülste bei Tieren. Ergebn. d. all. Path. u. path. Anat., 11: 1068–1122, 1907.

5. Eggeling: Quoted by Casper.

6. Ehlers: Sarcoma endotheliale am Psalter einer Kuh. Berl. tierärtzl. Wchnschr., 28, 1899.

7. Endotheliomata in a day-old colt. Am. Jour. Vet. Med. (Dept. of Lab. Diagnosis), 15: 390, 1920.

8. Fabris, A.: On so-called angiomatosis of the liver (cavernous degeneration). Sperimentale, Arch. di biol., 80: 219–227, 1926. Abstr. in: Cancer Rev., 2: 171 (April), 1927.

9. Fölger, A. F.: Geschwülste bei Tieren. Ergebn. d. all. Path. u. path. Anat., 18: 372–676, 1917.

10. Fröhner: Statistische und casuistische Mittheilungen über das Vorkommen und die chirurgische Behandlung der Geschwülste beim Hunde. Monatschr. f. prakt. Thierh., 6: 1; 79; 111; 1894–1895.

11. Fröhner, E.: Hundert weitere Geschwülste beim Pferde. Monatschr. f. prakt. Thierh., 13: 1, 1902.

12. Gebruth, J. A.: Endothelioma of the membrana nictitans in a horse. Vet. Jour., 66: 486, 1910.

13. Grebe, L.: Angioma cavernosum diffusum beim Pferde. Arch. f. wissensch. u. prakt. Thierh., 9: 356–362, 1882.

14. Hedrén, G.: Die Aetiologie der angiomatosis der Rindsleber (Teleangiectasia hepatis dissemimata des Verfassers). Arch. f. wissensch. u. prakt. Thierh., 37: 271–298, 1911.

15. Jaeger, A.: Die Teleangiektasis der Leber der Bovinen. Arch. f. wissensch. u. prakt. Thierh., 32: 71–112, 1907.

16. Johne: Quoted by Casper.

17. Kettler, J.: Quoted by Fölger.

18. Kingman, H. E. and Newson, I. E.: An interesting tumor. Case report. Jour. Am. Vet. Med. Assn., 52: 703–705 (Feb.), 1918.

19. Koch, M.: Quoted by Fölger.

20. Leisering: Quoted by Casper.

21. Liénaux, E.: Deux cas d'endotheliomes de la region parotidienne chez le chien. Ann. de méd. Vét., 48: 502, 1899.

22. Mallory, F. B.: The principles of pathologic histology. Philadelphia, W. B. Saunders Company, 1914, p. 309.

23. Markus, H.: Multiple lymphangiom van de pleura bij het paard. Tijdschr. v. veeartsenijk. Maandbl., **30**: 480–490, 1902–1903. Translated in: Monatschr. f. prakt. Tierh., **15**: 185–192, 1903.

24. Medwedew: Quoted by Fölger.

25. Montané: Rev. Vet., 633, 1890.

26. Ravenna, E.: Cavernoma multiplo in un cavallo. Il moderno zooistrio (parte scientif.), **22**: 267, 1911.

27. Ravenna, E.: Ectasia vasali ed emorrhagie multiple in un asino. Il moderno zooistrio (parte scientif.), **22**: 368, 1911.

28. Regenbogen: Ueber das Vorkommen der Hämangiome. Monatschr. f. prakt. Thierh., **18**: 293–298, 1907.

29. Rigot: Quoted by Casper.

30. Rühmekorf, K.: Über multiple disseminierte Kapillarektasien der Leber des Rindes und ihre Beziehungen zu den echten Angiomen. Leipzig, 1907, 49 pp.

31. Siedamgrotzky: Quoted by Casper.

32. Stenzel, W.: Ueber Angiome, Carcinome un Chondrome in der Milchdrüse der Hausthiere. Arch. f. wissensch. u. prakt. Thierh., **29**: 165–194, 1903.

33. Stephan, L.: Quoted by Fölger.

34. Stockmann: Quoted by Casper.

35. Stroh: Ueber die fleckige Kapillarektasie in der Leber der Wiederkäuer. Monatschr. f. prakt. Thierh., **14**: 133, 1903.

36. Suffran: Angiome caverneus sous-cutane. Rev. Vet., 229, 1904.

37. Trotter, A. M.: Angioma of the skin of a cow. Jour. Comp. Path. and Therap., **16**: 54 (March), 1903.

38. Trotter, M.: Cavernous angioma of the liver of a cow. Vet. Jour., **66**: 150, 1910.

39. Volland: Quoted by Fölger.

13

CHAPTER XII

MESOTHELIOBLASTOMA

DEFINITION AND TERMINOLOGY

Mesothelioblastoma is composed of cells of varied potentialities, the precursors of which are derived from the mesodermal elements lining the primitive celomic cavity. These cells normally cover the surface of all serous membranes. New growths in which the type cell is mesothelial are not common, and the literature yields little data concerning their occurrence in the lower animals.

Because of the variation in structure of the type cell of many of these tumors, and the difference of opinion as to embryogenesis, a great deal of confusion has existed in nomenclature and classification. Tumors springing from tissues covered with mesothelial cells, such as the pleura, pericardium, and peritoneum have been variously called mesotheliomas, endotheliomas, and alveolar sarcomas, and some consider new growths arising from the superficial cells of the serous membranes to be epithelial in nature, or carcinomatous. Part of the difficulty in properly classifying these growths, as Klemperer and Rabin recently have shown, is in determining whether the tumor in question arose from the superficial lining cells of the pleura (mesothelium), the connective tissue of the subserosa, or the endothelium of the subserous lymphatic structures.

HISTOGENESIS

In order properly to interpret the variable structure of many of these tumors, it is imperative to keep in mind the essential facts concerning the origin of normal mesothelial cells.

The studies of Hertwig have shown that in the embryo the mesoderm divides and forms the celomic cavity. From the cells that line this space are derived the lining cells of the serous membranes, whereas the vascular endothelium, the connective tissue, and the blood are derived from the adjacent mesenchyme. Klemperer and Rabin emphasized the fact that a basement membrane does not exist between the cells lining the celomic cavity on the one hand, and those of the underlying mesenchyme on the other, and that the close genetic relationship of these elements to the parent mesoderm is sufficient to account for the multipotent behavior

of immature mesothelial cells in a neoplasm. The experimental observations of Maximow in which he was able, by means of tissue cultures, to demonstrate the transformation of mesothelial cells to fibroblasts, lends further support to the contention that mesothelial cells
possess the potencies of mesenchyme, and that they may, under proper
stimuli, assume an appearance not dissimilar to certain connective tissue
cells.

With the foregoing facts in mind, the complex nature of many of these
growths becomes understandable. The structure of some may simulate
an epithelial growth; in others, connective tissue characteristics may
predominate, and it is not unusual that a combination of the two structures may occur within the same tumor.

INCIDENCE

Although mesotheliomas undoubtedly are rare, they must occur
more frequently in lower animals than is indicated by reported cases.
The lack of a uniform nomenclature would suggest that perhaps many
of these tumors have been designated as carcinomas, endotheliomas, or
as some form of sarcoma, and as a consequence they are difficult to
recognize in the literature.

Among the neoplasms in my collection, mesothelial tumors occurred
once among forty-three tumors of horses, and twice among 230 tumors
of cattle.

OCCURRENCE

A tumor diagnosed as endothelioma was reported by Gagliardi to
have occurred in a seventeen-year-old horse. The tumor consisted of
many small nodules scattered over the surface of the pleura and the
peritoneum and was composed of groups of round cells surrounded by
connective tissue. The anatomic distribution of the tumor, and its
general structure, perhaps justifies its inclusion with the mesothelioblastomas, although proof of its exact nature is not available.

A diffuse nodular tumor which resembled tuberculous peritonitis
was found by Purmann in a six- to eight-week-old calf. The process
was designated endothelioma and consisted, in addition to the main
portion of the growth which surrounded the stomach, of small growths
scattered throughout the abdominal cavity. As in the preceding case
there is a temptation to consider the tumor reported by Purmann of
mesothelial origin, but the data are not conclusive.

Two cases of primary neoplasm of the peritoneum were reported by
Scott as occurring in captive wild animals at the London zoo. One of

the tumors developed in a female gnu. During a period of two and a half years there was increasing enlargement of the abdomen, and at necropsy neoplastic masses were found affecting the omentum, the serosa of the liver, the spleen, and the diaphragm. The second tumor was found in a female hamster and involved the mesentery, visceral, and parietal peritoneum, and left lung. Scott considered the various views concerning neoplasms of the serous membranes and subscribed to the term "mesothelioma."

I obtained a mesothelioma from a ten-year-old horse which had been brought to a veterinary hospital because of pronounced edema of the ventral portion of the thorax. The animal was apparently in good condition otherwise, and continued to eat and drink as usual up to the time of death. The cause of the edema was obscure, and since the condition did not improve with treatment, but became progressively worse, the animal was finally killed for necropsy. A large, irregular, fleshy tumor was found at the anterior thoracic aperture. It involved, in a very intimate way, the esophagus, common carotid arteries, and jugular veins. The growth, which was difficult to separate from the adjacent tissues, weighed 900 gm. and measured 55 cm. in circumference. Small, flattened, nodular formations were also found firmly attached to the parietal pleura of the right side. These nodules were multiple, firm, and grayish white, and measured 0.5 by 1.5 cm. The pulmonary tissue was not affected. A similar case was reported by Douville, in which the trachea was also embedded in the tumor.

In two cases, mesotheliomas were obtained from the thoracic cavities of cattle. In one case the neoplastic process involved the pericardium, the parietal pleura, and the suprasternal lymph node, although the lungs were not affected. In the second case the tumors were multiple and were distributed generally throughout the serosa of the thoracic wall and pericardium of a cow. Many of the growths were pedunculated, polypus-like, and of a dirty yellow color resembling fat. Metastasis to the regional lymph nodes or adjacent organs had not occurred.

EFFECT ON THE HOST

From the meager data available concerning mesothelioblastomas, it seems that these tumors are more harmful because of their size and the situations they occupy than because of any marked tendency to invade and destroy vital tissues. The deleterious effects are largely mechanical, due to pressure exerted on the adjacent soft tissues. Those of the thoracic cavity may be expected eventually to encroach on the lungs, as a consequence of which the animal may experience respiratory embarrassment, especially when subjected to strenuous exercise.

The effect of pressure exerted by progressive enlargement of the neoplastic process was well illustrated in the case of mesothelioblastoma of the horse in my series. The main unit of growth encroached in a striking manner on the common carotid arteries and the jugular veins, and edema of the tissues of the ventral thoracic wall resulted.

METASTASIS

Available data afford little evidence of metastatic propensities on the part of these tumors. Certain observers claim that they never metastasize; others hold that metastasis does occur. Although a large number of immature cell forms may be present, many of which are undergoing mitosis, the tendency of these cells to enter the blood vascular system or the lymphatics is not comparable to that manifested by many other varieties of malignant growths. It is true that a nearby lymph node occasionally is invaded, and rarely there may be extensive invasion of an adjacent organ, but this is exceptional. The tumors ordinarily remain localized, although frequently multiple growths may be present which do not exhibit malignant aggressiveness comparable to what might be expected from the histologic structure of the mass.

Since multiplicity is one of the commonest characteristics reported, spread within a short radius perhaps occurs, although the exact mechanism of this phenomenon is somewhat obscure. However, it might be explained on the basis of transplantation caused by dissemination of the tumor cells over the surface of the serosa as a consequence of friction, or the multiplicity may be due to the simultaneous origin of new growths at a number of different points.

GROSS CHARACTERISTICS

Grossly these tumors are usually fleshy or fibrous, and grayish-white to yellow, although the color may vary with the degree of inflammatory exudation present. An occasional specimen has a yellowish, fat-like appearance. In shape they vary from irregularly rounded, nodular masses to smooth, flattened units of tissue attached over a broad base to the underlying serous membrane. In one of my cases the multiple growths were polypus-like. They are of rather firm consistence and do not yield readily to traction. In fact, they may contain sufficient connective tissue to insure rigidity comparable to that of some of the benign connective tissue tumors. For the most part, mesotheliomas are compact, closely knit masses of tissue that exhibit a diffuse relationship with the underlying serosa. A capsule may or may not be present, and the blood supply is generous but not excessive.

MICROSCOPIC DESCRIPTION

The inherent potencies of the type cell of mesothelioblastomas provide potential variations in the histologic appearance of these tumors. They may be composed of diffuse collections of epithelial-like cells, or sufficient connective tissue elements may be present to impart to the structure a marked resemblance to a sarcomatous neoplasm. A mix-

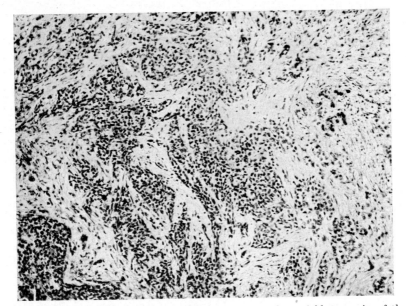

Fig. 81.—Mesothelioma of the pleura of a horse showing the variable potencies of the architectural elements ($\times$ 100).

ture of these different structural elements may occur (Fig. 81). In those tumors that contain much fibrous tissue it is not uncommon to find definite alveoli, within which are closely packed nests of irregularly spherical, or somewhat flattened cells, with a minimal amount of finely granular cytoplasm and nucleus that occupies a considerable portion of the cellular bulk. In some fields are irregular, compact rows of cells, in intimate relationship with adjacent strands of connective tissue, and one may merge almost imperceptibly into the other. The amount of connective tissue varies; it is scant in some regions and abundant in others.

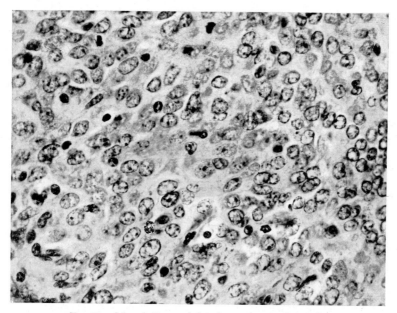

Fig. 82.—Mesothelioma of the pleura of a cow (× 525).

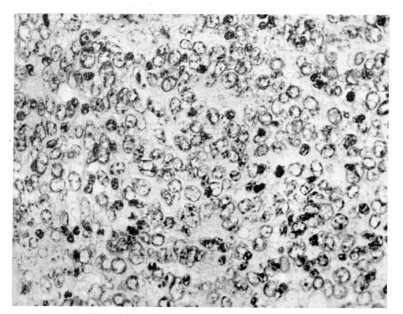

Fig. 83.—Mesothelioma of the pleura of a cow. The pale or clear nuclei predominate. Same cases as represented in Figure 81 (× 450).

Mesotheliomas in which there is predominance of epithelial-like cells are usually composed of broad expanses of closely arranged cells, of ovoid or polyhedral contour, which possess a rather large, pale staining or clear nucleus. Nucleoli are prominent. The cells are disposed in a manner suggestive of squamous epithelium, with a minimal amount of connective tissue fibers discernible (Figs. 82 and 83). Many of the cells frequently reveal evidences of immaturity, and mitosis is not uncommon even though the tumor remains localized. Numerous well-formed although small blood vessels usually can be seen. In some material I have examined, eosinophiles were distributed promiscuously throughout the tissue, and necrosis with early calcification was observed.

Deviations from the foregoing description are common. The cytoplasmic outlines of many of the cells are heaped up or overlap; spindle-

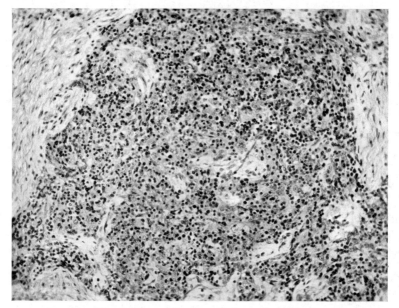

Fig. 84.—Mesothelioma of the visceral pleura of a sheep (× 150).

shaped forms may occur, in which it is possible to trace the gradual transition from the large, ovoid forms to those that are definitely elongated (Fig. 84). In material from one case which I studied, the formation of numerous duct or gland-like structures of different sizes had taken place. Each of these was composed of a single layer of cells, which was apparently derived from the cells constituting the surrounding neoplasms. A basement membrane was not discernible; the cells which made up the adenomatous structure apparently arose out of the adjacent cellular portion. The various spaces contained a homogeneous substance and considerable débris suggestive of an inflammatory exudate.

Thus a wide diversity of structures may occur in tumors derived from mesothelial cells, attesting to the multipotency of the mesodermal elements from which the type cell is developed.

DIAGNOSTIC CONSIDERATIONS

In the recognition of a tumor derived from mesothelial cells there are several points of significance. The tumors arise from the pleura, pericardium or peritoneum. The surface cells and not the subserous connective tissues give rise to the neoplasm. The tumors are diffuse, usually multiple, and exhibit a tendency to remain localized; metastasis is unusual. The presence of a primary tumor in some other portion of the body should make one extremely cautious in venturing a diagnosis of primary mesothelioma. Metastatic tumors of the serous membranes are not uncommon.

CLINICAL CONSIDERATIONS

Mesothelioblastic tumors are of such infrequent occurrence as to be of practically no significance to the clinician.

The presence of a primary neoplasm of a serous membrane may occasion complex symptoms, but the anatomic situation affected by these tumors usually precludes the possibility of their removal even though their presence were discovered, which is rather unlikely. The meat inspector should be more successful than the clinician in recognizing this condition. The presence of numerous diffuse tumorous masses on the surface of the serous membranes, in the absence of primary tumors elsewhere, would suggest the possibility of mesothelioma. The ultimate decision, however, must depend on the microscopic examination of sections prepared from the growth.

BIBLIOGRAPHY

1. Douville: Tumors of the anterior mediastinum. Editorial. Am. Vet. Rev., **31**: 166, 1907.

2. Gagliardi, G.: Endothelioma delle sierose in un cavallo. La Clin. Vet., **25**: 505, 1902.

3. Hertwig: Quoted by Klemperer and Rabin.

4. Klemperer, Paul and Rabin, C. B.: Primary neoplasms of the pleura. A report of five cases. Arch. Path., **11**: 385–412 (March), 1931.

5. Maximow, Alexander: Über das Mesothel (Deckzellen der serösen Häute) und die Zellen der serösen Exudate. Untersuchungen an entzündetem Gewebe und an Gewebskulturen. Arch. f. exper. Zellforsch., **4**: 1–42, 1927.

6. Purmann, T.: Über einen Fall von peritonealer Deckzellegeschwulst bei einen Kalbe. Beitr. z. path. Anat. u. z. allg. Path., **84**: 659–666, 1930.

7. Scott, H. H.: Two cases of peritoneal neoplasm (endothelioma). Proc. Zool. Soc. London, 1927, pp. 511–516.

CHAPTER XIII

LYMPHOBLASTOMA

Probably no diseases lead to so much confusion as those which arise from the lymphoid elements or from the cells of the lymphocytic series. Bewildering discussions deal with lymphadenoma, pseudoleukemia, lymphoma, leukemia, lymphocytoma, alveolar sarcoma, lymphosarcomatosis, round-cell sarcoma, lymphatic leukemia, lymphosarcoma, and Hodgkin's disease. In describing cases belonging to this group of diseases, writers have, with few exceptions, selected from these terms those which they thought most applicable to their particular cases, without making any real attempt to justify the use of the terms on the basis of fundamental pathologic changes. The literature dealing with this group of diseases as they affect animals reveals that in many cases the diagnosis was made on the basis of a general examination only, or, if necropsy was performed, histologic study was often omitted. Furthermore, there has been relatively little opportunity for comprehensive study of these diseases in the living animal, not because of infrequent occurrence, but rather because physical reasons have made it difficult, particularly in the larger mammals, to conduct proper studies for sufficient periods.

Although the concept that these conditions are neoplastic is not accepted by all, the unrestricted growth, the invasion and destruction of normal tissues, and the widespread metastasis which frequently occurs, are definite characteristics of a neoplastic process. Much of the confusion which has arisen concerning these conditions has been due to the insistence of many observers that they should be separated on the basis of clinical and morphologic criteria into several subdivisions or varieties. Others contend that they are so closely related genetically as to justify their classification in one group. This view was first advanced by Warthin[13] in 1904 and is gradually gaining support from pathologists engaged in the study of human and of comparative material.

The disease often differs in its clinical manifestations. The difference is due to the anatomic situation of the primary disturbance, the degree of differentiation of the type cells, and the extent of the metastatic involvement. However, regardless of variations in the clinical aspects of the disease, the different clinical varieties which may be encountered are simply different expressions of a fundamental cellular disturbance which is common to all.

DEFINITIONS

Although the conditions designated as lymphoblastoma have close genetic relationship, certain clinical and morphologic differences make at least two subdivisions justifiable.

Lymphoma.—This is a slowly progressive, benign tumor which arises within lymph nodes and other lymphoid tissues. It is strictly localized and replaces the normal lymphatic tissue by gradual expansion. Lymphomas do not exhibit tendencies to metastasize or to infiltrate the surrounding tissues, and the leukocytes in the blood are not disturbed. They frequently are the sites of extensive retrograde changes. If such a tumor should suddenly assume malign tendencies, it no longer could be considered as a lymphoma, but would become a lymphocytoma, the term used to designate the malignant forms of lymphoblastoma.

Lymphocytoma.—In this group should be placed all of the malignant types of neoplastic hyperplasia of which the immature lymphocyte or its forerunner is the type cell. Malignancy is evidenced by rapidity of growth, recurrence after surgical removal, infiltration and destruction of normal tissues, multiplicity of lesions, and metastasis. Although there may be wide variations in the extent of involvement, the main factor is the lawless and continuous overgrowth of lymphoid cells occurring primarily in preëxistent lymphoid tissue. The cells may invade the blood stream and multiply there to such a degree as markedly to change the proportions of its cellular content. The resultant leukemic state is essentially lymphatic, and the condition is often referred to as lymphatic leukemia. However, it should be emphasized that a diagnosis of lymphocytoma is not dependent on the presence of an excessive number of lymphoid cells in the blood stream, but on the neoplastic proclivities of the lymphocyte-producing tissues. In fact, in a considerable percentage of the cases, the customary blood picture of leukemia is lacking.

According to this view, the blood picture is of secondary importance; it is dependent on the primarily neoplastic process present extravascularly in the lymphoid tissues. In other words, this is a disease of certain of the blood-forming tissues, and not of the blood itself. The use of the words "leukemic" or "aleukemic," in a qualifying sense before the term "lymphocytoma," provides a fairly concise nomenclature which is descriptive of the pathologic changes concerned.

HISTOGENESIS

The type cell of this tumor, which is the lymphoblast, has its origin mainly in certain undifferentiated mesenchymal elements found in the various lymphoid deposits throughout the body. In the physiologic state, these cells pass through a succession of transitional or developmental stages, from relatively immature, undifferentiated forms, to that of the fully developed large and small lymphocyte. Since the adult forms are concerned chiefly in normal physiologic processes, they obviously are not implicated in lawless proliferations which characterize the neoplastic phenomenon. Neoplasia must depend on the continuous overproduction of immature cells for which there can be no physiologic utilization, and it is these undifferentiated forms which constitute, or are responsible for, the type cells of lymphoblastoma.

Little, if anything, is known as to factors which may influence the inception of these tumors. In man it is thought that certain of them possibly may have a relation to tuberculosis, although definite proof of the relationship being anything more than coincidental is difficult to assemble. Up to this time, no significant etiologic influence has been attributed to tuberculosis in the lymphoblastomas as they affect animals, nor has any other specific infectious agent been definitely implicated in their inception. In the present state of knowledge, there seems no valid reason to suppose that the disease is due to bacteria, and about all that can safely be said of its etiology is that it is probably due to an abnormal response of certain of the lymphocytic series of cells to a stimulus of unknown origin and nature. Perhaps the excitant factor which is responsible for the progressive overproduction of the cells in this disease is the same or closely related to that responsible for carcinoma and other lawless new growths.

INCIDENCE

If all species are considered, the lymphoblastomas probably occur with greater frequency than any of the other neoplasms which affect lower animals. In one series of 416 tumors in my collection, representing four different species of mammals, 104 (25 per cent) were malignant forms of lymphoblastoma. The relative incidence of occurrence in the different mammals was as follows:

Among 221 tumors in cattle there were fifty-nine malignant lymphoblastomas (35.6 per cent); among seventy-seven tumors in swine there were twenty-five malignant lymphoblastomas (32.4 per cent), and among forty tumors in sheep there were six malignant lymphoblastomas (15.5 per cent).

My material contains six cases of lymphoma; two were in cattle, two were in sheep, one was in a swine, and one was in a goat; the last was the only neoplasm I have observed in a goat.

In a series of 3,032 postmortem examinations, including mammals and fowls, Crocker listed only two cases that could be classified as instances of lymphoblastoma, and both occurred in dogs. Crocker's figures were compiled from records of a veterinary hospital, whereas much of my material was from slaughter houses.

Practically all domestic animals are susceptible to the disease, although unquestionably it occurs more frequently in some than in others. As early as 1858, Leisering, who first recognized leukemia in animals, stated that it is more common in dogs than other house animals, and certainly the literature on the subject contains more references to this animal than to any other. Here, as of most tumors of animals, it is extremely difficult to obtain accurate figures on the occurrence of the disease in the respective species, because of difficulty in collecting the material, as well as the paucity of published data that are reliable. Crocker's two cases in dogs occurred in a total of 1,548 dogs examined, which certainly does not present a high incidence. The disease has been observed in cats by Siedamgrotzky, and by Lellmann. Houdemer and Bablet described the only case I have found of generalized lymphoblastomatous involvement of the abdominal cavity and viscera in a mule.

Without question this disease is most common in the bovine species; the horse is rarely affected. The condition is responsible for condemnation of a large number of cattle yearly by veterinarians in the meat inspection division of the Bureau of Animal Industry. The reports of the Chief of the Bureau of Animal Industry of the United States De-

TABLE 4

CONDEMNATIONS FOR LEUKEMIA BY FEDERAL MEAT INSPECTION SERVICE OF THE BUREAU OF ANIMAL INDUSTRY*

Animals.	Necropsy.	Condemned for so-called leukemia.	Ratio.
Cattle	35,654,719	4,183	1 in approximately 8,500
Calves†	18,872,047	126	1 in approximately 149,000
Swine	204,870,269	924	1 in approximately 220,000
Sheep	54,953,621	32	1 in approximately 1,714,000
Horses	402,714	2	1 in approximately 201,000

* During the period over which these statistics were gathered necropsies were also performed on 94,004 goat carcasses, in none of which was there gross demonstrable evidence of leukemia.

† Aged one year or less.

partment of Agriculture for the four years prior to June 30, 1930, show lymphoblastoma, which is designated leukemia, to have been the cause of condemnations among the various classes of livestock, as given in Table 4.

The facts seem to justify the conclusion that primary lymphoid hyperplasia of a neoplastic nature is among the more common diseases of many of the domestic animals and undoubtedly is the cause of many more or less obscure deaths, for unless thorough necropsy is performed, the true nature of the disease may escape detection. From the available data, it seems that the disease most commonly affects cattle, dogs, swine, and chickens.

REGIONS OF THE BODY AFFECTED

Since this is a disease primarily of the lymphoid tissue it is natural to expect lesions to be present in these structures. When one realizes the extent of the distribution of lymphoid tissues throughout the body, the widespread distribution of the lesions frequently seen in this condition is not unexpected (Fig. 85). Although the lesions may be confined to the lymph nodes and the other deposits of lymphoid tissue, they are capable of extensive metastasis, and secondary involvement may occur in the lungs, adrenal glands, heart, liver, kidneys, and even the brain (Fig. 86). Strange as it may seem, and contrary to the opinion of many observers, the spleen, in many of my cases, was not demonstrably involved. Although the cardiac muscle and the voluntary striated muscles often are extensively invaded metastatically, smooth muscle seems to possess more or less stubborn resistance to advances of the neoplastic process. In cases of lymphocytoma it is not unusual, particularly in cattle and swine, to find every lymph node of the body exhibiting neoplastic hyperplasia, and in addition, each cavity of the body, and the diaphragm, may contain many large, irregular, more or less diffuse masses of tumorous tissue, constituting a degree of involvement which is truly remarkable (Fig. 87.)

Of the two lymphomas in my collection which affected cattle, one was situated in the deep inguinal region, and one was attached by a short pedicle in the region immediately adjacent to one kidney. One of the two lymphomas of the sheep was obtained from the dorsal aspect of the middle cervical region and the other from the mediastinum. The one lymphoma obtained from swine apparently arose in the left supramammary lymph node, and the one affecting the goat was situated in the thorax, near the thoracic aperture.

A summary of the lesions which occurred in a series of forty un-
selected cases of lymphocytoma in cattle, thirty-nine of which were

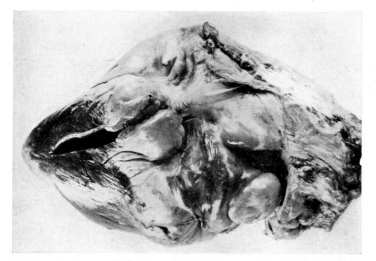

Fig. 85.—Lymphocytoma. Multiple tumorous nodules overlying the auricles of the heart
of a bovine.

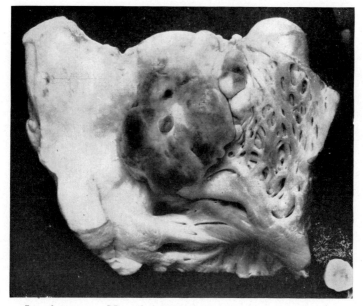

Fig. 86.—Lymphocytoma. Mass of neoplastic tissue in the right auricle. Same case as
represented in Figure 85.

females, showed that the spleen was affected in fourteen, the liver
in eleven, the lungs in nine, the digestive tract in twelve, the uterus in

eleven, and the cardiac muscle in twenty; the blood was leukemic in twenty-seven, as determined by cross sections of blood vessels. In only one of these was the parenchyma of the kidney violated, although in several animals extensive neoplastic masses were present at the hilum

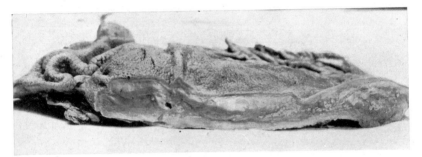

Fig. 87.—Lymphocytoma. Diffuse neoplastic accumulation in the submucosa of the abomasum of a bovine.

and in the subscapular region (Fig. 88). There was extensive or generalized involvement of lymph nodes in thirty-five of the cases, and in three cases the lymphoid hyperplasia was confined to one or several lymph nodes in a definitely localized region. In two cases involvement of

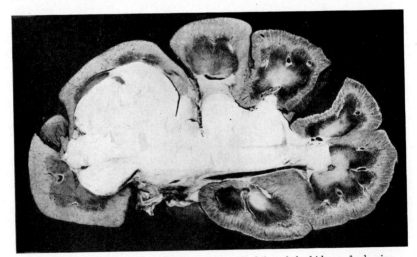

Fig. 88.—Lymphocytoma. Tumor occupying the hilus of the kidney of a bovine.

lymph nodes was not apparent; the lesions were confined in one case to the muscle of the heart, and in the other to the wall of the duodenum and the muscle of the heart. In the latter, the blood also was leukemic. In five of the cases the eyeballs were crowded out of their normal position by large masses of tumorous tissue in the orbital space. This involvement may be bilateral, and occasionally the eyeballs project markedly from their normal position. Knuth and Volkmann also observed involvement of the orbit in five of nineteen cattle affected with the disease.

The distribution of lesions in sixteen female and two male swine was as follows: The spleen in four cases, the liver in ten, the kidney in three, the lung in three, the digestive tract in three, and the ovary in one case; there were none in the uterus or in the muscle of the heart. In twelve of the eighteen cases the lymph nodes were extensively involved, and the blood was definitely leukemic. In four of the cases the hyperplasia of the lymph nodes was confined to a single or to a small, localized group, and in two cases there was no noticeable enlargement.

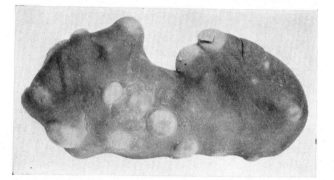

Fig. 89.—Lymphocytoma. Numerous neoplastic nodules in the kidney of a swine.

In one of these the lesions were confined to the digestive tract and the liver; in the other, the kidneys were the only tissues which were demonstrably affected (Fig. 89).

The distribution of lesions in the sheep is similar to that in the ox. In the dog the lesions consist of small, rather firm, rapidly growing nodular growths in the skin or subcutis of the neck, shoulder, or thoracic region, and metastasis to the regional lymph nodes frequently results. In most cases, however, the disease in the dog is characterized by progressive enlargement of the lymph nodes of the exterior of the body, which usually becomes evident first in the lymph nodes of the head and neck. The enlargements which may be bilateral, are not painful, and they may exhibit a tendency to become multiple or lobulated. At necropsy, lesions may be found in the spleen, kidneys, liver, and, rarely, in the lungs.

14

GROSS CHARACTERISTICS

Lymphoma usually appears as a single, firm to hard, nodular mass which may or may not be encapsulated. It is grayish-white and may be tough, due to the presence of variable amounts of fibrous connective tissue.

Lymphocytoma consists of nodular or diffuse, irregular, fleshy masses of tissue, flesh pink or grayish-white. The tissue is usually compact, but is seldom hard. If freshly cut, the exposed portion reveals a moist, glistening surface of soft, velvety texture. Not infrequently the tissue is markedly hemorrhagic, and occasionally the neoplastic elements and the adjacent nontumorous tissues present an edematous or water-logged appearance. Encapsulation does not occur, and the intimate, infiltrative relation of the metastatic, tumorous tissues with the adjacent nontumorous tissues is a feature of these malignant processes. If the masses are large, necrosis and other retrogressive changes may occur.

MICROSCOPIC DESCRIPTION

Microscopically the two varieties of lymphoblastoma present dissimilar pictures.

Lymphomas consist of rather circumscribed collections of closely packed lymphoid cells without the features usually associated with the appearance of malignancy. The cells are of a fairly uniform size, and mitosis is seen only occasionally. There is, however, unmistakable evidence of slow, progressive encroachment on the surrounding lymphoid tissue. Strands of fibrous connective tissue may be present and constitute an alveolar-like matrix of varying proportions. The chronicity of these tumors is favorable for the appearance of retrogressive changes; in one case which I studied in the ox, much of the tumor was involved in atypical amyloid degeneration.

The type cell of lymphocytomas has been designated "round cell" by many of the older writers, and either the large or small variety may predominate. The cell, which is lymphoid, is irregularly spherical, with a narrow zone of nongranular cytoplasm surrounding a slightly eccentrically situated nucleus. The nucleus, which constitutes most of the cellular bulk, is spherical and strongly basophilic. An abundance of chromatin is distributed as small granules throughout the nuclear substance. Nucleoli are seldom observed. Mitosis is often a striking feature, and frequently several cells showing different phases of this phenomenon may be observed in a single field. The cells vary considerably in size, as do those of most rapidly growing malignant tumors.

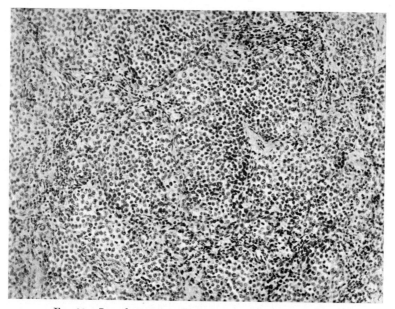

Fig. 90.—Lymphocytoma. Lymph node of a bovine (× 130).

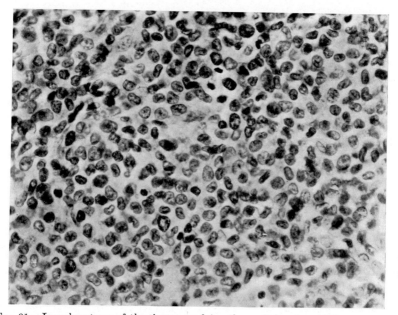

Fig. 91.—Lymphocytoma of the tissues overlying the medial surface of the metatarsus of a six-month-old fox terrier (× 660).

This is particularly characteristic of cells which are immature and undifferentiated (Fig. 90).

The cells which are infiltrative in the involved tissue are laid down in compact formation, occasionally with a tendency toward an alveolar type of structure. The cells rest in a fine reticulum, and a few delicate strands of fibrous stroma may be demonstrable, but this material is usually scanty in the more malignant forms (Fig. 91). Definite blood channels seldom are present; the blood appears to be in direct contact with the cells of the tumor. In the larger specimens small regions of necrosis occasionally may be present.

When lymph nodes are involved, the cells of the tumor soon replace the lymph tissue, and sections often reveal only the slightest traces of

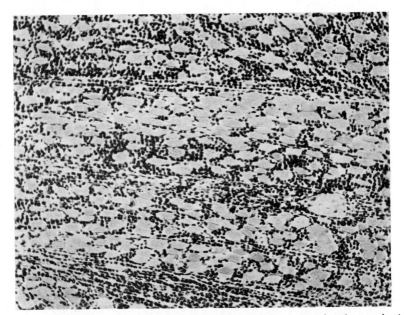

Fig. 92.—Lymphocytoma of a bovine. Infiltration and destruction by the neoplastic cells of striated muscle (× 180).

the original structure. Involvement of the musculature causes destruction of the muscle fibers, their replacement by compact masses of tumor cells, and hydropic degeneration often is seen in the muscle fibers adjacent to a region of invasion (Fig. 92). If pulmonary tissue is affected, frequently there is extensive perivascular and peribronchial infiltration of tumor cells throughout the parenchyma. The livers of cattle and sheep may possess foci of tumorous tissue distributed promiscuously throughout the organ, whereas in the livers of swine there usually is a perilobular infiltration by the neoplastic elements (Figs. 93 and 94). In the kidney, the tumor cells invade the interstitial spaces and eventu-

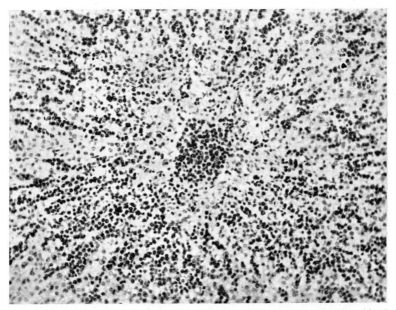

Fig. 93.—Lymphocytoma of the liver of a bovine. The leukemic state of the blood is apparent since the sinusoids of the liver are filled with neoplastic cells (× 160).

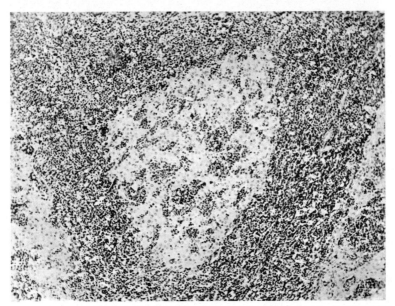

Fig. 94.—Lymphocytoma of the liver of a swine. The blood spaces show leukemia. Marked perilobular infiltration (× 110).

ally replace the tubules. The glomeruli seem somewhat more resistant, and these structures are the last to disappear. In the spleen the tumorous process appears as diffuse masses of closely packed cells which replace the normal parenchyma, or as subserous deposits of the splenic capsule. In one case in my series in which a calf, six months old, was affected with leukemic lymphocytoma, large multinuclear giant cells of uncertain significance were present in the involved spleen. In the gastro-intestinal tract and the uterus the majority of tumor cells are confined to the submucosa, which may be enormously expanded if the involvement is excessive (Fig. 95).

In cases in which there is invasion of the blood stream by the cells of the tumor, sections of the liver generally reveal variable numbers of

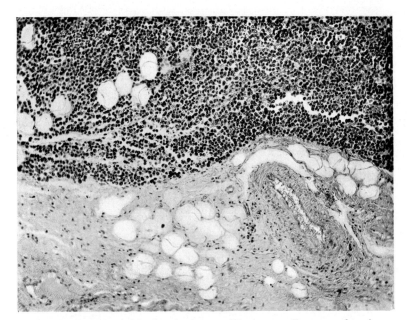

Fig. 95.—Lymphocytoma of bovine abomasum. The tumor cells occupy the submucosa with no tendency to violate the smooth musculature (× 200).

tumorous cells in the capillaries of the hepatic sinusoids. Cross sections of larger vessels, if they contain blood, usually reveal an excessively large number of lymphoid cells, which makes it possible to determine a leukemic state in many cases, even though smears of blood were not obtained in life (Figs. 93 and 96).

In livers of bovines affected with lymphocytoma, I have occasionally observed extensive thrombosis of the greatly dilated central veins, which was due, perhaps, to the passive congestion brought about by neoplastic involvement of the cardiovascular system.

In examining the blood of an animal affected with lymphocytoma it is important to keep in mind that alterations in the blood are secondary to a disease which has its inception in the blood-forming tissues and not in the blood itself. As I have mentioned, a leukemic state may or may not be apparent, depending on the ability of the tumor cells to invade the blood vascular channels and to multiply and thrive within the blood stream (Fig. 96). Leukemic blood usually discloses diminution of the concentration of hemoglobin, slowing of the coagulation time, and nucleated erythrocytes. The lymphoid cell, in various stages of its de-

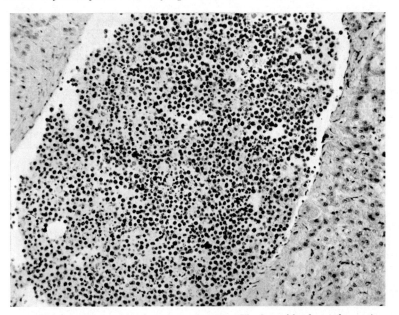

Fig. 96.—Lymphocytoma of liver of a bovine. The large blood vessel contains excessive numbers of immature lymphoid cells constituting circulating metastasis or leukemia (× 150).

velopment, dominates the blood picture so that the ratios between leukocytes and erythrocytes, instead of being approximately 1 to 400 or 1 to 600, as in normal blood, may be as low as 1 to 25 or 1 to 50. In cattle the total leukocyte count may vary between 100,000 and more than 200,000 for each cubic millimeter of blood, whereas in dogs the leukocyte count may reach 320,000 for each cubic millimeter.[15]

INFLUENCE OF AGE, SEX, AND BREED

The ages of forty cattle with lymphocytoma varied from six months to twelve years; six years was the average age for the entire group. So far as can be concluded from this relatively small series, the disease seems to show a predilection for adult cattle. Udall and Olafson recently described a case of aleukemic lymphocytoma in a Guernsey calf aged six weeks. Concerning the influence of age on the incidence of the disease, the statistics of meat inspection previously referred to are of particular interest. Although the disease was observed once in approximately 8,500 cattle aged more than one year, it was found in calves aged less than one year once in approximately 149,000.

Although the condition is observed most frequently among females, it is not proved that sex is of significance because more females than males are permitted to attain mature or adult life.

In thirty-seven of the forty bovine cases mentioned in which the breed was known, the disease affected twenty-three shorthorns, seven Holsteins, two Jerseys, and two Guernseys; animals of the Angus, Durham, and Hereford breed were each affected once. The respective breeds are perhaps represented in about the same proportion as they are presented for slaughter.

CLINICAL CONSIDERATIONS

Since the malignant form of lymphoblastoma among dairy cattle and dogs is not infrequent its recognition by practitioners is important. The insidious onset renders it difficult to describe what might be considered typical symptoms of lymphoblastoma as it occurs in animals, particularly in the early stages of the disease. In many of the cases reported, a tendency to tire easily has been noted, associated with increased appetite, although in cases in which the digestive apparatus is involved there is usually noticeable anorexia, bloating, and often diarrhea. There is frequently progressive loss of flesh, and if the animal lives long enough, a state of emaciation may result. The animal is usually disinclined to move, and appears listless and disinterested in its surroundings. The appearance of the disease in cattle which are lactating very often occasions sudden cessation of the flow of milk. As the disease progresses, and the animal becomes weaker, it prefers a recumbent position. If the heart is involved, as it so often is in cattle, cardiac irregularities may be detected; frequently the animal has difficulty in swallowing, and symptoms of respiratory distress are not uncommon.

The palpable lymph nodes may be enormously enlarged and firm, but they are not painful. Involvement of lymph nodes is frequently bilateral and those of the head and cervical region are usually the first to become noticeable, especially in dogs and cattle. However, I have observed cases in which lesions were extensive in the thoracic and abdominal viscera, but without any apparent increase in the palpable lymph nodes of the body. Such cases are exceptional.

The course of the disease is variable. An occasional case may terminate fatally within a week or so after recognition of symptoms. In the majority of cases the disease is of longer duration, and in some cases it may continue for many weeks, or even for a few months, before death ensues.

Of chief importance in the diagnosis of lymphoblastoma is the sudden appearance of tumorous enlargements which cannot be accounted for by infection or trauma. Obscure nodular swellings in the skin of the neck or thoracic region of dogs should be considered possible lymphoblastomas, and if they persist, biopsy should be obtained. Particular effort should be made to determine whether or not the more important lymph nodes are enlarged; bilateral enlargement is especially significant of the presence of lymphoblastoma. A history of increasing fatigue, preference for a recumbent position, and evidence of digestive disturbances should be looked on as suggestive of the disease. Enlargement of the spleen is of doubtful significance. If examination of the blood reveals a leukemic state in which the leukocytes are predominately lymphoid, a diagnosis of leukemic lymphocytoma is suggested, and confirmatory lesions usually can be demonstrated. It should be kept in mind, however, that demonstrable changes in the blood are absent in a large percentage of cases and may be transitory in others, and as a consequence the significance of the blood picture is diminished. However, for separation of this condition from myelogenous leukemia and so-called chloroma, study of the blood is most important. These conditions are not so common in the lower animals as are the lymphoid disturbances.

In distinguishing between lymphoblastoma and the condition known as chloroma, the green color of the tumorous tissue in the latter is characteristic, and should suggest the nature of the condition. There are several other conditions which may be confused with lymphoblastoma during general examination.

In dogs, there is cutaneous granuloma,[3] transmissible (so-called infectious) lymphosarcoma, which occupies a special place in the classification of tumors, other metastatic tumors which may invade the lymph nodes, and possibly tuberculosis.

In cattle tuberculosis should be excluded in the differential diagnosis of lymphoblastoma, and the possibility of coexistence of the two diseases must be considered. The tuberculin test would be helpful as would biopsy if it could be obtained. In some regards, cases of lymphoblastoma of cattle may suggest traumatic pericarditis. This is most likely to happen in those more or less acute cases in which evident enlargement of lymph nodes does not occur. However, in traumatic pericarditis there is usually more or less fever and significant polymorphonuclear leukocytosis, which are foreign to neoplastic disease. The friction sounds in the cardiac region, together with the splashing of the pericardial fluid, so often characteristic of traumatic pericarditis, are likewise absent.

In sheep, enlargement of lymph nodes due to nonspecific pyogenic bacteria, as well as the enlargement of caseous lymphadenitis, may be confused with lymphoblastoma. However, the disease is so seldom seen in this species as to make the necessity of a diagnosis during life improbable. Swine likewise are infrequently affected.

The lymphocytomas, because of their malignant nature, cannot be considered as being amenable to surgical interference in animals. Even when the operation is done early and most thoroughly, recurrence, with metastasis, may be expected. The widespread distribution in most cases of lymphocytoma precludes the possibility of successful surgical intervention. In human beings affected with the disease, Fowler's solution, sodium cacodylate, and, more recently, arsphenamine, have been used as treatment for the resultant anemia. For the destruction of the abdominal lymphoid cells, roentgen rays, benzol, and radium have been used. Although temporarily promising results are frequently observed following therapeutic application of these agents, the disease is practically always fatal. Although little can be offered of permanent benefit, in the treatment of lymphocytomas, the surgical removal of lymphomas situated in accessible situations should be attempted.

EXPERIMENTAL WORK

Up to this time very little experimental work has been reported which has dealt with malignant lymphoblastomas in the larger mammals. In 1929 Creech and Bunyea published an account of their attempts to transmit the disease from a spontaneously affected cow to an animal of the same species and to animals of different species. Bacteriologic studies were also made. The affected animal was kept under observation for a considerable time before its physical condition necessitated slaughter, and a series of blood counts, as follows, was made:

April 6, 1926, leukocytes numbered 102,400 and erythrocytes numbered 5,246,800; the ratio of leukocytes to erythrocytes was 1 to 51.

April 9, 1926, leukocytes numbered 117,000 and erythrocytes numbered 6,640,000; the ratio of leukocytes to erythrocytes was 1 to 56. April 14, 1926, leukocytes numbered 101,875 and erythrocytes 5,840,000; the ratio of leukocytes to erythrocytes was 1 to 57. April 19, 1926, leukocytes numbered 203,250 and erythrocytes 5,520,000; the ratio of leukocytes to erythrocytes was 1 to 27.

Using the Fleischl hemoglobinometer two determinations were made of the hemoglobin content of the blood during the same period that the counts of blood cells were made and it was found to be 35. The hemoglobinometer reading of a normal cow's blood with the same apparatus and technic was 60.

Guinea pigs, rabbits, a sheep, a weanling calf, and another cow were inoculated with portions of the jugular blood but the disease failed to develop. Likewise attempts to induce the disease in several species of animals by injection of emulsified hyperplastic lymph nodes were unsuccessful. Bacteriologic studies also failed of positive results.

HODGKIN'S DISEASE

In 1832 Hodgkin described a malignant disease of man which now bears his name, and which is characterized by a rather protracted, progressive, and painless enlargement of groups of lymph nodes. The condition occasionally has been reported as occurring in lower animals, although perhaps not so frequently as formerly. McFadyean, in 1903, described four cases in the dog and one in a hog, and Hodgson reported one case in a hog. From the published descriptions of these cases and of others, it is evident that they all had much in common with, or were identical with, the usual picture of lymphocytoma. In fairness, however, it should be mentioned that McFadyean was somewhat uncertain that his cases could properly be designated Hodgkin's disease, but he also wrote: "If the condition of which these cases are illustrative cannot be enrolled under the head of Hodgkin's disease, it is equally certain that they are not covered by any other recognized term and that a new name is required for them."

Although Hodgkin's disease no doubt exists as a separate disease of man, and is considered by many observers as granulomatous, with perhaps some obscure relationship to tuberculosis, and by others as true tumor, I seriously doubt its existence in lower animals. I have never encountered a case in a study of approximately 600 neoplasms from animals. Moreover, the descriptions of the cases recorded in the literature fail to impress one that the diagnosis was in keeping with the usual conception of what constitutes the histologic picture of Hodgkin's disease. My experience has been similar to that of Fox, pathologist to the Zoological Society of Philadelphia; he failed to see any case resembling that of Hodgkin's disease of man in the thousands of captive wild animals under his observation.

BIBLIOGRAPHY

1. Creech, G. T. and Bunyea, Hubert: Experimental studies of bovine leukemia. Jour. Agr. Res., 38: 395–404 (April 1), 1929.

2. Crocker, W. J.: Three thousand autopsies. Cornell Vet., 9: 142–161 (Jan.), 1919.

3. Feldman, W. H.: Kennel granuloma. Jour. Am. Vet. Med. Assn., 73: 617–622 (Sept.), 1928.

4. Fox, Herbert: Disease in captive wild mammals and birds, incidence, description, comparison. Philadelphia, J. B. Lippincott Co., 1923, p. 118.

5. Hodgson, J. F.: Hodgkin's disease in a pig. Jour. Comp. Path. and Therap., 16: 382, 1903.

6. Houdemer and Bablet, J.: Deux cas de tumeurs ganglionnaires malignes observées au Tonkin chez des animaux domestiques. Bull. Soc. Path. Exot., 20: 345–349, 1927. Abstr. in: Cancer Rev., 2: 402 (Nov.), 1927.

7. Knuth, P. and Volkmann: Untersuchungen über die Lymphozytomatose des Rindes. Ztschr. f. Infekt., 17: 395–467, 1915.

8. Leisering, A.: Quoted by Ordway, Thomas, and Gorham, L. W.: Leukemia. In: Oxford Medicine, New York, Oxford University Press, 1920, 2, pp. 681–762.

9. Lellmann: Quoted by Simonds, J. P.: Leukemia, pseudoleukemia and related conditions in the Slye stock of mice. Jour. Cancer Res., 9: 329–373 (Sept.), 1925.

10. McFadyean, J.: Five cases of Hodgkin's disease in the lower animals. Jour. Comp. Path. and Therap., 16: 379–382, 1903.

11. Siedamgrotzky: Quoted by Simonds, J. P.: Leukemia, pseudoleukemia and related conditions in the Slye stock of mice. Jour. Cancer Res., 9: 329–373 (Sept.), 1925.

12. Udall, D. H. and Olafson, Peter: Pseudoleukemia in a calf. Cornell Vet., 20: 81–84 (Jan.), 1930.

13. Warthin, A. S.: The neoplasm theory of leukemia, with report of a case supporting this view. Preliminary report. Tr. Assn. Am. Phys., 19: 421–432, 1904.

14. Warthin, A. S.: Diseases of the lymphatic glands. In: Osler, William: Modern medicine. Ed. 3, Philadelphia, Lea & Febiger, 1927, 5, pp. 199–225.

15. Weil and Clerc: Quoted by Hutyra, Franz and Marek, Josef: Special pathology and therapeutics of the diseases of domestic animals. Ed. 3, Chicago, A. Eger, 1926, 3: p. 126.

CHAPTER XIV

LYMPHOBLASTOMA (*Continued*): LYMPHOCYTOMA OF CHICKENS

Lymphocytoma of chickens belongs to a group of allied conditions, known as fowl leukosis, and bears close morphologic relationship to the various neoplastic conditions of mammals grouped as lymphoblastoma. The disease is frequently referred to rather loosely as fowl leukemia, but since there is usually no demonstrable change in the total leukocyte count, this term is somewhat misleading and fails to designate the disease properly.

The observations of Ellermann,[3, 4, 5] Ellermann and Bang,[6, 7] and more recently of Furth,[9, 10] have definitely shown the existence of three, or perhaps of four, pathologic entities under the collective term "leukosis." "Myeloid leukemia," "erythroleukosis," "myeloma," and "lymphoid leukosis" are terms used to designate these conditions of chickens. From the valuable data supplied by Furth, who observed these conditions experimentally, it is possible to summarize briefly the essential characteristics of the respective conditions included under the heading of leukosis.

Myeloid leukemia begins as a tumor-like hyperplasia of the myelocytic and myeloblastic elements of the bone marrow, with subsequent invasion of the blood stream by the immature myeloblastic cells, and the formation of heterotopic myeloid foci, usually in the liver. There is marked leukemia, and the number of leukocytes may exceed that of the erythrocytes. The disease is transmissible experimentally. The conditions referred to by Furth as "myeloma" (leukochloroma of Mathews) and "myeloid leukosis" seem to be sufficiently related in genesis to warrant the assumption that they are probably morphologic variations of the same disease (see Chapter XV).

Erythroleukosis is a disease peculiar to chickens, characterized by severe anemia and the appearance in the blood of hemoglobin-free precursors of erythrocytes, occasionally in such numbers as to constitute leukemia. The bone marrow, liver, and spleen contain an intravascular accumulation of primitive lymphoid cells which are considered to be progenitors of erythrocytes. It is transmissible to other chickens.

Lymphoid leukosis is characterized by the presence of diffuse or nodular, neoplastic, extravascular depositions in the various organs, particularly the liver, or large lymphocytes. The occurrence of leukemia is doubtful, and transmissibility has not been proved. I prefer the term "lymphocytoma" and this term will be used when I refer to the entity designated by some other observers as "lymphoid leukosis."

Although lymphocytoma of chickens was first reported by Butterfield in 1905, it remained for Warthin to give the first complete description of the pathologic changes characteristic of it. Kon, in 1907, also gave a complete gross and microscopic picture of what was probably a case of this disease; the blood changes were studied from stained sections of tissue and not from blood smears. Since Warthin's paper, in 1907, the condition has been studied by several investigators, none of whom has been able to identify an etiologic agent. Although some observers refuse to consider the condition as a true neoplastic process, I believe its characteristics justify such classification. The progressive malignant nature, characterized by accumulation of rapidly proliferating lymphoid cells in separate tissues and organs, the tendency of the cells to infiltrate and destroy the surrounding tissues, and perhaps in some instances to invade the blood stream, makes the process analogous in its pathologic aspects to other malignant tumors.

DEFINITION

Lymphocytoma of chickens may be defined as a fatal neoplastic disease of domestic fowls, the type cell of which is the undifferentiated lymphocyte. The most striking anatomic change is the presence, in the various organs, of diffuse masses or nodules, of pinkish-gray to grayish-white, fleshy tissue composed of cells which have an extravascular relationship to the blood spaces.

INCIDENCE

Reliable data concerning the occurrence of lymphocytoma among chickens are difficult to assemble.* The opinion is shared by most pathologists, however, that without question this is the most commonly encountered tumor of the domestic fowl. The disease is endemic in many localities, and there is some evidence that in certain flocks it may

---

* The possibility of confusing lymphocytoma with erythroleukosis, and failure to recognize the latter, may have resulted in the grouping by many observers of these two conditions under the one heading of fowl leukemia. Many of the reports in the literature are therefore of limited value in disclosing the frequency of occurrence of lymphocytoma.

assume an epizoötic form, with a morbidity of 10 to 30 per cent. That the disease is not rare is suggested by comparison of the number of tumors of this kind with the other varieties of tumors of chickens encountered.

In a report by Tyzzer and Ordway, in which nine tumors of chickens were described, seven were malignant lymphocytomas. In my series of fifty-five tumors of the common fowl, twenty (36.3 per cent) were of this variety. Further evidence as to the relative frequency of the disease is the paper by Pickens based on the study of twenty-two cases, and Pickens' statement that he had observed about thirty cases in his laboratory at Cornell University. Thirteen of the twenty-two cases constituting the basis of Pickens' study were observed during a period of five years among fowls from the same farm where a flock of between 1,500 and 2,500 birds was maintained. From another farm, where the flock consisted of 125 birds, within a period of two months, four deaths occurred as a result of the disease. Of much interest was the fact that the stock on the second farm originally came from the first farm.

Lentz reported the finding of eleven cases of the disease at postmortem examination of 356 chickens, 170 of which were dressed for market. The reports of the Department of Poultry Husbandry of the New Jersey State Agricultural Experiment Station show that fifty-seven cases of neoplastic disease were found in 1,219 postmortem examinations of chickens, and seventeen were classified as lymphocytomas (leukemia). Mathews and Walkey, at Purdue University, observed 168 cases in five years which they considered of a lymphoid nature, and recorded an instance in which 30 per cent of a flock of 240 chickens died in three months. A summary of the relatively few facts available concerning the incidence of this neoplastic process suggests that it is much more common than any of the other tumors of chickens.

Although Mathews and Walkey were of the opinion that the disease occurs with greater frequency in Barred Rocks than in all other breeds combined, the data seem too meager to state definitely what influence breed has on occurrence. Two of Tyzzer's cases occurred in Rhode Island Red hens from the same flock, and another was observed in a white Leghorn. Warthin's case was in a buff cochin bantam hen and my cases were distributed among the different breeds as follows: White Leghorn, six cases; Barred Rock, five cases; Rhode Island Red, five cases; bantam, one case, and breed not known, three cases. Breed may be a negligible factor in the susceptibility of chickens to this disease, although there is some evidence to support the contention that hereditary influences are not without significance in the pathogenesis of the condition.

SYMPTOMS

Since the anatomic alterations of this disease are usually confined to the tissues of the interior of the body, the disease is ordinarily not detected until serious functional derangement ensues. The symptoms are seldom pathognomonic at first. The insidious nature of the condition makes it difficult to determine how long a subject is affected before recognizable symptoms become apparent. Since the process is neoplastic, there is no demonstrable incubation period, such as many of the diseases due to infective agents pass through, and the condition becomes apparent symptomatically only in its later stages. Occasionally, however, nodular lesions affect the head or neck, the presence of which assists materially in earlier diagnosis. Ordinarily, the comb and wattles, and the mucous membranes of the affected chickens are pale or even light yellow, and the birds appear listless and disinclined to move. The chicken becomes progressively weaker, appears exhausted following the slightest unusual physical exertion, and prefers a recumbent posture. Production of eggs ceases.

Although the chicken loses flesh rapidly as the disease continues, the total loss in body weight is not always in keeping with the emaciation noted in the musculature. This is due to the excessive amount of neoplastic tissue which is often present in the liver, spleen, and kidneys, or as nodular accumulations along the intestines. Enormous masses of tumorous tissue are not infrequently observed in chickens which die of this disease, and the total weight of the tumors may be considerable. Pickens mentioned one instance in which the liver of an affected chicken weighed 237 gm., 24 per cent of the total body weight. In one of my cases the weight of the diseased fowl increased from 1,250 gm. one hundred thirty-four days before death to 1,630 gm. at the time of necropsy. The increase in weight in this instance was due to the great amount of tumorous tissue; the musculature had wasted. Often the affected chicken experiences periods of improvement. The appetite is good in the early stages of the disease; later it becomes precarious, and it fails entirely in the terminal phases of the condition. Most observers mention the presence of diarrhea, but it is doubtful if this is of any significance, since diarrhea occurs with many other more or less protracted diseases of fowls.

The information obtained from the symptoms alone usually is not sufficient to justify a definite diagnosis and in instances in which there is definite leukemia, examination of the blood is of the greatest assistance in the differential diagnosis, since lymphocytoma is seldom associated with a leukemic state of the blood. However, in practically all affected fowls there is a reduction of hemoglobin and the capacity of the blood to clot diminishes; as a consequence hemorrhage is difficult to control.

THE BLOOD

In considering the blood picture associated with lymphocytoma it should be borne in mind that in the majority of cases leukemia does not occur, and, consequently, if this phase of the examination of the blood is negative it does not eliminate the disease from diagnostic considerations. Many writers have, heretofore, divided the condition into two separate diseases on the basis of the condition of the blood; they have considered cases in which there was definite increase in proportion of lymphocytes as leukemia, and those without leukemia as pseudoleukemia. In view of the failure of many observers to recognize the existence of erythroleukemia and to distinguish the condition properly from the lymphoid condition considered here as lymphocytoma, little credence can be given those reported cases in which a leukemic state of the blood was described. Many of these were undoubtedly cases of erythroleukemia.

The disease probably originates as a result of some stimulus which incites the cells of the various lymphoid deposits to overactivity. As a consequence of their tremendous inherent reproductive ability, enhanced by the usual loss of restraint characteristic of neoplasms, the cells pile up in huge masses. Since the cells usually are infiltrative it would seem possible that occasionally some of them should find their way into the blood stream. If this happens, a blood count probably will reveal transitory leukemia, or at least the differential study may give evidence of an unusually large number of immature lymphoid cells.

Whether or not there is circulatory lymphocytosis, the blood of a chicken suffering from lymphocytoma practically always reveals some pathologic changes. There is a reduction of hemoglobin from normal of between 50 and 60 per cent (Dare) to 15 per cent or less. The blood coagulates slowly, and hemorrhage resulting from a small prick wound, made to secure blood for examination, may be extremely difficult to stop. The normal viscosity, so characteristic of normal chicken blood, is much reduced, and the blood appears thin and watery. The erythrocytes decrease from a normal count of approximately 3,000,000 in each cubic millimeter (Forkner) to well under 1,000,000.

GROSS CHARACTERISTICS

Although the most striking anatomic alterations are usually confined to the viscera of the abdominal cavity, cases often are observed in which

15

lesions are situated on the exterior of the body (Fig. 97). External lesions usually involve the tissues of the head and neck, although I observed one case in which large subcutaneous tumors were situated over the posterior aspect of the tibia, over the femoral-tibial articulation, in the inferior cervical or prescapular region, and over the sternum near the xyphoid process. Microscopically, the liver also revealed numerous irregular foci of neoplastic cells. In the region of the head and neck the masses may appear unilateral or bilateral, and their size and position may impart to the affected individual a strikingly grotesque appearance (Fig. 98). The tumors frequently appear as irregular nodular masses freely movable in the subcutis. They are covered with skin which becomes taut as the tumor expands, and the skin which covers

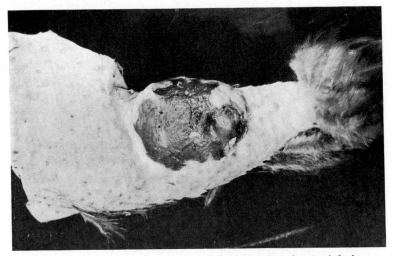

FIG. 97.—Lymphocytoma of a chicken. Nodule in the subcutis of the leg.

the new growth is usually devoid of feathers, and is yellow. The destructive, infiltrative character of the process, as it affects the tissues of the head, makes it impossible to separate the neoplasm from the tissues in immediate contact with it, and renders such an attempt useless as a therapeutic measure. It is relatively simple, however, to obtain a small bit of the tumor for biopsy. Unlike many other tumors on the surface of the body, lymphocytomas seldom, if ever, ulcerate. Apparently their subcutaneous situation affords sufficient protection against most external trauma.

Although the gross anatomic changes may be confined to lesions affecting the tissues of the exterior of the body, these lesions are frequently part of a more or less generalized process involving the organs and tissues of the interior of the body, few of which are exempt from the possibility of involvement. The process exhibits a predilection for the

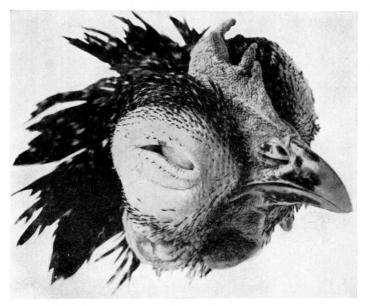

Fig. 98.—Lymphocytoma of a chicken. Bilateral involvement of the head.

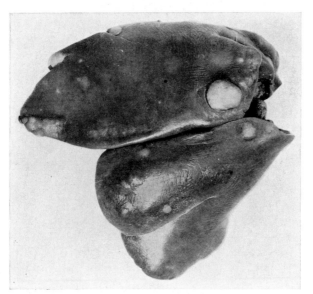

Fig. 99.—Lymphocytoma of a chicken. Multiple lesions in the liver.

liver. In one series of twenty cases, I observed the organ to be affected in twelve (Figs. 99 and 100). The spleen and kidney are also commonly involved simultaneously with the liver, and, occasionally nodular masses are found in the gizzard, proventriculus, intestines, mesentery, omentum,

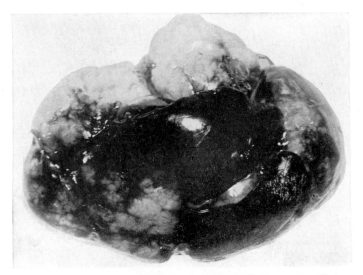

Fig. 100.—Lymphocytoma of the liver of a chicken.   Diffuse types of lesions.

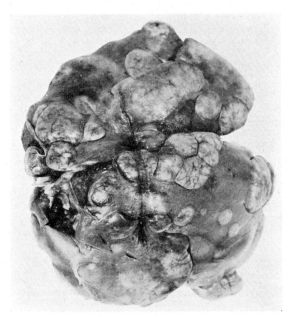

Fig. 101.—Lymphocytoma of a chicken.   Multiple nodular lesions.

ovary, pancreas, heart, and lungs (Figs. 101 to 104).   In some instances, small isolated masses may be found under the parietal peritoneum, and

Warthin mentioned the involvement of the bone marrow and the hemolymph nodes.

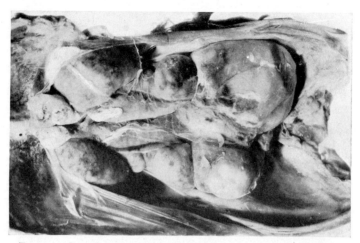

Fig. 102.—Lymphocytoma of a chicken.   Bilateral renal involvement.

The neoplastic tissue, which is grayish-pink or white, with an occasional yellow tinge, is very friable and well embedded in the substance of the affected organ or tissue (Fig. 101).   In birds which have died

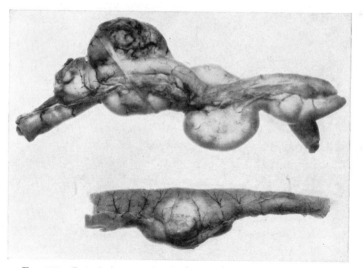

Fig. 103.—Lymphocytoma of a chicken.   Masses along the intestine.

from other causes, one not infrequently finds extensive microscopic involvement of the liver.   The infiltration and destruction may be so pronounced in organs such as the liver, spleen, and kidney, as to make it difficult or even impossible to demonstrate normal tissue, and, as a consequence, the tumors often attain considerable size (Fig. 102). In one of my cases the involved liver weighed 385 gm. and in three cases observed by Butterfield, they weighed 340 gm., 420 gm., and 270 gm., respectively. In some instances the liver may be so enlarged as to be distinctly palpable in life. The process in the respective organs may appear as small diffuse nodular masses, or the separate foci of neoplastic cells may coalesce and present a single, irregular mass of new tissue, the contour of which is often indistinct. If the birds die suddenly, a large amount of blood may often be found free in the abdomen, and it is usually possible to demonstrate rupture of the liver as the source of

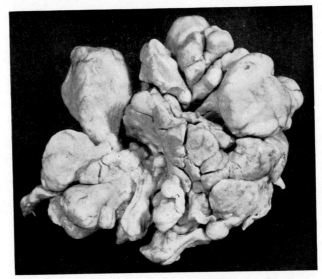

Fig. 104.—Lymphocytoma of the ovary of a chicken.

the fatal hemorrhage. The increased friability of an organ possessing a tumor of this kind renders the involved tissues susceptible to fracture from causes that would be of no consequence if the tissues were normal.

MICROSCOPIC CHARACTERISTICS

The tumor consists of compact masses of proliferating lymphoid cells supported by irregular strands of fibrous stroma, and a delicate reticulum. The amount of fibrous tissue varies and is dependent on the structure involved by the tumor and the rate of growth of the latter (Fig. 105).

The type cell is usually comparable in size to the large lymphocyte of normal fowl's blood, although an occasional case is seen in which it is somewhat smaller.   In fresh, unfixed tissue the cells are spherical, although in fixed tissue many present a polyhedral appearance.   Because of pressure, many of the cells in compact masses may be slightly elongated or ovoid.   The largest portion of the cellular bulk consists of the nucleus, which occupies a slightly eccentric position.   The cytoplasm is nongranular and presents a rim-like appearance.   The nucleus has strong basophilic tendencies, and a highly granular, chromatin substance.   The number and size of the chromatin granules varies in different cells in the same field and seems to have some relation to the degree of differentiation achieved by the respective cells.   A nucleolus

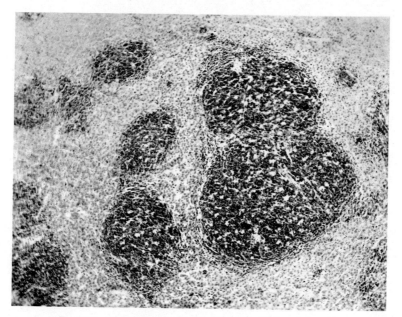

FIG. 105.—Lymphocytoma of the liver of a chicken (× 110).

occasionally can be seen, although it is seldom prominent.   In most tissue mitosis is easily demonstrated.

Definite blood channels are absent, although it is not uncommon to find free erythrocytes in direct contact with the tumor cells.   The intimate relationship of the tumor cells to blood channels in such organs as the liver, spleen, and kidney provides ample opportunity for the neoplastic cells to find their way into the general circulation (Fig. 106). The fact that leukemic blood is seldom seen is presumptive evidence that the blood is perhaps antagonistic to the tumor cells, and they perish soon after entering the circulation.

The involved tissues are gradually destroyed and replaced by the

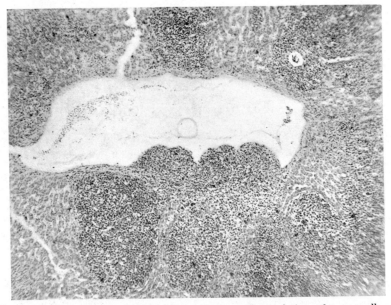

Fig. 106.—Lymphocytoma of the liver of a chicken. Accumulations of tumor cells advancing into the lumen of a vein (× 90).

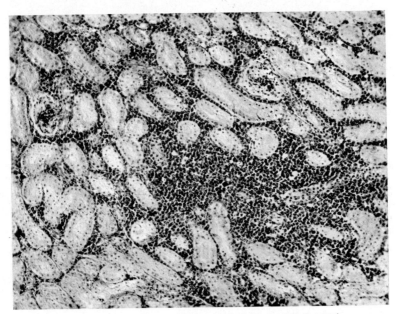

Fig. 107.—Lymphocytoma of the kidney of a chicken (× 150).

tumor cells. But few structures appear to be exempt from the destructive encroachment of the proliferating neoplastic elements, although the more specialized parenchymatous organs, such as the liver and kidney, offer a more favorable situation for their unrestricted growth than muscle tissue, which is seldom extensively involved. Nerve tissue is likewise very resistant, and I have never seen a nerve invaded by the cells of a lymphocytoma. The remaining parenchyma of involved organs is atrophic and pushed out of normal position by the advancing neoplasm (Fig. 107).

Tumor cells possess remarkable vitality, and it is unusual to find any considerable number undergoing necrosis or other retrogressive changes.

DIAGNOSTIC CONSIDERATIONS

The diagnosis of lymphocytoma, like that of many neoplasms, is made with greatest certainty after death. However, typical cases may be detected while the bird is living, if a careful study is made. The most significant clinical features of the disease are progressive weakness, disinclination to move, paleness of the comb and wattles, loss of flesh, and inappetence. Occasionally, if the disease is well advanced, the enlarged liver and other neoplastic masses can be palpated through the abdominal wall. The occurrence of multiple, fleshy tumors over the head and along the neck are significant. External tumors offer opportunities for biopsy, and microscopic examination of the tumor is possible as a consequence. The blood should always be examined, for even if a leukemic state is absent, there is usually a lowered concentration of hemoglobin and diminished coagulability. If a leukemic state is found it will be necessary to distinguish between erythroleukosis and myeloid leukosis. A differential count may show a predominance of lymphocytes, many of which are immature. A bird dying suddenly from internal hemorrhage should be examined with lymphocytoma in mind, since fatal hemorrhage from rupture of the diseased liver is a common termination of this malady. At necropsy the internal tumors are usually strikingly evident as pinkish or yellowish-white fleshy masses, involving the liver, spleen, kidneys, intestines, or ovary. Occasionally, however, a bird dies and the lesions can be demonstrated only by the aid of the microscope.

Other diseases with which lymphocytoma may be confused are fowl typhoid and tuberculosis. In attempting to distinguish lymphocytoma from these two diseases one should bear in mind the possibility of each or both of them occurring in association with lymphocytoma. These conditions represent some of the most common diseases of poultry, and the simultaneous occurrence of two or more of them is occasionally demonstrated. In their differential diagnosis Table 5 may be of assistance:

TABLE 5

DIFFERENTIAL DIAGNOSIS OF LYMPHOCYTOMA, TYPHOID, AND TUBERCULOSIS OF FOWLS

	Lymphocytoma.	Typhoid.	Tuberculosis.
Age	Seldom in the very young, usually in young adults and old birds	Any age	Usually more than one year
Duration of disease	Seldom more than two months	Four to twelve days	Many months
Course of disease	Often periods of improvement with sudden death	Rapidly fatal	Prolonged, with progressive emaciation
Kidney	Often contains nodular masses	Pale, not enlarged, urates present	Seldom involved
Liver	Usually enlarged; soft, diffuse, or nodular masses	Grayish focal necrosis	Enlarged, discrete, yellowish, firm, hard lesions
Spleen	May be enlarged with grayish-white masses	Enlarged and congested	Enlarged, irregular, yellowish nodules
Erythrocytes	Marked decrease	Marked decrease	Slight decrease
Differential blood count	Possibly increase of lymphocytes	Principally polymorphonuclears	Of no significance
Temperature	Normal	Elevated 3 to 5°	Normal
Blood cultures	Negative	Positive for Bacillus sanguinarium	Negative
Bacterial smear from lesion	Negative	Uncertain	Acid-fast bacilli
Appetite	Slight	Absent	Ravenous
Tuberculin test	Negative	Negative	Positive
Histology of lesions	Extravascular accumulations of lymphoid cells	Necrosis, congestion	Tubercles
Transmissibility	Not proved	Occurs	Occurs

The distinction of lymphocytoma from the other forms of so-called leukosis of fowls is not ordinarily difficult, although the occasional occurrence of the entity known as erythroleukemia may confuse the inexperienced observer. Myeloid leukosis and myeloma are characterized by a myelocytic or myeloblastic type of cell that is dissimilar to the lymphoid character of the elements present in lymphocytoma.

In erythroleukemia* blood smears contain developmental forms of erythroblasts, frequently in sufficient numbers to constitute a condition of leukemia. Microscopic examination of the tissues, particularly the liver, reveals a marked intravascular accumulation of these immature cells; often they are so numerous within the capillary spaces of the organ as to reduce the intervening hepatic parenchyma to mere strands of atrophic hepatic cells. The type cell of the process exhibits a charac-

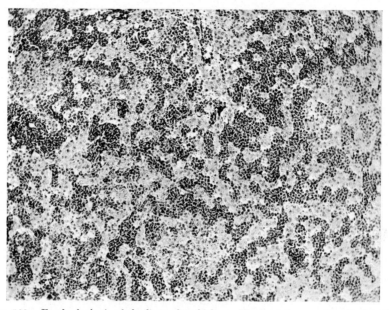

FIG. 108.—Erythroleukosis of the liver of a chicken. The immature erythroblastic cells are situated intravascularly ($\times$ 140).

teristic predilection for the vascular spaces and seldom produces extravascular accumulations, such as occur in lymphocytoma (Fig. 108).

CONTROL OF THE DISEASE

In the control of lymphocytoma the individual bird is of little significance, except to provide material for a correct diagnosis. Treatment is futile. Sanitary measures should be instituted in order to promote the general welfare of the flock, although there is as yet insufficient evidence

---

* Whether erythroleukosis should be considered a neoplastic disease is problematic. Although it possesses certain features suggestive of neoplasia, so little is known of its pathology as to make one hesitate in subscribing to the neoplastic concept concerning it. On the other hand, the condition described by Mathews as leukochloroma (myeloma) is perhaps properly designated a neoplasm (see Chapter XV, page 238).

to justify the belief that lymphocytoma is a contagious disease. If the loss is unusually high it may be necessary to dispose of the entire stock and obtain a different and unrelated strain in order to minimize possible hereditary factors that may be of etiologic significance in the occurrence of the disease. Certainly inbreeding should be avoided in a flock in which the condition occurs even infrequently. The hereditary predisposition to lymphocytoma is suggested, and care should be taken when introducing new breeding stock into a flock in which the disease seldom, if ever, occurs.

TRANSMISSIBILITY

The recent studies of Furth,[9] Stubbs and Furth, and of Jarmai permit of little doubt that myeloid leukosis and erythroleukosis can be transmitted to normal fowls. The disease can be induced by the injection of emulsions of infiltrated organs, whole blood cells, blood plasma, and by the bite of blood-sucking parasites. These authors also have ample proof that myeloid leukosis and erythroleukosis are capable of transmission by cell-free material and that their causative agents are filtrable.

In claiming transmissibility for fowl leukosis exception must, however, be made for the lymphoid variety or lymphocytoma. Up to this time there has been no properly controlled experiment conducted in which it could be conclusively shown that material from fowls affected with lymphocytoma induced the disease in inoculated chickens. The experiments of Andersen and Bang, of Mathews and Walkey, and of Furth, would indicate that this disease is not transmissible. I have also tried repeatedly to transmit the disease to normal fowls by inoculation of material from spontaneously affected chickens, and have likewise failed in every instance. Undoubtedly, many of those who have insisted that the lymphoid variety of leukosis is transmissible, have failed to take into account the possibility of the spontaneous occurrence of the disease in experimental animals, or have confused the condition with one of the other forms of leukosis, particularly erythroleukosis.

The relatively high incidence of spontaneous lymphocytoma in certain flocks makes the question of its experimental transmission one of uncertainty and doubt. Until it is possible to determine by appropriate studies something more of the incidence of the spontaneous appearance of the disease, claims as to transmissibility must be viewed with skepticism. The apparent differences in the incidence of the disease in various flocks would suggest the desirability of approaching the problem from the standpoint of heredity. Although this would necessitate a project of considerable proportions, it is nevertheless essential before a convincing experiment can be consummated concerning transmission of the disease from one chicken to another.

For the present, it must be concluded that experimental transmission of lymphocytoma of chickens has not been proved.

BIBLIOGRAPHY

1. Andersen, C. W. and Bang, O.: La leucémie ou leucose transmissible des poules. Festsk. B. Bang, Kopenhagen, 1928, pp. 355–389. Abstr. in: Centralbl. f. Bakt., Ref., **92**: 283, 1929.

2. Butterfield, E. E.: Aleukemic lymphadenoid tumors of the hen. Folia haematol., **2**: 649–657, 1905.

3. Ellermann, V.: Experimentelle Leukämie bei Hühnern. Verhandl. d. deutsch. path. Gesellsch., **12**: 224–225, 1908.

4. Ellermann, V.: Quoted by Furth.[9]

5. Ellermann, V.: Histogenese der übertragbaren Hünerleukose. IV. Zusammenfassende Betrachtungen. Folia haematol., **29**: 203–212 (Nov.), 1923.

6. Ellermann, V. and Bang, O.: Experimentelle Leukämie bei Hühnern. Centralbl. f. Bakt., Orig., **46**: 4–5, 1908.

7. Ellermann, V. and Bang, O.: Experimentelle Leukämie bei Hühnern. Centralbl. f. Bakt., Orig., **46**: 595–609, 1908.

8. Forkner, C. E.: Blood and bone marrow cells of the domestic fowl. Jour. Exper. Med., **50**: 121–141 (July 1), 1929.

9. Furth, J.: Observations with new transmissible strain of leucosis (leucemia) of fowls. Jour. Exper. Med., **53**: 243–267 (Feb.), 1931.

10. Furth, J.: Erythroleukosis and the anemias of the fowl. Arch. Path., **12**: 1–30 (July), 1931.

11. Jarmai, K.: Beiträge zur Kenntnis der Hühnerleukose. Arch. f. wissensch. u. prakt. Tierh., **62**: 113–131 (Oct. 4), 1930.

12. Kon, Jutaka: Über Leukämie beim Huhn. Virchow's Arch. f. path. Anat. u. Physiol., **190**: 338–349 (Nov. 18), 1907.

13. Lentz, J. W.: A study in the control of poultry disease. Poultry Sc., **2**: 33–38, 1922–1923.

14. Mathews, F. P.: Leukochloroma in the common fowl, its relation to myelogenic leukemia and its analogies to chloroma in man. Arch. Path., **7**: 442–457 (March), 1929.

15. Mathews, F. P. and Walkey, F. L.: Lymphadenomas of the common fowl. Jour. Cancer Res., **13**: 383–400 (Dec.), 1929.

16. Pickens, E. M.: Leukemia and pseudo-leukemia in the common fowl. Report of the New York State Veterinary College, pp. 226–251, 1915–1916.

17. Reports of the Department of Poultry Husbandry, New Jersey State Agricultural Experiment Station, New Brunswick, June 30, 1924, to June 30, 1926, p. 3.

18. Stubbs, E. L. and Furth, J.: Transmission experiments with leucosis of fowls. Jour. Exper. Med., **53**: 269–276 (Feb.), 1931.

19. Tyzzer, E. E. and Ordway, Thomas: Tumors in the common fowl. Jour. Med. Res., **21**: 459–477 (Oct.), 1909.

20. Warthin, A. S.: Leukemia of the common fowl. Jour. Infect. Dis., **4**: 338–369 (June 15), 1907.

CHAPTER XV

MYELOBLASTOMA

DEFINITION

Myeloblastoma is made up of cells derived from elements of the myeloid tissue. The cells possess varied potentialities and exhibit a tendency to differentiate in a manner similar to those derived from normal myeloblasts. The main interest, in this chapter, is directed to myelocytoma.

INCIDENCE AND OCCURRENCE

Neoplastic overgrowth of the myeloblastic series of cells seldom has been recognized in lower animals, although the disease is frequently seen in human beings and is variously designated myeloblastoma, myelogenous leukemia, and chloroma. Although opportunities to study the disease in live animals have been extremely meager, tumorous conditions in which the type cell unquestionably was of myeloblastic derivation occasionally have been found at necropsy, particularly of meat-producing mammals. Mathews described in chickens a myeloblastic tumorous process, which he considered resembled in many respects so-called chloroma of man; he found it frequently associated with leukemia of the myeloid type.

Comprehensive statistical data pertaining to the incidence of myeloblastoma of mammals and fowls have not been compiled. The disease apparently is more common among fowls than among mammals. However, the use of the collective term "leukosis," as applied to several diseases of fowls, and failure of many to recognize the characteristic pathologic changes of myelocytoma, make it difficult to obtain information concerning prevalence of the disease.

Myelocytoma occurred seven times among 535 tumors of mammals and fowls in my collection, distributed among the different species as follows:

Among 230 tumors of cattle, three were myelocytomas; among fifty-five tumors of fowls, three were myelocytomas; and among forty-three tumors of horses, one was a myelocytoma.

Mathews, who contributed the first comprehensive pathologic study of myelocytoma of fowls, observed thirty-six cases (0.9 per cent) of the disease among 3,938 chickens examined at necropsy in a period of five years. Pentimalli, who seems to have been the first to describe the pathologic changes of the disease as it occurs spontaneously in chickens, included two cases in a report of eighteen cases of tumor of the common fowl. One of Pentimalli's cases was that of a bird that had been inoculated experimentally with chondroma, and in the second case the liver only was received from another laboratory.

Claussen found in a well-nourished pig chloromatous growths that he diagnosed histologically as myeloid chloroma. The process consisted of nodular and diffuse proliferations of tumors involving the bone marrow, liver, kidneys, and lymph nodes. The case of Kucsera, which Henschen considered an example of multiple chloromyeloma, is of interest. The process, which affected the flat or spongy bones, and had a peculiar greenish color, consisted of myeloblasts and myelocytes. The tumors projected somewhat above the periosteum, were sharply circumscribed, and were not difficult to remove. The long bones were not affected, and metastasis was observed in the lymph nodes of the lumbosacral region, and in the zone adjacent to the periphery of the right kidney. In a well-nourished cow that had been slaughtered for food, Weaver observed lesions of a myeloid, neoplastic process, involving the ribs of the left side, lungs, and liver. There was also enlargement of the mediastinal, left precrural, and portal lymph nodes. The spleen was considered normal. The lesions were bright green, and soon faded when exposed to the air. Treatment of the tissues with hydrogen peroxide restored the green color. Microscopically, myeloid cells in different stages of differentiation predominated. Blood smears were not made.

The disease in dogs has been studied by Weil and Clerc and by Wirth, and each of these workers has contributed to the knowledge of hematology associated with this condition.

In my series of neoplasms, one myelocytoma was found in a twenty-year-old Percheron gelding, on which necropsy was performed following accidental death. From the meager data obtained it was ascertained that a large tumor occupied the anterior portion of the thoracic cavity and that there were a few flattened, elongated growths on the parietal serosa. Circumstances pertaining to the necropsy precluded the possibility of examining the remainder of the tissues for study.

Each of the three cattle affected was aged approximately ten years, and in every instance the condition was first observed at the time of necropsy, following slaughter of the respective animals for food. In each of the cases the lesions were green and rather widespread. In one case the growths were present in the uterus, lungs, spleen, kidneys, muscles, and in practically all lymph nodes. In another case the main tumor, which weighed approximately 15 kg., was situated in the muscles of the inferior cervical region, with a rounded nodule 7 cm. in diameter in the musculature of the abdominal wall. The lymph nodes of the anterior thoracic and cervical regions were also involved. In the third animal were flattened, green tumors just beneath the skin of the flank. Although the major growth was in the region of the right flank, the tissues of the left flank were also somewhat affected. The internal organs and regional lymph nodes were not involved. In none of these was there evidence in the bones of gross alterations. The blood was not studied and the microscopic examination was confined to portions of the tumor.

Two of the chickens affected with myelocytoma in my series were white Leghorns and one was of the Barred Rock breed. All were aged more than one year. Although the histologic picture of the neoplastic process in each of these was similar in essential details to that described by Mathews, the gross pathologic changes were somewhat at variance with the lesions he described. The lesions I observed were confined to the pelvic and lumbar regions. In no case were lesions observed in association with bones of the sternum or ribs which Mathews reported to be affected with remarkable regularity. The process was characterized by the presence of bilateral, diffusely attached, irregularly rounded or nodular, fleshy masses of soft tissue. In one case both kidneys were affected and in none of the birds were the livers or spleens involved even microscopically. The chickens had died without noticeable symptoms of disease; the blood was not examined.

GROSS CHARACTERISTICS

Tumors of mammals made up of cells derived from myeloblastic elements frequently are a bright pea-green color that has a tendency to fade on exposure to air, but which may be restored even in formalin-fixed material by treatment with peroxide of hydrogen. The green color possessed by many of these tumors is not sufficient, however, to justify a diagnosis of myelocytoma without the benefit of a microscopic examination of the tissues. In the bone marrow, particularly of the long bones, fat may be diminished and replaced by tumorous tissue of firm consistence. A thorough examination should be made of the marrow of all the bones of animals with tumors suspected of being derived from myeloid elements, to ascertain if possible the site of the primary lesion.

A greenish discoloration of the neoplastic tissue of fowls has not been reported. The new growth consists of white to grayish-white masses of tissue of a friable nature, attesting to the great cellularity of the structure. As mentioned, Mathews found that in the majority of the cases he examined, the neoplasms were associated with some portion of the skeletal system, the sternum and the ribs exhibiting a predilection for the process; this was not noted in the few cases I observed. Mathews also frequently found the spleen involved, and in about 65 per cent of the cases gross evidence of the disease was discernible in the liver. The ovary usually was affected, and other organs mentioned by Mathews as occasionally involved were the kidneys, small intestines, pancreas, heart, lungs, and lymph nodes.

MICROSCOPIC CHARACTERISTICS

The cellular constituents of a myelocytoma vary with the degree of differentiation attained by the type cell or myeloblast. Under normal circumstances there are derived from this cell, by a series of developmental transitions, the specific granular leukocytes known as polymorphonuclear neutrophilic leukocytes, eosinophilic leukocytes, and basophilic leukocytes. The evolution of these mature cells is dependent on the occurrence of several intermediate forms which are conveniently referred to collectively as myelocytes. These unripe cells vary greatly in structural design in their transition from the parent myeloblast to adult leukocytes, and much experience is necessary in order to recognize many of the developmental forms.* It is the myelocyte or its immediate precursor that usually predominates in the neoplastic process known as myelocytoma.

The myeloid descendants of the myeloblast have the capacity to produce an oxidizing ferment which can be demonstrated within the cytoplasm as deep blue granules by the oxidase reaction of Schultze. Cells of the lymphocytic series do not give this reaction.

The materials I obtained from mammals revealed a much greater variation in the structure of the type cell than that obtained from chickens. The tumor consists of diffuse, infiltrating collections of myeloid cells, enmeshed in a rather delicate reticulum. The type cell, which is

---

* In the recognition of the various cellular constituents of the blood of mammals, the description by Downey of human blood cells is helpful. For a description of the cells of chicken blood see the report of Forkner.

16

usually rather large and polygonal, or rounded, possesses a prominent nucleus which is eccentrically situated and is usually irregularly oval in contour (Fig. 109). Slightly elongated, indented or crescentic nuclei may occasionally be observed and a nucleolus is frequently apparent. The nucleus contains a considerable amount of rather coarse chromatin material and the structure often has a vesicular appearance. The cytoplasm is rarely basophilic; usually it is neutrophilic or markedly acidophilic. The numerous cytoplasmic granules may be almost infinitesimal in size, or of such proportions as to render the individual component readily discernible. Mitosis is common. One may frequently

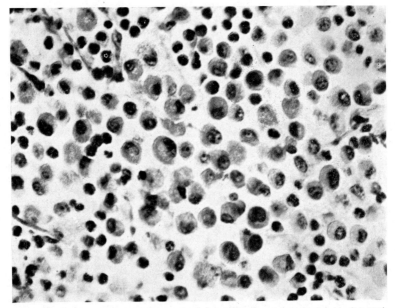

Fig. 109.—Myelocytoma involving one of the skeletal muscles of a bovine (× 660).

find, within a single field, different gradations in the transition of cells from the most immature forms that exhibit little if any differentiation, to those that approach adult leukocytes in appearance. In some of the material it is not uncommon to find areas in which cells similar to eosinophilic leukocytes predominate. A few lymphocytes may occur. Large blood vessels are seldom seen and although capillaries usually can be demonstrated they are by no means numerous.

Myelocytoma of fowls is composed of compact accumulations of myeloid cells which are strikingly similar. The cells are rounded or spherical, although in fixed preparations they may be polygonal. The irregularly ovoid nucleus is large, eccentrically situated, and possesses numerous, irregularly disposed, rather coarse chromatin granules. Occasionally clear nuclei occur, with the chromatin granules arranged at the periphery of the nuclear structure. Many of the nuclei possess nucleoli. The cytoplasm is characteristically filled to capacity with rather large, globular eosinophilic granules (Fig. 110). The demonstration, by appropriate stains, of a few small basophilic granules in the cytoplasm was mentioned by Pentimalli. Mitotic figures are commonly observed and small groups of lymphoid cells are often present. A delicate fibrous reticulum provides a matrix for the neoplastic cells, and a generous blood supply is insured by capillaries and other ill-defined

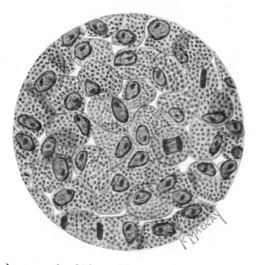

Fig. 110.—Myelocytoma of a chicken. The tumor was situated in the lumbar region.

blood channels of variable dimensions. The tumor infiltrates into the adjacent normal tissues which are gradually replaced by the neoplastic process.

THE BLOOD

Since myeloblastoma is primarily a neoplastic overgrowth of the myeloblastic elements of the bone marrow, it is to be expected that some or many of the vigorously proliferating cells would often find their way into the blood stream in sufficient numbers to constitute a condition of leukemia. This frequently happens in human beings, hence the term "myelogenous leukemia." Although it is generally believed that myeloid leukocytosis occurs in at least some of the cases of myelocytoma in animals, the opportunity to make comprehensive studies of the phenomena in spontaneous cases has been limited. Weil and Clerc found the

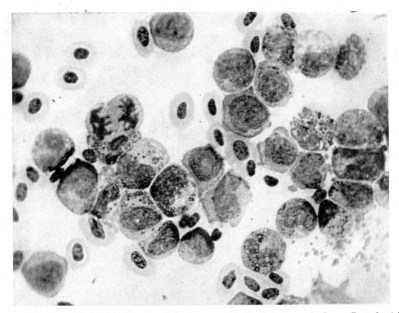

Fig. 111.—Myeloid leukemia. Blood smear prepared from a chicken affected with myelocytoma. Slide obtained through the courtesy of Dr. J. Furth of Philadelphia (× 1,100).

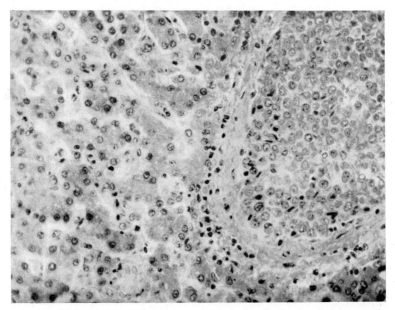

Fig. 112.—Myelocytoma of the liver of a chicken. The large vessel contains large numbers of immature myeloid cells. Prepared from a slide obtained through the courtesy of Dr. J. Furth.

leukocytes increased in a dog to 165,000 for each cubic millimeter. Wirth, however, found much less. In the majority of dogs he found that the leukocytes varied from 14,000 to 40,000 for each cubic millimeter, and in one case the number was increased to 87,000 for each cubic millimeter. Henschen stated that polymorphonuclear leukocytes completely dominated the blood picture in Weil and Clerc's cases, whereas the various organs were infiltrated with basophilic, nongranular myelocytes.

In chickens, secondary leukemia, particularly during the latter course of the disease, may be expected (Figs. 111 and 112). The data Mathews secured from examination of six fowls affected with the spontaneous form of the disease indicated a definite increase in the leukocytic elements in five. The total number of leukocytes varied from 40,000 to 125,000 for each cubic millimeter (normal, approximately 24,000, Forkner). Although Mathews contended that an aleukemic stage of the disease had not been demonstrated, Furth's recent experimental observations would suggest that in some instances involvement of the blood may be slight or absent.* More information is needed concerning this.

CLINICAL CONSIDERATIONS

The infrequent occurrence of myeloid tumors among domesticated mammals makes them of little clinical significance to the average practitioner. Veterinarians engaged in meat inspection may occasionally observe an affected carcass and the bright green of certain myelocytomas may be of assistance in suggesting their true nature. The rarity of the disease, and the paucity of information concerning certain phases of it, should provide a stimulus for more detailed study of the lesions. Recognition of the disease in the living animal which would provide the opportunity to study the blood, would be invaluable. The appearance of a case of myelocytoma should prompt thorough postmortem examination which should include careful examination of the bone marrow.

Myelocytoma constitutes one of the more serious neoplastic diseases of chickens, and there is reason to believe that the disease is transmissible to normal fowls. Its early recognition in a flock is desirable in order that proper measures of control may be instituted. Sick fowls should be isolated at once for observation or killed for necropsy. The gross appearance of lesions alone is not sufficient to justify a designation of

---

* The leukosis referred to by Furth as myeloid leukemia I believe to bear a close relationship to the myeloid neoplastic condition designated as myelocytoma in the context (leukochloroma of Mathews). These conditions perhaps represent different morphologic expressions of a fundamental disturbance that is common to both.

myelocytoma, and material must be prepared for microscopic examination. The premises should be made as sanitary as practicable, and the fowls rid of external parasites, since transmission of the disease by blood-sucking parasites seems possible. A hereditary predisposition to the condition is suggested and it may appear with greater frequency in a particular strain of fowls than in others. Inbreeding should be practiced only judiciously, and new blood lines introduced with caution. Treatment is of no avail; the disease is best controlled by developing a strain of fowls in which the incidence of myelocytoma is minimal. This would at least seem possible by intensifying individual resistance.

BIBLIOGRAPHY

1. Claussen: Ein Fall von Chlorom beim Schwein. Ztschr. f. Fleisch. u. Milchhyg., **38:** 175–178 (Feb. 15), 1928.

2. Downey, Hal: Diseases of the blood. In: Bell, E. T.: A text-book of pathology. Philadelphia, Lea & Febiger, 1930, pp. 569–612.

3. Forkner, C. E.: Blood and bone marrow cells of the domestic fowl. Jour. Exper. Med., **50:** 121–141 (July 1), 1929.

4. Furth, J.: Observations with new transmissible strain of leucosis (leucemia) of fowls. Jour. Exper. Med., **53:** 243–267 (Feb.), 1931.

5. Henschen, Fokke: Blutbildende Organe. In: Joest, Ernst: Handbuch der speziellen pathologischen Anatomie der Haustiere. Ed. 3. Berlin, R. Schoetze, **5:** 248, 1929.

6. Mathews, F. P.: Leukochloroma in the common fowl; its relation to myelogenic leukemia and its analogies to chloroma in man. Arch. Path., **7:** 442–457 (March), 1929.

7. Pentimalli, F.: Ueber die Geschwülste bei Hühnern. I. Mitteilung Allgemeine Morphologie der spontanen und der transplantablen Hühnergeschwülste. Ztschr. f. Krebsforsch., **15:** 111–153, 1915–1916.

8. Schultze: Quoted by Mallory, F. B. and Wright, J. H.: Pathological technique. Ed. 8. Philadelphia, W. B. Saunders Co., 1924, p. 522.

9. Weaver, C. H.: Chloroma in a cow. Jour. Am. Med. Vet. Assn., **59:** 766–768 (Sept.), 1921.

10. Weil and Clerc: Quoted by Hutyra, Franz, and Marek Josef: Special pathology and therapeutics of the diseases of domestic animals. Chicago, A. Eger, **3:** 127, 1926.

11. Wirth: Quoted by Hutyra, Franz, and Marek, Josef: Special pathology and therapeutics of the diseases of domestic animals. Chicago, A. Eger.

CHAPTER XVI

MELANOBLASTOMA

DEFINITION AND GENERAL DESCRIPTION

Melanoblastomas consist of definitely specialized cells known as melanoblasts which produce pigment called melanin. This product often is so excessive as to impart to the growth a characteristic, smoke gray to black color. If the tumor is malignant it is known as a malignant melanoma; if benign, simply as melanoma.

The natural color of the skin of domestic animals is due to a heaping up of small pigment granules in the basal layer of the epidermis, and, to a smaller degree, to the pigment-containing cells in the upper zone of the corium. This pigment, which is known as melanin, resembles small, needle-like crystals, or more frequently small, brownish granules. The pigment usually is situated intracellularly; it is insoluble in acids and alkalies and does not contain iron, sulphur, or fat. It may be bleached by exposure to peroxide of hydrogen whereas it becomes black by contact with silver nitrate. Melanin is the product of the metabolic activity of certain specific cells. Its formation, according to Dawson, is accomplished by conversion of protein material into pigment by means of an enzyme. Besides those in the skin, the pigment-producing cells are found in the choroid of the eye and in the pia mater of the medulla. Melanoblastomas arise as a consequence of the progressive and unrestrained proliferation of the melanoblast, or pigment-producing cell, which is normally concerned with the production of pigment for physiologic purposes. The occasional appearance of melanomas as congenital tumors suggests prenatal disturbances in development that result in excessive production or misplacement of the melanoblastic cells, as responsible for certain of these new growths. Melanotic tumors of the skin of man not infrequently have their inception from pigmented moles or nevi, but this relationship has not been demonstrated in horses, in which the majority of melanotic tumors of animals occur. In view of the fact that white horses are notoriously prone to melanotic tumors, Jaeger's observations are significant. He was unable to find pigmented nevi of the skin in the examination at necropsy of sixty-three white horses. However, benign melanotic nonelevated pigmented areas are frequently seen in the skin of calves and swine; the condition is usually designated as melanosis (Fig. 113). A nodular growth is not evident and the condition has none of the characteristics of a neoplasm. In calves, the pigmented spots of the subcutis, which are known as melanosis maculosa, have a tendency to disappear with advancing age and are usually absent in adult cattle.

Melanotic areas of variable size may occur in the subcutis of dogs, most frequently on the abdomen. Occasionally there is a more or less generalized distribution of melanin, with deposits of pigment in the lungs, liver, kidneys, peritoneum, and so forth. Since the various foci of pigmentation in these cases are nothing more than excessive accumulations of melanin within phagocytic cells, or within tissue spaces, such phenomena are not examples of neoplasia.

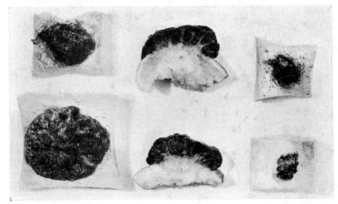

Fig. 113.—Benign melanomas and melanosis of the skin of hogs.

Whether benign pigmentation may give rise to a potentially malignant melanotic tumor is problematic. Histologically, it would at least seem possible.

HISTOGENESIS

The histogenesis of the type cell of melanoblastomas long has provided a complex problem. Although many views have been advanced of the genesis of the pigment-producing cell, or melanoblast, there is as yet no agreement concerning the character of the specific elements which are directly responsible for these cells. Some authors state that the tumors are of epithelial origin; others insist that they are derived from certain mesodermal elements, such as immature connective tissue or endothelium; still others contend that they arise from a definitely characterized cell, known as the chromatophore, which has its origin in the mesoderm. A neurogenic derivation has also been suggested for the type cell of melanoblastoma.

The comprehensive work of Jaeger, who studied the development of melanotic tumors in the gray horse, should be mentioned. Jaeger was convinced that these tumors were not related in their genesis to the epithelium of the skin, and although limited to the corium at the time of their inception chromatophores are not concerned. He concluded that the cell responsible for the process is the fibroblast which has undergone functional degeneration, and finally morphologic differentiation, as a consequence of which the cell assumes a capacity for abnormal pigment metabolism. Jaeger therefore considered the malignant melanotic tumors to be genuine spindle-cell sarcomas (fibrosarcomas). Although Jaeger's conclusions were based on impressive evidence, the histologic aspects of these tumors, as they occur in the different species, do not substantiate the theory that their origin is fibroblastic. Certainly the majority of them have little in common with so-called spindle-cell sarcoma.

Until the origin of the specific cell constituting the melanoblastoma is definitely determined, it would seem desirable to avoid the use of such terms as "melano-epithelioma," "melanocarcinoma," and "melanosarcoma," since these names imply specific histogenesis. Melanotic tumors which remain localized, with none of the characteristics of malignancy, can properly be called melanomas, whereas those which exhibit a tendency to infiltrate and destroy the surrounding tissues and to metastasize can be designated malignant melanomas.

INCIDENCE

Among animals, most melanotic tumors are observed in the horse; they are particularly common in old gray horses. In fact most, if not all, old gray or white horses seem to have these tumors. Martel,[11] in one of his annual reports, stated that it was extremely rare to find white or gray horses entirely free from melanotic growths, and van Dorssen, who studied the incidence of these tumors, came to the conclusion that all old gray horses were affected.

Van Dorssen studied the incidence of melanotic tumors among 235 gray horses belonging to the Amsterdam Street Railway. When arranged in seven age groups the occurrence of melanoblastoma was as follows:

Among seventeen horses aged less than six years, there was none with melanoblastoma; among forty-five horses aged from six to eight years, five (11 per cent) had tumors; among fifty-two horses aged from eight to ten years, nine (36 per cent) had tumors; among sixty horses aged from ten to twelve years, thirty-seven (61 per cent) had tumors; among thirty-eight horses aged from twelve to fourteen years, twenty-seven (71 per cent) had tumors; among seven horses aged fourteen to fifteen years, five (7 per cent) had tumors, and among fifteen horses aged more than fifteen years, twelve (80 per cent) had tumors.

These data indicate definite increase in incidence with advancing age which in gray horses is associated with gradual loss of pigment of the hair, and they become white. Fölger[15] reported that 42.82 per cent of 527 malignant tumors of horses were malignant melanomas. Peyronny examined at necropsy sixty-nine gray to white horses of an average age of twelve years; the oldest was aged twenty-eight years. All had melanotic tumors, whereas five brown or red horses similarly examined at necropsy did not have pigmented growths. Budnowski found malignant melanomas in ninety-two (12 per cent) of 771 white horses used in the army.

It should be pointed out that these tumors do occur in brown horses, and they have been observed in black horses.[20] It is not clear what influence the depigmentation of the hair has on the appearance of melanoblastomas, although there is evidence that the predominance of the disease in gray or white horses may have some relationship to the fact that in dark horses the pigmented cells of the cutis are absent, whereas in gray horses, of middle to old age, they are always present.[10] Their presence provides a genesis for potential melanoblastic tumors.

Reliable statistics concerning the incidence of melanotic tumors in the other species of domestic animals are not available. Suffice to say that the disease occurs in other animals. It is occasionally observed in dogs, cattle, and swine. Among 507 animal tumors in my collection eighteen were melanoblastomas:

Among 214 tumors of cattle there were four melanoblastomas; among seventy-eight tumors of dogs there was one melanoblastoma; among seventy-six swine there were six melanoblastomas; among fifty-three fowls, there were no melanoblastomas; among forty horses there were six melanoblastomas; among thirty-nine sheep there were no melanoblastomas; among five mules, there was one melanoblastoma, and of one goat there was no melanoblastoma. Nine of the tumors were considered clinically and histologically benign and ten were considered to be malignant. The incidence of melanotic tumors in my collection is in no sense considered to be a correct index of their actual occurrence, since pigmented melanomas are easily diagnosed grossly, and the curiosity which might have prompted sending other tumors to the laboratory for a diagnosis was absent in the case of most of these pigmented growths.

OCCURRENCE AND POINTS OF ORIGIN

Horse.—By far the greatest number of melanomas occurs in the horse, with the highest incidence, as has been suggested, in old gray animals which have undergone depigmentation of the hair. This observation was made as early as 1813 by Gohier. Anatomically, the sites of predilection of these tumors are the skin of the ventral surface of the tail,

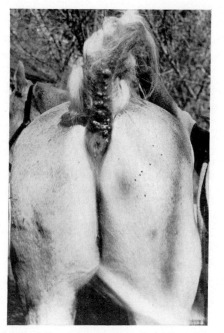

Fig. 114.—Small, multiple, malignant melanomas of the ventral surface of the tail of a horse.

the anal region, the vulva, the sheath, the scrotum, the region of the perineum, and the skin over the mammæ (Fig. 114). The tumors are not uncommonly seen on the anterior surface of the lips, and they sometimes arise from the skin of the concha. Occasionally the skin of the shoulder and of the parotid region is the point of origin. Those in the regions of the pelvis and shoulder frequently extensively infiltrate the adjacent musculature, and metastasis to the regional lymph nodes usually occurs. Although it is possible for a melanoblastoma to originate from the tissues of the interior of the body, usually when they are found in these tissues it may be considered that they have metastasized from a primary lesion elsewhere. It is not uncommon for extensive metastasis to occur internally, from a small, primary lesion in the skin which might easily escape detection. For this reason it is not uncommon to observe at necropsy many large tumorous nodules in the interior of the body of an animal in which tumors of the exterior were not detected in life. Malignant melanomas are capable of widespread metastasis, and practically every organ of the body may become a repository for secondary growths. The literature pertaining to melanoblastoma in the horse is replete with such cases. Goldberg described a typical case in a gray mare. The primary tumor was considered to have arisen in the mammary gland, and metastasis had occurred to the lymph nodes, lungs, spleen, liver, pancreas, bones, muscles, diaphragm, peritoneum, pleura, kidneys, myocardium, and adrenal glands. Goldberg thought that the widespread dissemination of the neoplastic processes probably implicated both the blood and lymph streams in the process of dissemination. The promiscuous scattering throughout the body of tumorous foci in malignant melanoma not infrequently occasions encroachment on important nerves with serious consequences. Nerves in the lumbar and sacral regions are most frequently involved.

A melanoma of the brain of an old gray mare was reported by Scott; both cerebellar hemispheres were involved. Siebert observed a malignant melanoma in the spinal canal in the lumbar region of a fourteen-year-old gelding, and cases in which the disease affected the skeleton were recorded by Fröhner, Messner, and Nicolas.

The melanotic tumors obtained from the horse in my collection include three benign melanomas, one of which was obtained from the ventral surface of the tail of an eight-year-old black gelding, and the other two from the skin of one upper eyelid of old gray mares. The malignant melanomas were from the following animals: (1) An eighteen-year-old gray mare, in which there was extensive involvement which included a growth extending outward from the pelvis through the obturator foramen with serious encroachment on the great sciatic nerve; tumors were also present in the liver, spleen, and lungs, and many lymph nodes were affected; (2) an old gray gelding; the tumors were in the skin of the neck and anal region, with widespread metastasis to internal organs, and (3) a fourteen-year-old sorrel horse, sex not given, in which the primary tumor was in the dorsal cervical region; metastatic tumors were present in both sides of the neck ventrally from the primary growth. The initial growth had been removed surgically, after which recurrence had resulted, and following second removal the tumor reappeared and grew with increased rapidity. Because of inanition and respiratory distress the animal was killed, and at necropsy metastasis was observed in the lungs, liver, parietal and visceral pleura and the pericardium. The muscles of the forearm and shoulder were also extensively involved. This case is of particular interest because of the absence of demonstrable pigment in the gross specimen. Microscopically, however, a few neoplastic cells were observed, in the cytoplasm of which were melanin granules.

Bovine.—Melanotic tumors are uncommon in cattle. In my series of 214 tumors of cattle only four were melanotic. In the literature an occasional case is recorded. Imminger, who observed that melanotic

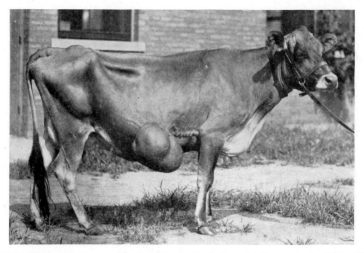

Fig. 115.—Melanoblastoma. Photograph obtained through the courtesy of Dr. W. L. Boyd, University Farm, St. Paul, Minnesota.

tumors occur more frequently in albino than in dark cattle, recorded a case of melanoma of the inner canthus of the eye. Fölger[14] quoted Sluis as having observed generalized melanotic malignancy in a four-year-old cow; the skin, lungs, bronchial lymph nodes, and pericardium were involved. A melanoma about 12 cm. in diameter, at the anus of a three-week-old calf was reported by Görig, who also observed a tumor of the same character, about 8 cm. in diameter, involving the rumen of a cow. A malignant melanoma of the dura mater of the left cerebral hemisphere was observed in a six-year-old cow by Adrendt. Clinical evidence of the presence of the tumor was not observed. Boyd recorded the presence of a large, malignant melanoma in a four-year-old cow (Fig. 115). The growth was on the right side, close to the distal attachment of the posterior ribs, near the juncture of the abdominal and thoracic cavities. It was first observed while the animal was still a calf, and it gradually increased in size until its weight caused the adjacent skin to be drawn badly out of position. The tumor was removed surgically, and at the time of Boyd's report the animal had passed through three pregnancies successfully without evidence of recurrence of the primary tumor or of metastasis.

The four melanotic tumors affecting cattle in my series were benign, and had their origin in the skin. Anatomically they were distributed as follows: (1) Region of the knee of right foreleg; (2) slightly distal to the right ear; (3) over the lower third of the metatarsus, and (4) the region of the flank. Two of the animals were Shorthorns, one was a

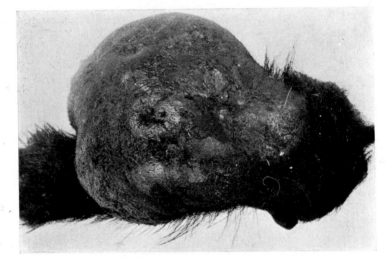

Fig. 116.—Melanoma of the tail of a bovine.

Hereford, and the breed of the fourth was listed as grade. The age of the animals varied from four months to twelve years (Fig. 116).

Although melanoblastoma is occasionally encountered among cattle the information available would indicate that the tumor occurs much more frequently in horses than in cattle. The disease in cattle apparently is less often malignant than in horses, and if the tumor is in operable situations the possibility of successful removal is worthy of trial.

Dog.—Melanotic tumors are rarely observed in dogs. The majority of those which have been reported have been characterized by marked malignancy with recurrence following operative interference in practically every case in which surgery has been attempted. Most of these growths occur in the skin and the tissues of the digital regions seem to yield a considerable percentage. Sammon reported a primary tumor in this region that was productive of generalized metastasis in which the liver escaped involvement. Ball and Cuny noted a malignant melanoma of the tissues of the paw of a dog, which was associated with secondary tumors on the skin over the body, but there was no visceral metastasis. A melanotic tumor of the tissues of the foot of a three-year-old dog was reported by Rautmann. Metastasis occurred to the joint cavity of the knee, the deep inguinal lymph nodes, lungs, kidneys, pancreas, pleura, myocardium, and omentum.

Petit and Germain observed a case suggestive of the influence of trauma in subsequent metastasis of malignant melanoma from a primary tumor that looked innocent. A black French poodle had two small, black, hairless, wart-like tumors in the skin at the base of the tail. These had been bruised and cut by a hair clipper. They refused to heal and persisted as bleeding, granulomatous areas. Following amputation of the tail the animal's condition gradually declined and death eventually occurred. At necropsy metastasis was observed in the sub-cutaneous and intramuscular tissues, extending for a considerable distance anteriorly from the caudal vertebræ. Secondary tumors were also observed in the lungs, heart, spleen, liver, adrenal glands, pleura, omentum, and kidneys. An interesting case of malignant melanoma of an Irish setter was reported by Seddon. The animal had been treated for several years for eczema, and pigmented warts or other tumors of the skin had never been noticed. Necropsy revealed metastatic melanomas in the lungs, spleen, pleura, mesentery, omentum, pericardium, endocardium, and kidneys. Seddon mentioned that in Victoria, Australia, generalized malignant melanoma is commonly associated with primary ulcerations of the skin and cutaneous warts.

Leon removed a malignant melanoma from the scrotum of a dog; the melanoma recurred one year later, with subsequent metastatic involvement of the parietal peritoneum.

A melanoma of the base of the brain of a dog was reported by Bruchmüller, and my collection contains one case in which a malignant melanoma primary in the mammary gland induced generalized metastasis including involvement of the meninges of the spinal cord in the lumbar region.

Swine.—Considering the relatively short span of life permitted the majority of swine, melanotic tumors are not uncommonly seen in this animal, and widespread dissemination of the disease sometimes occurs. In many swine affected with melanoblastoma, the tumor is first observed when the animal is a suckling; this suggests that certain congenital influences may be factors in the inception of some of the tumors. The disease may arise from any portion of the skin, although a considerable percentage of tumors is seen in the region of the flank (Fig. 117). Although the greater number of melanoblastomas which occurs in swine is definitely malignant, two of the six in my series were benign. One was from the skin of the abdomen near the umbilical scar; the other was obtained from the region of the poll. Multiple tumors may be widely separated and of such character as to preclude the possibility of determining which growth antedated the others. In one of these cases in my series the tumors were in the skin of the regions of the hip, loin, and shoulder, with involvement of the prescapular and precrural lymph nodes.

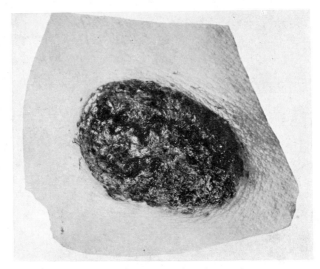

Fig. 117.—Melanoma of the skin of a hog.

Pickens also reported a case in which multiple tumors occurred. The animal was a Duroc pig that was aged between six and eight weeks when the tumors appeared. They were situated cutaneously and subcutaneously above the eye, posterior to the base of the ear, over the anterior border of the scapula, at the angle of the jaw, slightly anterior to the sternum, and on the posterior surface of the carpus. There were also cutaneous nodules above the angle of the ilium and in the right flank. Metastatic nodules were present in the lungs, liver, and kidneys. A melanotic tumor was also found in the right sublumbar region, ventral to the last two lumbar vertebræ.

Caylor and Schlotthauer observed malignant melanomas in the region of the flank in three young Duroc swine in one of which generalized dissemination of the disease occurred throughout the lungs, liver, and kidneys in addition to many of the lymph nodes (Fig. 118).

Although melanoblastoma does not occur in swine as frequently as in some of the other species, the occasional appearance of the condition in relatively young swine is generally characterized by excessive malignancy and the occurrence of early metastasis. The surgical elimination of such a disease is usually futile, owing to the multiplicity of lesions, the malign character of the process and the tendency to early metastasis.

Other species.—Apparently all species of common domestic animals are susceptible to melanotic tumors. A malignant melanoma which developed in a defective eye of a syphilitic rabbit was described by Brown and Pearce. The appearance of the tumor coincided with the

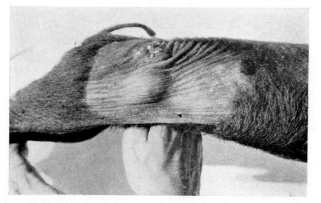

Fig. 118.—Malignant melanoma of the skin of a young hog. The adjacent prefemoral lymph node is much enlarged. Photograph obtained through the courtesy of Dr. Caylor and Dr. Schlotthauer.

development of a syphilitic lesion in the same eye, and this suggested possible relation between the occurrence of the two lesions. Although the iris and ciliary body were virtually replaced by the infiltrating growth metastasis was not observed on complete postmortem examination. In view of the very definite histologic appearance of malignancy in this case, failure of the tumor to metastasize seems unusual. In my review of the literature I failed to find mention of a case of melanotic tumor in rabbits except the instance described by Brown and Pearce. Polson did not find any among reports of fifty-two tumors of this animal which he reviewed in the literature. Polson also contributed the results of a study of fourteen tumors of rabbits, none of which was melanoma.

The paucity of reported cases of melanoblastoma affecting cats would suggest that these animals are seldom victims of this neoplasm.

17

However, Mulvey observed a malignant melanoma in an old black and white cat which was brought to him for treatment of "a sore on the side." The primary tumor, which had ulcerated and was discharging black, pigmented fluid, was situated in the skin on the lateral aspect of the thorax, just posterior to the elbow joint. From the initial lesion a chain of small nodules could be traced forward into the axilla. At necropsy, metastatic tumors were to be seen in the lungs, liver, spleen, kidneys, and mesentery. Most of the lymph nodes were also involved.

Melanoblastoma is also seen in the mule. A malignant melanoma in a sixteen-year-old mule was described by Aubry. The thoracic aperture, the lungs, and the regional lymph nodes were involved. Death resulted from hemorrhage into the thoracic cavity as a consequence of degenerative changes of the tumors in the lungs. One of the malignant melanomas in my collection was also obtained from a mule. The animal was aged seventeen years, and the initial tumor extended from the anterior limit of the brisket, for a considerable distance up the neck. At necropsy, besides many small tumors distributed irregularly over the skin, metastatic growths were observed in the lungs, liver, spleen, kidneys, mesentery, and brain.

The unusual occurrence of malignant melanoma in a chicken was reported by Goldberg. One large pigmented mass, measuring 8 by 6 by 4 cm., and several smaller ones were situated in the mesentery. Similar growths were also observed on the serous surface of the intestines, preventriculus, gizzard, and liver. An ovary was also involved. In the absence of complete data Goldberg was unable to determine the situation which gave rise to the primary growth in this case. His report constitutes the only case reported in the literature consulted of malignant melanoma of the fowl.*

METASTASIS AND MALIGNANCY

Generally speaking, among the melanoblastomas are to be found the most malignant of all neoplasms. It is indeed remarkable that in certain instances a small, innocent-appearing nodular lesion should suddenly assume malignant behavior and initiate widespread metastasis within a relatively short time. The extensive distribution of secondary tumors in a case of malignant melanoma indicates that the metastatic movement of the cells of this tumor is accomplished by every means

* Several cases of melanotic tumors of chickens recently have been described by McGowan, who expressed the belief that in the fowl, these tumors may have either a mesoblastic or an epithelial origin.

available. Not only do the cells infiltrate and destroy the tissues immediately adjacent to the primary growth, but by pushing into tissue spaces and invading the blood stream and the lymph stream, secondary tumors may occur in any part of the body served by the blood and lymph vascular systems. Although the lungs, liver, and kidneys are the organs most frequently affected, apparently no tissue is exempt from the possible presence of metastatic melanomas (Fig. 119). Metastasis undoubtedly accounts for the majority of melanomas found internally; yet it is possible that these growths may occasionally develop from aberrant collections of melanoblasts. Ewing has expressed the feeling that melanoma of the spleen of man probably has this origin.

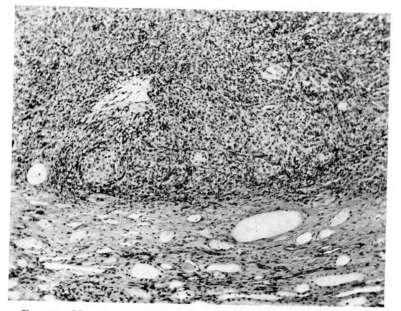

Fig. 119.—Metastatic, malignant melanoma of the kidney of a mule (× 120).

The occurrence of melanotic pigment in an organ is not in itself definite evidence of the presence of metastatic melanoma. Not infrequently melanotic deposits occur in organs such as the lungs and liver, as a consequence of transportation by the blood stream of melanin from a repository elsewhere in the body. Melanotic deposits found at a distance from the primary tumor can be claimed as evidence of definite metastasis when it can be demonstrated that the pigmental portions in question represent a collection of pigment-producing tumor cells (Fig. 120).

The majority of the benign forms of melanoblastoma, as they occur

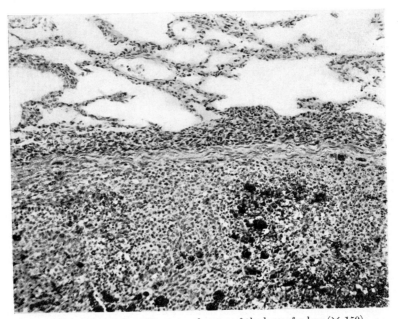

Fig. 120.—Metastatic malignant melanoma of the lung of a hog ($\times$ 150).

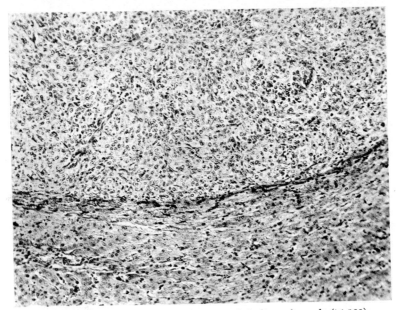

Fig. 121.—Metastatic malignant melanoma of the liver of a mule ($\times$ 120).

in the skin of hogs and in the skin of cattle, are black, firm nodules of variable size (Fig. 117). These may persist as localized tumors for years, with little evidence of growth and with no demonstrable effect on the well-being of the animal harboring them. In the skin, the malignant variety is frequently multiple within a small region, often soft to the touch, and, if rapidly growing, the content of pigment may be so reduced as to be visible only with the microscope. Involvement of the regional lymph nodes, or sudden and often rapid decline in the state of the animal's health, are presumptive evidences of a malignant process in which metastasis has occurred (Fig. 121).

In the horse, secondary tumors affecting the large vessels and nerves are not uncommon.

GROSS CHARACTERISTICS

Most melanoblastomas present a striking and characteristic appearance. They are usually moderately firm, although some are distinctly hard and others are fairly soft. The consistence depends on the amount of fibrinous connective tissue present, the degree of vascularity, and retrogressive changes such as ulceration, infection, and so forth. Most of them are brownish black to coal black, although smoke gray specimens are sometimes seen, and rarely a tumor may occur in which pigment is not demonstrable grossly. As a rule, however, they are so saturated with pigment as to discolor the fingers in handling them, and fluids in which they are preserved assume a brownish hue.

The shape of the melanomas which arise from the skin varies somewhat with the species in which they occur. Those of the horse are nodular, ovoid, or dome-like structures invested with skin, whereas those of swine usually are flattened, elevated and nodular, irregularly circular, and devoid of skin. Those of cattle are often dome-like, nodular masses, and those of the dog frequently are papillary and wart-like. The tumors may be single or they may be in large numbers of all sizes, particularly in the horse.

If the surface of the growth is ulcerated, the discharge is frequently foul-smelling, dark, and blood-stained.

The size of the tumors varies within wide limits. They may be 0.5 cm. or less in diameter, or they may be huge. Petit observed one on the back of a horse which he described as being the size of a human body. In one of my cases a benign melanoma on the skin just above the knee of a four-month-old calf weighed 7.2 kg. (approximately 6 pounds) and resembled a football in size and shape. Fitch, Boyd, and Billings observed at necropsy a malignant melanotic spleen of a horse which weighed 22.8 kg. (approximately 50 pounds). It was 80 cm. long, 55 cm. wide and 18 cm. thick. Newsom observed a similar condition in a horse in which the spleen weighed approximately 8 kg. (about 17 pounds). The normal spleen of the horse weighs between 1 and 1.5 kg.

These cases represent unusually large tumors; the average melanotic tumor is much smaller, and many of them are so small as to be partially if not entirely hidden by the hair of the animal.

MICROSCOPIC DESCRIPTION

The structure of melanoblastomas usually is richly cellular, consisting largely of closely packed, diffuse collections of melanoblasts, and variable amounts of fibrous connective tissue. In the benign forms the

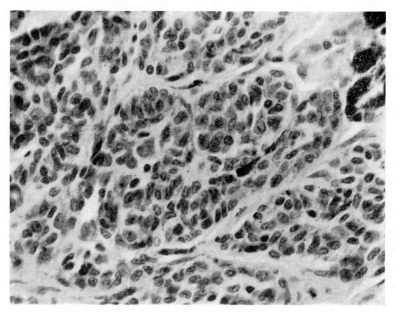

Fig. 122.—Malignant melanoma of the skin of a hog (× 525).

stroma presents a rather adult appearance and is usually more abundant than in the aggressive or metastatic forms. The most characteristic feature of the microscopic appearance of the majority of melanotic tumors is the presence of clump-like accumulations of brown melanin granules. The pigment, which is largely intracellular, is seldom distributed uniformly throughout the structure (Figs. 122 and 123).

Excessive accumulations of pigment may occur in some parts, whereas other parts may be practically free of pigment. Usually the pigment completely fills the interior of the cells that contain it. Apparently the cytoplasm of the cell becomes filled with pigment granules first, with the nucleus taking up the excess so far as its capacity permits. That which cannot be provided for within the cells which produce it is taken up by phagocytes, although, if the production of pigment is unusually large, a considerable amount of melanin may be carried away by the blood stream, to be deposited elsewhere in the body or excreted with the urine. The large amount of melanin in many of the cells may make it difficult to observe the finer details of their structure. Observation is best in places in which the amount of pigment is small and in which many of the cells contain none (Fig. 123). Occasionally a malignant melanoma is seen which is almost, if not entirely, devoid of melanin granules.

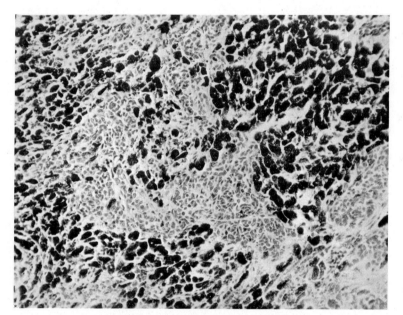

FIG. 123.—Metastatic malignant melanoma of a lymph node of a hog. Both pigmented and nonpigmented cells are present ($\times$ 150).

The absence of pigment is frequently associated with a rapid, aggressive type of growth of immature cells which exhibit little if any tendency to differentiate as do normal, adult melanoblasts (Fig. 124).

The type cell of melanoblastoma is usually polyhedral or oval, although elongated, spindle-shaped forms are not uncommon. There is considerable variation in the size of the type of cell of different melanotic tumors, and an occasional specimen is encountered in which the cell is unusually large. Generally the cells are somewhat larger in the malignant forms than in the benign forms, and intercellular substance is absent. The nucleus constitutes approximately half the cellular bulk, and its position may be slightly eccentric. The nuclei contain considerable fragmented chromatin material, and nucleoli usually can be seen. In benign and less malignant tumors, the nuclei exhibit less affinity for the basic stains, and characteristically stain a rather pale blue with hematoxylin. In the less mature forms, or those of aggravated malignancy, the nuclei stain more intensely.

In malignant melanomas, mitotic division of the tumor cells is often a striking feature, and it is not unusual to view many different phases of this phenomenon in the same microscopic field. The dividing cells do not contain demonstrable melanin.

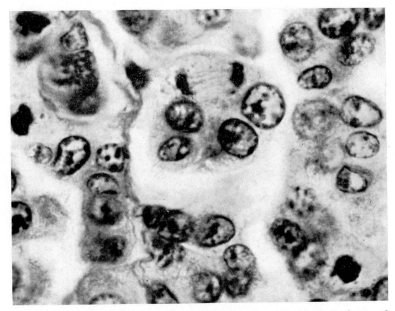

Fig. 124.—Nonpigmented metastatic malignant melanoma of the lungs of a horse. One cell is undergoing mitosis (× 1,350).

In the benign tumor a plentiful supply of blood is insured by the presence in the stroma of well-developed blood vessels, and in the highly cellular malignant varieties of this tumor it is not unusual to find large amounts of free extravascular blood in direct contact with the adjacent tumor cells. The intimate relation of the parenchyma of many of these tumors with the blood vascular system probably enhances the opportunity for early metastasis by way of the blood stream. In rapidly growing tumors extensive regions of necrosis may occur.

The malignant variety of melanoblastoma reveals, definitely, an infiltrative type of growth, with tumor cells arranged either in diffuse sheets, simulating an alveolar type of arrangement, or as slender columns of cells which tend to infiltrate the adjacent tissue in a destructive manner.

DIAGNOSTIC CHARACTERISTICS

Melanoblastomas may usually be recognized clinically by their black color. Most of the tumors appear in old, gray or white horses; they are relatively uncommon in cattle. The benign form occurs commonly in the skin of hogs, but is sometimes seen in the other domestic animals. These points on the occurrence of the tumor are important to the clinician who may venture a diagnosis without the aid of microscopic sections. Melanoblastoma of the skin should not be confused with diffuse, nonelevated deposits of melanin that are so often seen in the skin of hogs. These apparently are comparable to the pigmented nevi of man, and they are properly classified under the heading melanosis. Although it must be recognized that these deposits are potential seats of true tumor, they should be considered as such only when definite nodules develop (Fig. 113).

Microscopically the diagnosis offers few difficulties except perhaps in metastatic situations in which they often appear carcinomatous. The presence of melanin, even in small quantities, in the form of a brownish, granular pigment, usually will assist in the diagnosis. Occasionally, however, much skill and experience will be necessary in order to distinguish between the malignant and benign forms. The following may prove helpful in this regard:

Grossly benign melanomas are usually single, and encapsulated. Cattle and adult swine are most often affected. The tumor remains localized. It will not recur if properly removed. Grossly malignant melanoma is frequently multiple; usually it is not encapsulated. It is most common in horses, mules, and young swine. Metastasis is common. Recurrence after removal is likely to occur and metastasis is probable.

Microscopically, most cells of the benign melanomas contain much melanin. The cells are usually ovoid or spindle shaped and not large. Much stroma is present. Mitotic figures are not seen. Microscopically malignant melanomas contain many cells free of pigment. The cells are polyhedral and larger than is usual in the benign form. A minimal amount of stroma is present. Mitosis is common.

As I have mentioned, the finding of melanin in lymph nodes, or in the liver, lungs, or kidneys does not prove that metastasis has taken place. The deposition of pigment in these tissues must occur frequently if the tumor is heavily charged with pigment and has a generous blood supply. It is only when the melanoblasts have been metastatically transported and have reached an environment conducive to their growth and multiplication that secondary tumors become established.

CLINICAL CONSIDERATIONS

Although simple benign melanomas that occur singly, or even as multiple tumors, over the exterior of the body affect the well-being of the animal only slightly, the occurrence of malignant melanoma, externally or internally, is usually followed by grave consequences. The symptoms induced by these neoplasms depend largely on their size and the significance of the anatomic situation. Those which affect the pelvic, rectal, and anal regions of horses not infrequently seriously obstruct the passage of fecal material. The capacity of malignant melanoma to invade the various tissues may result, particularly in the horse, in serious involvement of portions of the central nervous system. Partial or complete paralysis may ensue. Establishment of the disease by metastasis in any of the vital organs, is usually followed by gradually progressive constitutional disturbances, which eventually cause complete incapacitation and death. Sudden death may occur following rupture of an internal malignant melanoma. If the kidney is affected, melanuria may be of some diagnostic significance. If the tumor involves the brain or its meninges, the subsequent effects will be serious or not serious depending on the physical characteristics of the growth and its exact anatomic situation.

If a benign melanoblastoma is situated in an operable region, surgical treatment is frequently successful and is worthy of consideration. One must be cautious, however, in selecting cases of melanoblastoma for operation, to be certain that the tumor in question is benign and not malignant. The tendency of many melanomas to assume malign aggressiveness following trauma makes it unwise to perform biopsy. For the clinician, the benign or malignant nature of these neoplasms is best determined by careful consideration of the history and close scrutiny of the physical characteristics of the growth. Loss of weight, the presence of multiple tumors, and enlargement of the regional lymph nodes are particularly significant in the recognition of malignancy.

The fact that most benign forms of the tumor grow slowly makes it possible for an affected animal to remain useful for months or even years, and finally to die or to be killed on account of old age or general uselessness. On the other hand, malignant melanoma may progress rapidly and incapacitate the animal within a comparatively short time.

Every melanoblastoma is potentially malignant. The type cell of the benign variety has the same histogenesis as that of the malignant form; the difference is essentially one of differentiation.

HEREDITY

There is evidence to suggest that certain melanoblastomas are influenced in their occurrence by heredity. Virchow recorded a case in which a young white stallion with melanomas of the anal region transmitted the disease to all of its white descendants, whereas those of a dark color escaped. The continued breeding of the descendants of the original sire was thought to be responsible for the increased occurrence of melanotic tumors among horses throughout the vicinity. Caylor and Schlotthauer reported three cases of spontaneous malignant melanoma in pure-bred Duroc hogs belonging to the same herd. The three swine had a common sire, and two of them the same mother. The mother of the third was a sister of the sow which had farrowed the first two. The fact that in all three of the animals the tumors had a similar anatomic origin is indeed unusual. In each, the tumor developed in the skin of the right flank. Transplantation experiments were unsuccessful.

BIBLIOGRAPHY

1. Adrendt: Ein Melanosarkom an der harten Hirnhaut einer Kuh. Ztschr. f. Fleisch. u. Milchhyg., **38**: 154, 1928.

2. Aubry: Quoted by Fölger.

3. Ball, V. and Cuny, C.: Secondary cutaneous melano-sarcomatosis in a dog. Abstr.: Am. Vet. Rev., **39**: 72–73, 1911.

4. Boyd, W. L.: Melanosarcoma of cow in which good results were obtained by surgical interference. Cornell Vet., **8**: 125–126 (Jan.), 1918.

5. Brown, W. H. and Pearce, Louise: Melanoma (sarcoma) of the eye in a syphilitic rabbit. Jour. Exper. Med., **43**: 807–813 (June 1), 1926.

6. Bruchmüller: Quoted by French, Cecil: Surgical disease and surgery of the dog. Chicago, A. Eger, 1923.

7. Budnowski: Das Melanosarkom des Pferdes. Ztschr. f. Veterinärk., **15**: 417–438, 1903.

8. Caylor, H. D. and Schlotthauer, C. F.: Melano-epitheliomas of swine; transplantation and cultural experiments. Arch. Path. and Lab. Med., **2**: 343–351 (Sept.), 1926.

9. Dawson, J. W.: The melanomata: Their morphology and histogenesis. Edinburgh Med. Jour., **32**: 501–732 (Oct.), 1925.

10. van Dorssen, J.: Quoted by Fölger.

11. Editorial. Cancer in horses. Am. Vet. Rev., **44**: 299–300 (Dec.), 1913.

12. Ewing, James: Neoplastic diseases. Ed. 3. Philadelphia, W. B. Saunders Co., 1928, p. 938.

13. Fitch, C. P., Boyd, W. L., and Billings, W. A.: Melanosis. Cornell Vet., **9**: 56–57 (Jan.), 1919.

14. Fölger, A. F.: Geschwülste bei Tieren. Ergebn. d. all. Path. u. path. Anat., 18: 372–676, 1917.

15. Fölger, A. F.: Quoted by Lubarsch, O.: Zur vergleichenden Pathologie der melanotischen Gewächse. Med. Klin., 1: 195–199 (Feb. 22), 1920.

16. Fröhner: Quoted by Fölger.

17. Gohier, J.-B.: Memoriés et observations sur la chirurgie et la médicine vétérinaires; ouvrage couronné en grande partie par la société d'agriculture du département de la Seine, Lyons, 1813, 450 pp.

18. Goldberg, S. A.: The differential features between melanosis and melanosarcoma. Jour. Am. Vet. Med. Assn., 56: 140–153 (Nov.), 250–264 (Dec.), 1919.

19. Görig: Melanom bei einer Kuh und einem Kalb. Deutsch. tierarztl. Wchnschr., 9: 130, 1901.

20. Hall: Quoted by Kitt, Theodor: Text-book of comparative general pathology. Chicago, Chicago Medical Book Co., 1906, p. 378.

21. Imminger: Quoted by Fölger.

22. Jaeger, Alfred: Die Melanosarkomatose der Schimmelpferde. Virchow's Arch. f. path. Anat. u. Physiol., 198: 1–61 (Oct. 2), 1909.

23. Leon, G. A.: Quoted by Fölger.

24. McGowan, J. P.: On rous, leucotic and allied tumours in the fowl. New York, Macmillan Co., 1928, p. 45.

25. Messner, E.: Quoted by Fölger.

26. Mulvey, W. S.: Melanosis in a cat. Vet. Rec., 18: 614, 1905–1906.

27. Newsom, I. E.: Personal communication to the author.

28. Nicolas, J.: Quoted by Fölger.

29. Petit: Énorme sarcome mélanique de la cuisse chez un cheval; considérations sur la melanose en général. Bull. et mém. Soc. anat. de Par., 78: 377, 1903.

30. Petit and Germain: Generalized melano-sarcoma in a dog. Abstract: Am. Vet. Rev., 42: 228–229, 1912–1913.

31. Peyronny: Quoted by Fölger.

32. Pickens, E. M.: Generalized melanosis in a pig. Jour. Am. Vet. Med. Assn., 52: 707–713 (Feb.), 1918.

33. Polson, C. J.: Tumours of the rabbit. Jour. Path. and Bacteriol., 30: 603–614 1927.

34. Rautmann: Quoted by Fölger.

35. Sammon, M.: Melanotic sarcoma with cutaneous and polyvisceral metastasis in a dog. Abstract: Am. Vet. Rev., 44: 255, 1913–1914.

36. Scott: Quoted by Goldberg.

37. Seddon, H. R.: Melano-sarcoma in the dog. Am. Vet. Med. Assn., 50: 894, 1916–1917.

38. Siebert, W.: Melanosarkomatose der Dura mater beim Pferde. Deutsch. tierarztl. Wchnschr., 638, 1907.

39. Virchow, R.: Quoted by Williams, W. R.: The natural history of cancer, London, W. Heinman, 1908, p. 363.

CHAPTER XVII

EPITHELIOBLASTOMA

To the epithelioblastomas, as a group, belong the majority of neoplasms which afflict domestic animals.

It is convenient to group the new growths arising from the epithelium of the skin, mucous membrane, and glandular organs under three heads: Papilloma, adenoma, and carcinoma. Although the first two usually are not malignant, it is not uncommon to observe a papillary new growth which structurally is papilloma, but which exhibits aggressive tendencies; it is then designated papillary carcinoma. The same is true in case of adenoma. These are looked on as benign growths but those with an adenomatous type of structure which are histologically and clinically malignant are correctly spoken of as adenocarcinomas.

PAPILLOMA

Definition.—Papillomas are warty, roughened, brush-like papillary structures. They are often horny or spiny to the touch. They contain fibrous cores or projections covered to a variable depth by epithelial cells.

Incidence.—The greater number of papillomas seem to occur in young animals. Goldberg considered papillomas to be the most common epithelial tumor, but my experience suggests that papillomas are less commonly encountered than the malignant forms of epithelial new growths. In my series of more than 500 tumors of animals, seven were papillomas and two were papillary carcinomas. Perhaps the fact that the benign papilloma progresses so slowly, and seldom gives rise to symptoms severe enough to excite attention, accounts for the relatively few cases in the literature, and the infrequency with which such tumors reach the laboratory.

These growths may occur anywhere on the cutaneous and mucous surfaces, particularly at the points of juncture of the skin and mucous membranes.

Horse.—Occasionally an animal is seen with the mucosa of the gums and lips covered with hundreds of small papillomas. The skin, eyelids, and penis may likewise be the points of origin of these tumors, which frequently are multiple. Leese reported a papilloma from the bladder of a mare, and Kinsley mentioned finding a collection of these tumors at the cardiopyloric juncture in the stomach of a horse used for dissection.

Bovine.—In cattle these growths frequently occur in the skin around the eyes, and ears, and, particularly in calves, over the shoulders and back. One tumor which I had occasion to study was removed from the rumen of a cow. Papillomas may arise in the mucosa of the esophagus of the ox, and Lisi reported a papilloma of the urethra and bladder of a cow. No doubt there are more tumors in these situations than one would infer from the cases reported; the majority naturally escape de-

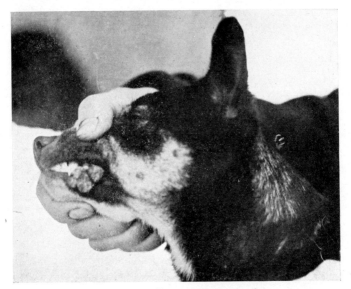

Fig. 125.—Papilloma of the lip of a dog.

tection unless discovered at necropsy. The teats and teat canals of the ox often give rise to papillomas. Kinsley[6] recorded a case in which a tumor of this kind was removed from the eyelid of a cow.

Dog.—In this animal, papillomas most frequently arise from the lips, buccal mucosa, and tongue (Fig. 125), and they are usually multiple. The skin of the sheath and of the anal region also seems to favor the development of papillomas. Hobday mentioned that although papillomas of the region of the larynx and throat are not common, they do occur; he described a case of a toy Yorkshire terrier in which a papilloma was found in the vulva. Hobday also mentioned a case recorded by Petit and Germain, in which a bulldog died suddenly and was found to have a small papilloma arising from the right ventricle of the larynx. Similar tumors were present on the surface of the right vocal cord, and on the left cord were small, multiple tumors. In my series I found the skin of the sternum affected twice, the lips once, and in one case the interdigital spaces of the foot.

Other species.—Kinsley[7] noted that the mucosa of the bladder of sheep and hogs may be the origin of multiple papillomas, and Eve reported a somewhat unusual case in which a three-year-old cat was found with a papillomatous mass in each side of the back of the tongue. The orifice of the larynx was almost completely occluded by the growths. Papillomas are sometimes seen on the combs, feet, and wattles of fowls, but I have not found instances reported in which the tumor has been seen in the interior of the chicken. Joest recorded a case of multiple papilloma which affected the feet of a crow. Polson recorded a papilloma of the sacculus rotundus in a rabbit.

Effects on the host.—Unlike the malignant growths, papillomas seldom actually menace life. They are objectionable largely because of mechanical interference with the physiologic function of a part. For instance a papilloma of the esophagus of sufficient size will seriously interfere with the passage of food, whereas one on the lip might make the prehension of food and water difficult. Papillomatous growths of the pharynx or larynx may cause troublesome dysphagia or fatal dyspnea. If they are on the penis, and the involvement is extensive, most strenuous efforts to urinate may result in the passage of only a few drops. If the animal is used for breeding purposes it is obvious that the presence of such a tumor would constitute a serious impediment. The presence of a papilloma in the bladder may result in occlusion of the urethral passage, with serious consequences. It is evident that the degree of seriousness resulting from a papilloma depends, to a great extent, on the position it occupies. Furthermore, a small percentage of papillomas suddenly assume malignant tendencies and become papillary carcinomas or true carcinomas, which, of course, are potentially dangerous.

Origin and malignancy.—The true papilloma never metastasizes, but remains fixed at the point of origin. The fact that many of these growths appear multiple may perhaps give the impression of the formation of secondary foci, but the multiplicity undoubtedly is due to independent multicentric origin and not to metastasis. Formation of multiple papillomas strongly suggests the influence of predisposition on the part of the tissues involved. Certainly the frequency of multiple papillomas on the mucosa of the lips and gums of the dog and the horse cannot be considered a chance manifestation. Irritation of various kinds has been suggested, but this factor alone seems inadequate in offering a complete explanation.

Contagiousness of multiple papillomas of the dog's mouth has been suspected by many observers. Hobday has expressed the feeling that the disease is disseminated among puppies by their frolicsome habits of taking hold of each other's mouths. McFadyean and Hobday's transplantation experiments with this tumor are summarized as follows: "The experiments conclusively proved that the common papillomas of the dog's mouth are transmissible, and they support the clinical evidence in favor of contagion being the common cause of such growths. They also show that without any treatment whatever such papillomas may disappear, by a process of gradual shrinking and absorption, and they suggest the thought that the credit claimed for some methods of treatment may be undeserved. Lastly, the experiments indicate that after disappearance of a first crop of papillomas the animal is left in a measure protected against a second infection of the same kind."

Creech also has demonstrated the transmissibility of common warts of the skin of cattle. Definitely positive results were obtained in fifteen of twenty-two cattle inoculated with filtered or unfiltered emulsions prepared from wart tissue. Creech demonstrated that filtrates prepared from the tissue of warts from cattle, which were free from microorganisms that could be cultivated, were capable of producing papillomas when injected intracutaneously into healthy cattle, and, further, that the experimentally produced growths could be successfully transmitted in the second generation by inoculation of filtrate. Creech concluded, "The causative factor in common warts of cattle is probably of the nature of a filtrable virus."

Apparently certain aspects of the biology of papilliferous epithelial proliferations of cattle and dogs is significantly similar if not identical.

Gross characteristics.—If one keeps in mind the papillary structure of these growths and their usual situations, a correct diagnosis usually can be made from the gross specimen. The majority of growths vary in size from about 1 to 10 cm. in diameter. Some are attached by short, constricted necks of tissue, and others may present a pedunculated appearance, but the majority are attached to the underlying tissues rather broadly. The surface is always roughened and occasionally presents a great number of small spine-like projections, but is devoid of hair. Others have a cauliflower-like appearance, with the surface broken irregularly by deep rugæ. They are grayish white to pink, horny to the touch, and usually firm. Those that occur externally are subject to considerable trauma, and as a result they may become infected. Hemorrhage is not common, although suppuration may be seen in some of the larger external specimens which have been subjected to trauma.

Microscopic description.—Microscopically, the papillomas present a simple type of structure. It usually consists of a number of separate units or projections, each of which is composed of a fibrous core covered to a variable depth by epithelial cells. The stroma is firm and carries the blood vessels of the tumor. The epithelial cells vary in size and are compactly arranged. The cells nearest the stroma are less mature, and it is from them that new cells are formed (Fig. 126). Papillomas arising from the skin or mucosa of the mouth or esophagus frequently

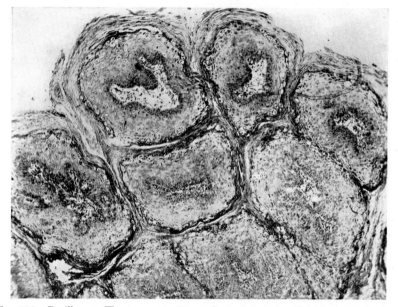

Fig. 126.—Papilloma. The separate units, each consisting of a fibrous core covered by epithelial cells, are characteristic (× 60).

present a horny deposit on the surface, between the various papillæ. This substance is keratin, and is the product of the more mature squamous epithelial cells. If the tumor has been subject to trauma, the more superficial cells may show evidence of necrosis, and leukocytes may be present.

Diagnostic characteristics.—Clinically, these growths are readily recognized by a warty-like projecting, or outward form of growth, a horny exterior, and a tendency to occur at the point of transition of skin and mucous membrane. Histologically, the tree-like projections of fibrous stroma covered by epithelial cells, which show no inclination

18

to infiltrate, but which grow in an outward rather than an inward direction, are typical of this tumor.

Clinical considerations.—The clinical diagnosis of papillomas of the interior of the body is seldom made, and their removal by operation is not feasible in the lower animals. In fact, this holds true for most internal neoplastic diseases, if subjects other than man are affected. Growths that occur externally in operable situations are usually removed without difficulty. Surgical removal of papillomas, if they are extensively multiple, is not practical. Occasionally, mild cases of papillary formations may be seen to disappear spontaneously in calves and colts.

Hobday has suggested that use of a saturated solution of tannic acid three times a day for several days is worthy of trial in cases in which tumors are multiple.

BIBLIOGRAPHY

1. Creech, G. T.: Experimental studies of the etiology of common warts in cattle. Jour. Agr. Res., 39: 723–737 (Nov. 15), 1929.

2. Eve, Henry: Quoted by Hobday.

3. Goldberg, S. A.: The occurrence of epithelial tumors in the domesticated animals. Am. Vet. Med. Assn., 58: 47–63 (Oct.), 1920.

4. Hobday, F. T. G.: Surgical diseases of the dog and cat. Chicago, Chicago Medical Book Co., 1925, pp. 144–147, and 158–159.

5. Joest, Ernst: Spezielle Pathologische Anatomie der Haustiere. Berlin, R. Schoetz, 3: 510, 1924.

6. Kinsley, A. T.: Ocular tumors with case reports. Am. Vet. Rev., 43: 291–294 (June), 1913.

7. Kinsley, A. T.: A text-book of veterinary pathology. Chicago, A. Eger, 1917, pp. 322–324.

8. Leese, A. S.: Papilloma in the bladder of a mare. Abstract: Am. Vet. Med. Assn., 50: 239, 1917.

9. Lisi, Garibaldi: Papilloma of the urethra and bladder in a cow. Abstract: Am. Vet. Rev., 37: 256–257 (May), 1910.

10. McFadyean, J. and Hobday, F.: Note on the experimental transmission of warts in the dog. Jour. Comp. Path. and Therap., 11: 341–344, 1902.

11. Polson, C. J.: Tumors of the rabbit. Jour. Path. and Bacteriol., 30: 603–614, 1927.

CHAPTER XVIII

EPITHELIOBLASTOMA (*Continued*)

ADENOMA

Definition.—An adenoma is a nonmalignant tumor consisting of epithelial cells and fibrous stroma, with the epithelial cells so arranged as to simulate a glandular structure.

Incidence.—These tumors seem to occupy an intermediate position between papillomas and true carcinomas. Available data tend to show that the majority of adenomas occur in the dog. In my fourteen cases, the tumor occurred nine times in the dog, twice in the common fowl, once in the sheep, and twice in cattle; the two cases in cattle occurred in a series of more than 200 neoplasms of this species, which suggests the comparative rarity of adenoma in this species and is hardly in accord with Kitt's statement that it is not infrequently seen in the liver of the ox. In my experience most of the epithelial tumors of the liver of the ox are malignant; they are either hepatic cell carcinomas or adenocarcinomas of the epithelium of the bile ducts. Among approximately forty neoplasms of the horse, none was an adenoma.

Since tumors of this type arise from glandular structures, they may be expected to appear in practically any of the situations in which a glandular type of epithelium normally occurs.

Bovine.—Aside from the adenomas of the liver mentioned by Kitt, these tumors are seldom observed in the ox. Boyd, Fitch, Grinnels and Billings reported a case of multiple adenoma of the pancreas in a ten-year-old cow, and a similar case was reported by Messner. Adenoma of the adrenal cortex is not uncommonly seen in cattle. I had the opportunity to study a mucoid type of papillary adenoma of the urinary bladder associated with calculi in a four-year-old cow.[9] The tumor consisted of a fleshy mass which was firmly attached to the mucosa of the body of the bladder by a rather broad base. Many small, yellowish, cystic foci were present throughout the tumor. A second tumor, that arose from the mucosa of the urinary bladder of a bovine, which was also designated papillary adenoma, presented a most remarkable appearance (Fig. 127). The interior was literally filled with hundreds of flattened, string-like prolongations of neoplastic tissue, many of which were approximately 5 cm. long. The bladder was enlarged at least four times normal size, and the walls were thick and somewhat edematous. These cases are of particular interest because of the comparative rarity of neoplasms affecting the urinary bladder in cattle. Adenoma of the urinary bladder of the bovine also has been reported by Berg and by Grips. A tumor which occurred in my series arose from the mucosa of the neck of the gallbladder, and projected in a papilliferous fashion into the interior of the gallbladder. Gallstones were absent, although the liver was infested with flukes. The literature also contains references to cases of adenoma of the gallbladder by Joest, Gozzini, and Zellhuber.

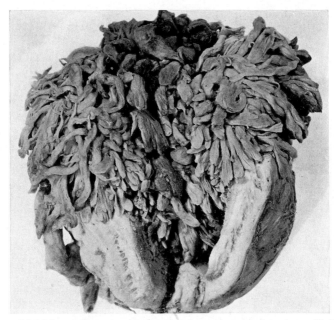

Fig. 127.—Multiple papillary cystadenoma of the mucosa of the urinary bladder of a bovine. The organ has been opened to show the neoplastic content.

Dog.—The glandular tissues of the dog are very susceptible to adenomatous tumors. They are particularly common in the mammary gland, where they are frequently characterized by an excessive amount of fibrous tissue (fibro-adenoma) (Fig. 128). Certain observers believe that these benign tumors may undergo progressive transition and become carcinomas.[12] The epithelial tumors of the mammary gland of the dog are not uncommonly associated with other neoplastic elements of a connective tissue character, such as fibrous tissue, cartilage, and bone. Adenomas sometimes originate in structures such as the sweat glands and sebaceous glands. The sebaceous glands of the concha, and the perianal glands, exhibit a special predilection for these growths. Adenomas not uncommonly originate in the intrapalpebral gland of the

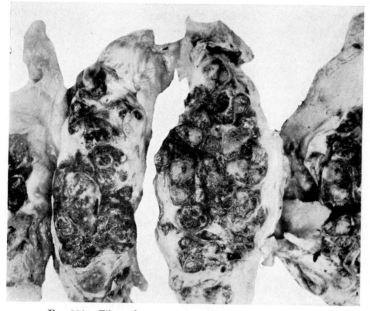

Fig. 128.—Fibro-adenoma of the mammary gland of a dog.

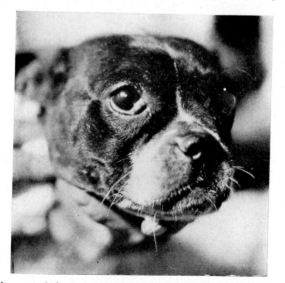

Fig. 129.—Adenoma of the intrapalpebral gland of the membrana nictitans of a dog.

membrana nictitans of young dogs, and are frequently bilateral (Fig. 129). In a rare case reported by Penberth an adenoma was found in the right lateral ventricle of the brain of an old bulldog. In male dogs aged more than ten years, hypertrophy of the parenchyma of the prostate gland is common and many of these become definitely neoplastic. Some of the specimens attain considerable size. Wooldridge described adenoma of the prostate gland of a dog, which weighed 840 gm. Such adenomas are often papillary, and exhibit a strong tendency to form cysts. I observed an adenoma of the dog which clearly had its forerunner in the mucosa of the small intestine. Three other tumors of the sebaceous type arose, respectively, from the skin of the eyelid, the skin of the metatarsal region, and the skin of the concha. Another specimen was obtained from the margin of the liver. Although there was no doubt about the histologic character of the growth, its exact histogenesis was not definitely determined. Cohrs, in a case of multiple neoplasms in a fourteen-year-old dachshund, found an adenoma of the right testis, and a papillary adenoma of the lung.

Other species.—I have observed a tumor in the lung of a sheep which probably arose from the bronchial mucous glands. In sheep, the possible relations to pulmonary infection, of tumor-like adenomatous changes in the lungs, has been the subject of considerable investigation. In this connection, mention should be made of the adenomatous epithelial proliferations, of neoplastic type, which have been described as occurring in the lungs of South African sheep affected with a specific form of catarrhal pneumonia, known as jagziekte. Such lesions which have been described by Mitchell, Cowdry, and by deKock are characterized in the early stages by multiple papillary proliferations of epithelium derived, in the majority of instances according to deKock, from the alveolar epithelium, although the epithelium of the bronchioles may also contribute to the proliferative foci. As the growth continues, definitely circumscribed nodules result, which may become confluent, and eventually the lesions resemble, according to Cowdry, adenoma of the mammary glands. Although grossly and microscopically the lesions have many of the features associated with malignancy, mitotic division is rarely observed, and metastasis even to the regional lymph nodes does not occur. As the disease progresses, acute catarrhal pneumonia may become evident, to which the animal succumbs. DeKock concluded that the process represents true neoplasia.

The observations of Cowdry and Marsh would indicate that lesions comparable to those which are characteristic of jagziekte occur in the lungs of sheep affected with progressive pneumonia.

Multiple adenomas in the fourth stomach of a sheep were described by Zietzschmann.

Adenoma of the horse has been reported infrequently. Aveston reported an adenoma of the kidney in a horse, and Kinsley mentioned a case of adenoma of the sebaceous glands of the tail of a horse. Kinsley also recorded the presence of an adenoma in the frontal sinus of a mule. Lüerseen reported an adenoma of the right ureter of a horse, and Jantze described a fibro-adenoma of the rectum of a horse.

Adenomatous overgrowths in the thyroid glands of horses which are without question of a neoplastic nature are not uncommon. In Litty's study of 300 horses in western Europe, he noted benign adenomatous changes in the thyroid glands of 27 per cent. These included 170 geldings, of which fifty-seven (33.5 per cent) were affected, and 130 mares, of which thirty (23 per cent) were affected. Leth found, in a study of

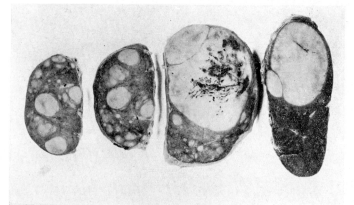

Fig. 130.—Adenomas of the thyroid gland. The material was derived from two different horses. The first three specimens were obtained from one animal, whereas the specimen on the right was secured from another.

200 horses, that approximately 50 per cent of all horses aged more than ten years had adenomas of the thyroid gland (Fig. 130).

More recently Schlotthauer, in an examination of the thyroid glands of 100 horses in southeastern Minnesota, found adenomas in 37 per cent of the animals (Fig. 131).

An adenoma from the mammary gland of a sow is reported by Allen. Koyama reported a case of multiple adenoma of the uterus of a rabbit in which there was one tumor in the right horn and three tumors in the left. The mammary gland of the affected animal became large, and milk was secreted. Polson found the uterus the most common site of tumors in rabbits; the majority were either adenomas or adenocarcinomas. He also noted an adenoma of the pituitary gland in a rabbit.

Fox, in material from captive wild mammals, observed a papillary adenoma of the gastric mucosa in a baboon; papillary adenoma of the prostate gland of a ring-tailed lemur; fibro-adenoma of the uterus and bile ducts in a jaguar; adenoma of the bile ducts in two foxes, and adenoma of the pancreatic ducts in one fox; adenoma of the pancreas in a racoon; adenoma of the liver in a woodchuck; fibro-adenoma of the bile ducts in the common deer, and adenoma of the kidney in an opossum. He also reported several adenomas of the kidney in birds. I found a cystadenoma in the abdomen of a chicken; the exact point of origin was not determined, and Calvanico reported an adenoma of the intestines of a fowl.

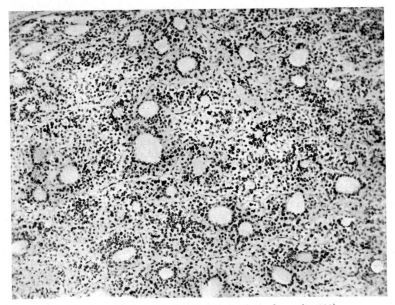

Fig. 131.—Adenoma of the thyroid gland of a horse (× 120).

Effects on the host.—In a manner comparable to papilloma the true adenoma exerts an objectionable influence through mechanical interference with the proper functioning of the part. Simple adenomas do not invade and destroy tissue like carcinoma. However, they may assume malignant aggressiveness, in which case, of course, they are known as adenocarcinomas. When these tumors occur in the intrapalpebral gland of the eye, they interfere with vision to some extent.

The involvement of a vital organ is always grave, particularly in the lower animals, because of the difficulties of surgical procedures in the larger cavities of the body. Adenomas in the liver or lung consequently must be considered serious. External tumors are disfiguring. Large adenomas of the mammæ may interfere with the movements of the animal, and because of their pendulous character, they are subject to considerable trauma. Cystic degeneration may result in considerable pressure exerted on adjacent tissues. This will be serious or not, depending on the importance of the part which is encroached on. In the case of adenoma of the brain reported by Penberth the animal gave evidence of mental deterioration and slight deafness; the pupils were dilated, and although appetite continued good, the animal rapidly became emaciated. In Wooldridge's case of adenoma of the prostate gland of a dog associated with adenocarcinoma of the liver, the animal was able to urinate in a normal manner even though the prostatic tumor weighed 840 gm. It is possible that horses with adenoma of the thyroid gland may suffer vague metabolic disturbances. This condition is worthy of serious clinical investigation.

Metastasis and malignancy.—Simple adenoma never infiltrates or gives rise to secondary foci by metastasis. When adenomas take on malign tendencies they are known as adenocarcinomas and must be considered with the true carcinomas. The possibility of certain adenomas being the point of origin of true carcinoma is of sufficient significance to justify the earliest possible removal of all operable adenomas, particularly those of the perianal glands and the mammæ.

Appearance.—Generally, adenomas are encapsulated, nodular, firm to soft swellings, depending on the proportion of stroma to parenchyma and on the presence or absence of cystic cavitations. They possess a generous blood supply, which often imparts to the tumor a flesh-pink color. They vary from less than 1 cm. to several centimeters in diameter. The size is often dependent on formation of cysts. They usually occur singly, but occasionally multiple forms are observed. Those that arise from the cells of the sweat and sebaceous glands often present a dirty, greasy appearance due to the secretion of the type cell and the absence of excretory ducts (Fig. 132).

Microscopically, the typical adenoma consists of a neoplastic overgrowth of epithelial cells arranged in a manner suggestive of a gland, a duct, or a tubular structure. The mimicry, however, is never complete, and functional excretory ducts are not provided. Alveolar spaces are frequently formed, although in many portions of the tumor these spaces may be obliterated, as a consequence of which the cells appear in compact masses (Figs. 133 to 137). The type cell will depend, of course, on the character of the parent epithelial cell from which the tumor cell arose. The parenchyma of the tumor rests on a fibrous stroma, which also

carries the blood supply. Evidence of an infiltrating, destructive type
of growth is missing (Fig. 134).

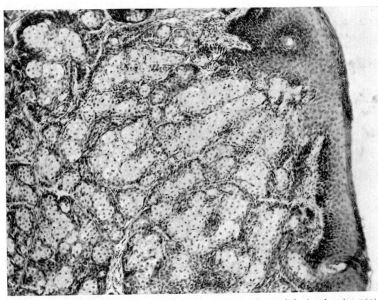

FIG. 132.—Adenoma of the sebaceous cell type, from the eyelid of a dog (× 100).

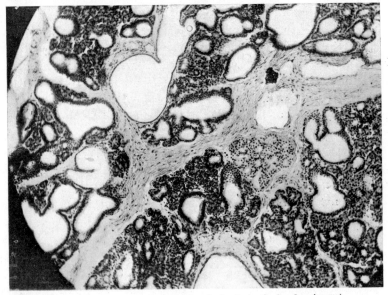

FIG. 133.—Adenoma of the intrapalpebral gland of a dog (× 75).

It often happens that the connective tissue elements of the stroma
of an adenoma grows more rapidly than the parenchyma of the tumor,

and as a consequence the fibrous stroma predominates and the epithelial cells are compressed into tortuous rows, or into small, compact nests. This form of adenoma is conveniently designated fibro-adenoma, and is most often seen in the mammary glands of bitches. Again, the epithelial elements may proliferate so rapidly as to exhibit an overwhelming tendency to form irregular, cyst-like cavities of variable size. An adenoma of this type is conveniently termed a cystadenoma (Fig. 135). Because the excretory ducts are absent, the cysts of such a tumor may be tremendously dilated, and of such a size as to be plainly visible to the unaided eye. The nature of the cystic content depends on the type of cell responsible for its production, and varies from fluid to gelatinous

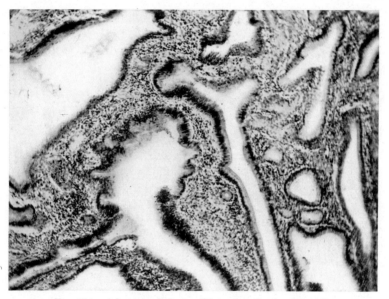

Fig. 134.—Adenoma of the small intestine of a dog (× 100).

consistence. The lining cells of a cystadenoma are often projected at irregular intervals into the interior of the cysts, in slender, finger-like fashion. This type of adenoma is called a papillary cystadenoma (Fig. 136). Examples of this variety of adenoma are often seen in the prostate glands of dogs. The term "papillary adenoma" or "papillary cystadenoma," may be properly applied to tumors that arise from the mucosa of hollow organs, and which are characterized by the occurrence of multiple adenomatous prolongations of tissue, with or without formation of cysts which project into the lumen of the organ.

Clinical considerations.—Although histologically the true adenoma is noninfiltrating and benign, clinically it must be considered as potenti-

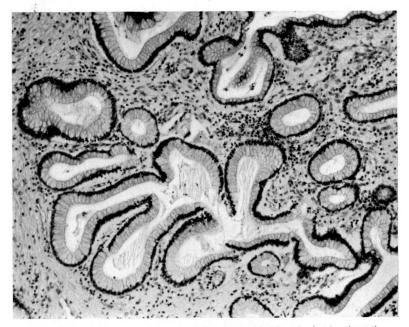

FIG. 135.—Papillary cystadenoma of the urinary bladder of a bovine (× 75).

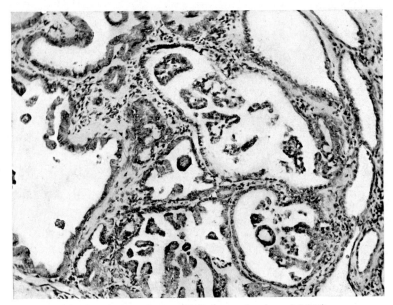

FIG. 136.—Cystadenoma of the lungs of a sheep (× 130).

ally dangerous, for, as previously mentioned, true carcinoma may arise, in some instances, from simple adenoma. For this reason, early sur-

gical removal is desirable in every case, if the tumor is in an operable
position. Because of encapsulation, removal of most adenomas is attended with very little difficulty, and with slight danger to the patient.
The exception is mammary adenomas of the dog. In such cases a high
percentage of fatalities may be expected following operation, due, no
doubt, to so-called surgical shock. A great many adenomas are very
vascular, and the control of hemorrhage which occurs as a consequence
of their surgical removal is often difficult. Adenomas seldom recur
when properly removed.

   Diagnostic characteristics.—Adenoma may be confused with carcinoma, and clinically it will be of assistance if it is kept in mind that

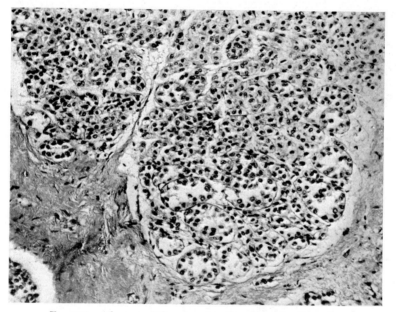

Fig. 137.—Adenoma of the adrenal cortex of a bovine (× 150).

adenomas are usually encapsulated and do not infiltrate the surrounding
tissue or give rise to metastasis.

   Tumors of dogs which occur at the inner canthus of the eye, or the
concha, or around the anus, usually are adenomas. However, the possibility of simple adenoma undergoing malignant change makes it
imperative to resort to the microscope for diagnosis in every case.
Microscopically, it is necessary to distinguish between adenoma, which
is benign, and adenocarcinoma, which is malignant, and capable of
causing grave consequences. In adenoma is found a more or less adult
type of epithelial cell, with few, if any, mitotic figures, and although the

epithelial elements represent an atypical overgrowth, the tumors grow by expansion, and evidence of infiltration and destruction of the adjacent tissue is not seen.

BIBLIOGRAPHY

1. Allen, I. W.: Adenoma from mammary gland of sow. Case report. Am. Jour. Vet. Med., **11**: 896 (Nov.), 1916.

2. Aveston, J. J.: Adenoma of the kidney in a horse. Abstract: Am. Vet. Med. Assn., **53**: 414–415 (June), 1918.

3. Berg, V.: Quoted by Fölger.

4. Boyd, W. L., Fitch, C. P., Grinnels, C. D., and Billings, W. A.: Cavernous hemangioma of the liver together with multiple adenoma of the pancreas. Case report. Cornell Vet., **9**: 169–170 (Jan.), 1919.

5. Calvanico, R.: L'adenoma de pollo. Policlinico (Sez. chir.), **33**: 1–12, 1926. Abstr. in: Cancer Rev., **2**: 153–154 (April), 1927.

6. Cohrs, Paul: Über primäre Multiplizität von Geschwülsten bei Haustieren. Ztschr. f. Krebsforsch., **24**: 156–221, 1926–1927.

7. Cowdry, E. V.: Studies on the etiology of jagziekte. I. Primary lesions. Jour. Exper. Med., **42**: 323–333 (Sept.), 1925.

8. Cowdry, E. V. and Marsh, Hadleigh: Comparative pathology of South African jagziekte and Montana progressive pneumonia of sheep. Jour. Exper. Med., **45**: 511–586 (April 1), 1927.

9. Feldman, W. H.: Papillary adenoma of the urinary bladder in the ox. Report of a case. Am. Jour. Path., **6**: 205–208 (March), 1930.

10. Fölger, A. F.: Geschwülste bei Tieren. Ergebn. d. all. path. u. Path. Anat., **18**: 372–676, 1917.

11. Fox, Herbert: Disease in captive wild mammals and birds; incidence, description, comparison. Philadelphia, J. B. Lippincott, 1923, pp. 477–482.

12. French, Cecil: Surgical diseases and surgery of the dog. Chicago, A. Eger, 1923.

13. Gozzini: Quoted by Fölger.

14. Grips: Quoted by Fölger.

15. Jantze: Quoted by Fölger.

16. Joest: Quoted by Fölger.

17. Kinsley, A. T.: A text-book of veterinary pathology. Chicago, A. Eger, 1917, p. 330.

18. Kitt, Theodor: Text-book of comparative pathology. Chicago, Chicago Medical Book Co., 1906, p. 392.

19. deKock, G.: Are the lesions of jagziekte in sheep of the nature of a neoplasm? Fifteenth Annual Report of the Director of Vet. Service, Union of South Africa, 611–641 (Oct.), 1929.

20. Koyama, Masamichi: Ein Fall von Uterusadenom bei Kaninchen. Nebst einen Befund über Hypertrophie und Fettsekretion der Milchdrüse dieses Tieres. Gann, **21**: 7–8 (March), 1927.

21. Leth, C.: Quoted by Fölger.

22. Litty, A.: Quoted by Fölger.

23. Lüerssen: Adenome in rechten Ureter eines Pferdes. Ein Beitrag zur Kenntnis des Vorkommens der Tumoren bei den Haustieren. Deutsch. tierärztl. Wchnschr., **19**: 596, 1911.

24. Messner, E.: Notiz über multiple Pankreasadenome beim Rinde. Deutsch. tierärztl. Wchnschr., **17**: 396, 1909.

25. Mitchell, D. T.: Investigations into jagzietke. Third and Fourth Reports of the Director of Vet. Research, Union of South Africa, 585–614, 1915.

26. Penberth, J.: Tumours in the brain of a dog. Jour. Comp. Path., 10: 75, 1897.

27. Polson, C. J.: Tumours of the rabbit. Jour. Path. and Bacteriol., 30: 603–614, 1927.

28. Schlotthauer, C. F.: The incidence and types of disease of the thyroid gland of adult horses. Jour. Am. Vet. Med. Assn., 78: 211–218 (Feb.), 1931.

29. Wooldridge, G. H.: Adenoma of the prostate and adeno-carcinoma of the liver in a dog. Abstr.: Am. Vet. Rev., 42: 223 (Nov.), 1912.

30. Zellhuber: Über die Zottengeschwülste der Gallen blase beim Rind. Monatschr. f. Tierh., 13: 97, 1902.

31. Zietzschmann, H.: Quoted by Fölger.

CHAPTER XIX

EPITHELIOBLASTOMA (*Continued*)

CARCINOMA

Carcinoma is so widespread, and its presence is such a menace to life that it must be properly considered the most important neoplasm affecting lower animals.

Definition.—A carcinoma is made up of epithelial cells which proliferate in an atypical and lawless manner, exhibit a tendency to infiltrate and destroy the surrounding tissues, and are likely to set up distant foci by metastasis. It will be convenient, in consideration of carcinoma, to include the malignant adenomatous tumors usually designated as adenocarcinomas. An adenocarcinoma is a true carcinoma, which is characterized by an adenomatous, glandular, or duct-like arrangement of the parenchymatous cells. In the remarks which follow, the word carcinoma refers to malignant epithelial tumors in general, unless otherwise indicated.

Incidence.—Hutchinson, in 1901, wrote: ". . . the most striking thing about cancer is its rarity in the lower animals, whether wild or domesticated." Since this was said at a period before a great deal was known concerning the occurrence of neoplasms in the different species of animals, Hutchinson's opinion was perhaps justifiable. However, the proved ubiquity of carcinoma in vertebrates, including fish and rodents, and the data which have been collected since then make it clearly evident that instead of carcinoma being a rarity in lower animals it is rather common.

The apparent rarity of the disease can well be explained: As has been said before, the great majority of meat-producing animals are killed before they attain carcinoma age. Dogs, dairy cattle, and horses are generally permitted to attain what would be considered middle or old age for the respective species. In these animals the incidence of carcinoma is perhaps comparable to that for man. However, tumors of animals have not incited the same interest among the laity as have tumors of man. Even the veterinarian has not always shown the proper interest in this phase of comparative medicine, and as a consequence much of value which might have been contributed has been lost. In my collection of more than 500 neoplasms, carcinoma constitutes about a third of all neoplasms encountered in eleven different species.

Reliable statistics bearing on incidence of carcinoma in domestic animals are too meager to justify drawing definite conclusions as to what portion of the animal population may be affected with the disease. The only data that can be given with confidence is the relative incidence or frequency of the respective types of tumor in the various species, although the comprehensive figures contributed by Sticker on the frequency of the disease in different species are perhaps significant. Murray's figures are of interest. Of forty-nine malignant new growths affecting the dog, twenty-three were carcinomas, and he found seven malignant epitheliomas in a total of eleven malignant new growths in the cat. Of twelve malignant tumors in the horse, nine were carcinomas, and twenty-two of twenty-four malignant growths in cattle studied by Murray were carcinomas. Attesting to the relative infrequency of carcinoma in horses are the statistics of Sticker. Of 215,037 horses observed in a period of twenty-two years at the Berlin Veterinary High School, only 103 cases of carcinoma were encountered. Since these figures were obtained from a study of animals which were presented for treatment they cannot be accepted as indicative of the correct incidence of carcinoma in horses as a whole. Crocker's statistics are more exact. In a total of 768 postmortem examinations of horses, twenty-two (2.9 per cent) were found to have carcinomas. Crocker reported finding eight carcinomas at necropsy of 1,548 dogs (0.51 per cent).

The use of horse flesh for food has made it possible to obtain additional data concerning the incidence of carcinoma in this animal. Martel[22] studied this problem from material secured from 39,800 horses slaughtered in the abattoirs of Paris; 184 animals (0.50 per cent), the majority of which were aged more than fifteen years, were affected with carcinoma.

In a series of 177 carcinomas encountered among 510 neoplasms of lower animals, I found the various species affected as follows: Bovine, eighty-nine; horse, eighteen; dog, twenty-eight; chicken, fifteen; sheep, twenty-three; hog, three, and guinea pig, one. Fadyean, in the clinic of the Royal Veterinary College, studied sixty-three malignant epithelial tumors in a period of six years. The tumors were distributed among the different species as follows: Horse, thirty-one; dog, twenty-three; bovine, five; cat, two, and sheep, two. Fröhner[36] observed twenty carcinomas (18 per cent) among a series of 107 neoplasms obtained from horses presented at the Veterinary Clinic in Berlin, and Sticker reported carcinoma in 5.5 per cent of 1,306 dogs examined. Semmer, in

19

an examination of 3,525 dogs, found carcinoma in 8 per cent. Fröhner,[39] at the Berlin Veterinary High School, reported carcinoma in 1,154 (1.9 per cent) of 60,471 canines. In a study of 300 cattle affected with malignant disease, the majority of which were classified as "aged," Trotter[121] found 279 carcinomas. Trotter's figures suggest the marked susceptibility of older cattle to malignant epithelial neoplasms.

Ehrenreich, in approximately 2,000 adult chickens prepared for cooking, found seven malignant tumors, five of which were carcinomas.

I found three carcinomas among seventy-six tumors from swine. Of fifty-three tumors of chickens fifteen were carcinomas. Tumors of sheep are not common, yet of the forty such tumors which I examined, twenty-three were carcinomas. An adenocarcinoma of the thyroid gland of a guinea pig was found in 1,053 postmortem examinations of this animal. Of forty tumors of the horse, eighteen were carcinomas. Of 214 tumors of cattle, eighty-nine (approximately 40 per cent), were true carcinomas. Of seventy-eight tumors of dogs, twenty-eight were carcinomas.

It is obvious, from the foregoing, that the incidence of carcinoma in lower animals differs in the respective species; carcinomas occur, perhaps, with greatest frequency in horses, dogs, and cattle. Swine are seldom affected. In Fadyean's series of sixty-three malignant epitheliomas, none was observed in a hog, and in Sticker's list of approximately 1,200 malignant neoplasms of common domestic animals, only twelve were obtained from swine. This number included seven tumors of the kidney, and since the majority of such tumors in swine are not carcinomas, but embryonal neoplasms of a mixed type, it is possible that all those in Sticker's series were not true carcinomas. These data substantiate the common conception that aside from tumors which arise as a result of a congenital anomaly, such as embryonal nephromas, swine are relatively free from tumorous growths. It is unnecessary to call attention, again, to the effect which slaughter of swine at a comparatively early age may have on apparent incidence. The same holds true for sheep in the United States. There can be no question, however, that the incidence of tumor increases as the age of a given population is extended.

Relation to age.[32]—The majority of carcinomas are observed in older animals. Ten to fifteen years is a common age for carcinoma of the horse. In one series of thirteen horses with carcinomas I found the average age to be approximately eleven years. Figures from a French source[22] show that of 39,800 horses slaughtered for food, and hence subject to careful postmortem examination, only four of the 184 carcinomas observed occurred in horses aged less than twelve years. In this study, most of the animals were old, which is usually the case if horses are slaughtered for food. Sticker gave the age incidence in ninety horses affected with malignant epithelial new growths as follows: Less than four years, 2.2 per cent; five to six years, 4.2 per cent; seven to eight years, 10 per cent; nine to ten years, 15.5 per cent; eleven to twelve years, 9 per cent; thirteen to fourteen years, 11 per cent; fifteen to sixteen years, 17.7 per cent; seventeen to eighteen years, 12.2 per cent; nineteen to twenty years, 14.4 per cent, and twenty-three to twenty-five years, 5.3 per cent.

Most dogs that have carcinoma can no longer be considered young. The age distribution of seventy dogs with carcinomas reported by Sticker was as follows: Two to three years, 14.3 per cent; five to six years, 25 per cent; seven to eight years, 28.5 per cent; nine to ten years, 20 per cent; eleven to twelve years, 5.7 per cent, and twelve to fifteen years, 5.7 per cent. In 100 cases of malignant epithelial neoplasia of dogs observed by Cadiot and Almy the age distribution was as follows: One to three years, 6 per cent; three to five years, 18 per cent; six to nine years, 33 per cent; nine to twelve years, 26 per cent; twelve to fifteen years, 14 per cent, and fifteen to twenty years, 3 per cent.

In cattle perhaps younger age incidence is observed than in horses or dogs, although the majority of carcinomas of cattle occur during or after what might be considered middle age. In Trotter's[121] series of 300 cattle with tumors, the majority of which were carcinomas, only three were aged less than three years; the other 297 were aged. The earliest age at which I have observed carcinoma to occur in cattle was one year. This was a case of carcinoma of the eye.

The possible influence of age on the occurrence of carcinoma in chickens is suggested by the observations of Ehrenreich who found five carcinomas in examination of 2,000 adults. In 3,000 cockerels aged less than one year tumors were not found.

Although the majority of tumors may appear in a certain period of life, nevertheless, there is evidence to justify the conclusion that most carcinomas in lower animals occur after the animal has passed from young into adult life or old age.

Anatomic inception.—The widespread distribution of epithelium provides generous possibilities for the development of tumors, and it is not surprising that so many epithelial tumors are observed. Carcinomas may arise from the following types of epithelium: Epithelium such as constitutes the integument of the body and makes up certain mucous membranes, and different varieties of simple columnar epithelium such as lines the uterus, the gastro-intestinal tract, and various excretory ducts, and that which constitutes different glandular structures such as the thyroid gland and the mammary gland. Carcinoma may arise from embryonic epithelium which has been misplaced or not utilized in fetal development, and the germinal epithelium of the ovary constitutes a possible origin for certain ovarian carcinomas.

Horse.—In this animal the eye and its appendages appear to be particularly prone to carcinoma; there were eight among eighteen carcinomas of horses in my collection. Most carcinomas of the eye arise in

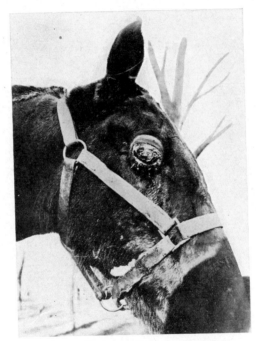

Fig. 138.—Carcinoma of the eye of a horse.

the membrana nictitans, although any of the related epithelial tissues may be implicated (Fig. 138). The penis also gives evidence of predilection for carcinoma, and next to the eye it is, perhaps, the most common site. In Sticker's series of 119 carcinomas of the horse, involving the integument, fifty-two affected the penis and eleven the vulva. The prepuce may be the point of origin of carcinoma that also frequently arises from the tissues of the alveoli of the molar teeth, the gums, and the maxillary sinuses (Fig. 139). The mucosa of the nasal passages is frequently involved.

Carcinoma of the stomach of the horse has been reported several times, although it must be considered rare. Sticker's compiled series of 311 primary carcinomas of the horse contained eight which affected the stomach. He called attention to the fact that although approximately a third of all carcinomas of man affect the stomach, only about 3 per cent of carcinomas of the horse affect this organ. The distribution in Sticker's series of 311 carcinomas of the horse was as follows: Penis, fifty-two cases; nose and nasal passage, fifty-two cases; kidney, twenty-nine cases; skin, twenty-two cases; vagina, eighteen cases; eye, fourteen cases; urinary bladder, fourteen cases; testis, thirteen cases; lung, thirteen cases; gums, eleven cases; stomach, eight cases; mammary gland, eight cases; uterus, eight cases; thyroid gland, eight cases; anus, eight cases; larynx, seven cases; intestines, five cases; adrenal gland,

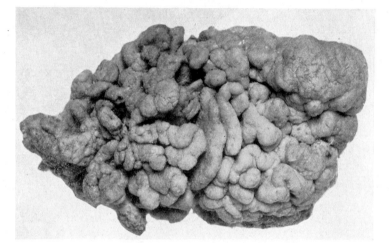

FIG. 139.—Papillary carcinoma of the prepuce of a horse.

five cases; upper lip, four cases; ovary, four cases; liver, three cases; pharyngeal cavity, three cases; prostate gland, one case, and thymus, one case. Friedberger and Fröhner mentioned Petit and Faget's case, in which a large ulcerating cauliflower-like carcinoma was found in the cardiac end of the stomach. They also mentioned Fadyean's case of primary carcinoma in the stomach, with metastasis to the liver, peritoneum, and mesentery. Fadyean found three gastric carcinomas in twenty-six tumors of horses. They arose from the cardiac portion of the stomach, which in the horse is lined with squamous epithelium, and exhibited marked local destructiveness; two of the tumors had metastasized. The remainder of the carcinomas arose as follows: seven from the penis; three from the tail; four from the antrum; two from the urinary bladder; one from the vulva and one from the mammary gland (adenocarcinoma). Fadyean also encountered five cases of adenocarcinoma of the kidney, in all of which there was metastasis to the omentum. Krammell also reported a case of carcinoma in the stomach of a horse. Ball and Lombard described a primary papilliferous carcinoma of the urinary bladder of a mare, with secondary nodules in the uterus, and Law quoted Cadéac to the effect that carcinoma of the urinary bladder of the horse may metastasize to all the abdominal organs. Ehlers observed an adenocarcinoma of the colon, and Kitt mentioned a primary carcinoma of the ovary, with secondary foci in the serous surface of the liver and omentum. According to Siedamgrotzky, adenomatous polyps of the intestine of the horse may undergo transitional changes and become definitely adenocarcinomatous.

A somewhat unusual case of multiple epithelioma in a nine-year-old mare was described by D'Arcy Power.[73] The tumors, which were of variable sizes, involved both the skin and subcutaneous tissue and were distributed on the outside of the hind legs from the hocks to the croup. They were also found over the abdomen and on the forelegs.

Quentin reported an extremely interesting case of carcinoma of the pancreas in a fifteen-year-old gelding. The pancreas was practically destroyed by the growth, which was also adherent to the stomach. Death resulted from hemorrhage from a perforated stomach. According to D'Arcy Power,[73] carcinoma of the tongue has been known to occur in the horse, and Crocker reported a carcinoma of the spermatic cord. A carcinoma of the clitoris was reported by Eberlein.

A most unusual case of carcinoma in the horse is that reported by Fröhner.[37] The animal had died with symptoms of internal hemorrhage and a carcinoma of the adrenal cortex was found which was "twice the size of a man's head." A tear in the anterior portion of the tumor was responsible for the hemorrhage which resulted in the animal's death.

Cunningham described a case of mammary carcinoma in an eleven-year-old mare which had experienced five pregnancies. The tumor had been noticed for a year, and weighed 30 pounds. There was much sloughing of the tissue, with ulceration and serious hemorrhage. Cunningham mentioned metastasis to the lungs, but did not make this point definite.

Udall, Fincher, and Gibbons reported carcinoma of the duodenum of a fifteen-year-old gelding. The tumor, which was approximately 15 cm. in diameter, was associated with ascites and peritonitis. A carcinoma of the bile duct of a horse was described by Grüttner.

Carcinoma of the thyroid gland, although rather commonly seen in dogs and occasionally in cattle, seems to occur but rarely in the horse. Although simple adenomas are present in the thyroid gland of a considerable percentage of old horses, epithelial malignancy is seldom seen. In view of Schlotthauer's failure to find carcinoma in a careful study of thyroid glands of 100 horses, 37 per cent of which were adenomatous, the case described by Pfeiffer is of much interest. The animal was a mare aged sixteen years in which a tumor about 12 cm. in diameter (kindskopfgrossen) developed in the region of the thyroid gland. The growth infiltrated the adjacent tissues and completely surrounded the trachea. Metastasis occurred to the lungs and the bronchial lymph nodes. Woundenberg also reported four cases of carcinoma of the thyroid gland of the horse. The animals were all old and the tumors had metastasized.

It is evident that the majority of malignant epithelial neoplasms of the horse originate externally from cells of the integument. The greater percentage of tumors arise from the skin proper, the penis, the eye and its appendages, the vulva, the mucosa of the nasal passages, the tissue lining the maxillary sinuses, and that of the gums and the alveoli of the molar teeth. Internally the kidney is most often affected. Carcinoma of the gastro-intestinal tract, and of the uterus, lungs, and thyroid gland is rarely observed. The stomach is rarely affected; carcinoma of this organ arises from the squamous epithelium of the cardiac portion.

Ox.—In my experience carcinoma in the ox is most common in the region of the eye and its appendages (Fig. 140). Carcinoma of the eye, in fact, is the most common of external tumors of cattle; in my series it constituted about 31 per cent of carcinomas obtained from this species.

The apparent susceptibility of the Hereford breed to carcinoma of the eye has been noted many times. Among stockmen in the western part of the United States the Hereford breed particularly is known to be affected with carcinoma of the eye, although no satisfactory explanation is made of the relatively high incidence in this breed. It is of interest to note that Voges, in reporting the occurrence of carcinoma of the eye of South American cattle, observed that the disease occurred only in animals of the Hereford breed. He also noted that those affected had white heads and that the disease never occurred in animals with a zone of red hair around the eye. Among the possible etiologic factors advanced by cattlemen as responsible for this tumor is the prolonged irritation of the mucosa of the eye by sand and other irritants, and the lack of pigment in the surrounding mucosa. Neither factor appears adequate to explain this apparent predilection.

In one group in my series of twenty-five cattle affected with carcinoma of the eye, fifteen were Herefords. In the same group carcinoma of the eye was found in seven Holstein cattle. Carcinoma of the eyes of cattle has also been observed in the following breeds: Jersey, shorthorn, Guernsey, Durham, and brown Swiss. Apparently breed does not confer immunity to this rather prevalent neoplasm, and the explanation of its occurrence must be sought elsewhere.

As regards the possible influence of pigmentation on the occurrence of carcinoma of the eye, it is apropos to give here the results of an in-

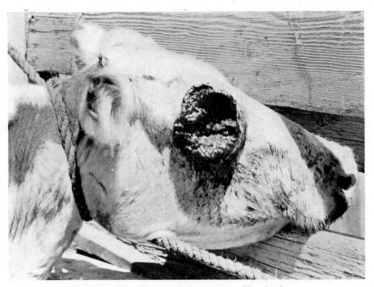

Fig. 140.—Carcinoma of the eye of a Hereford cow.

vestigation conducted by Davis and Leeper concerning the presence of pigment in the eyes of the various breeds of cattle slaughtered at a Denver, Colorado, packing house. They wrote: "The eyes of some five hundred cattle were examined, the majority of them being Herefords. From our observations we came to the following conclusions: The typical white face Herefords show no visible pigmentation. In several instances we have noted that in some lots of Hereford cattle where an animal has red spots on the face, especially around the eyes, there is some pigmentation either in the membrana nictitans or the lacrimal gland and sometimes in both. In the Shorthorn breed the majority of those examined showed pigmentation, while in some there was no evidence of it especially in the few roans we had occasion to examine. All other breeds of cattle showed more or less pigmentation, this condition being more pronounced in the Holstein breed."

From the foregoing it is difficult not to recognize pigmentation or the lack of it as of significance in the incidence of carcinoma of the eye, since the disease is without question more commonly found in the pigment-free mucosa of the eyes of Herefords than in the same tissues of other breeds which possess pigment to a greater degree.

Concerning the possible influence of lack of pigmentation on the occurrence of carcinoma of the skin of cattle, Drabble[18] recorded some interesting observations. He described the intense dermatitis which is set up in white skin only by sensitization to sunlight following ingestion of certain skin-sensitizing plants which grow in Australia. The lesions cause intense itching and considerable scabbing as a consequence of the animal's frequent rubbing the affected parts against any available object to allay the irritation. From some of these areas papillomatous formations develop, and a certain number is definitely carcinomatous. Drabble, in a period of four years, found 190 carcinomas of the skin of 955,798 cattle examined; 137 (72.1 per cent) of the tumors occurred in nonpigmented portions of the skin. In addition, the thirty roan animals which were affected were considered so lightly pigmented as to be approaching white. These observations seem to suggest that chronic dermatitis due to photosensitization of unpigmented or lightly pigmented skin, must be regarded as significant in the inception of certain carcinomas of the skin of cattle. Drabble was of the opinion that the term "brand cancer" has often been used incorrectly for conditions which are unrelated to branding. Only three of the carcinomas in his series were considered as having arisen from old brand scars.

It is possible that the explanation offered by Drabble for the inception of carcinoma of nonpigmented skin may suggest a clue to the etiology of carcinoma of the eye which occurs with greatest frequency in tissue deficient in pigment, particularly in Hereford cattle.

Carcinoma of the eyes and their appendages usually begins in the mucosa of the lower lid or the membrana nictitans. Rarely both eyes are affected. In the initial stages the eye proper is seldom involved, although later it may be completely destroyed. Occasionally the surrounding osseous structures may be affected. Metastasis to the regional lymph nodes and to the lungs is common.

From the available data based on the observations of Federal meat inspectors, from pathologists who study animal tissue, and from my own experience, I must conclude that carcinoma of the tissues of the orbital space is perhaps the most common epithelial malignant neoplasm of the ox. I believe that it occurs more often than the figures of Loeb would indicate. Loeb mentioned the discovery of only forty-eight cases of carcinoma of the eye during the examination of more than 2,500,000 cattle.

Carcinoma has been observed in cattle in other, widely separated organs. In Sticker's series, seventy-three carcinomas of cattle were distributed among the respective organs and tissues as follows: Uterus, sixteen cases; kidney, ten cases; urinary bladder, nine cases; ovary, six cases; stomach (probably rumen), six cases; liver, four cases; lung, three cases; vagina, three cases; skin, two cases; eye, two cases; penis, two cases; nasal passage, two cases; larynx, two cases; upper lip, one case; parotid gland, one case; mammary gland, one case; adrenal gland, one case; prostate gland, one case, and intestine, one case. Kitt[64] also mentioned squamous-cell carcinoma of the urinary bladder of a cow, and Goldberg reported a "granulose-celled" ovarian carcinoma in a two-year-old Holstein cow. The tumor had metastasized to the adjacent lymph nodes, peritoneum, and mammary gland. In a similar case reported by Goldberg the tumor was removed surgically before metastasis had occurred. Scheidt found a large carcinoma, about 8 cm. in diameter, in the urinary bladder of a cow which for two years had had hematuria.

Trotter[118] observed three cases of carcinoma of the rumen, all of which had metastasized. In one case in which the tumor was described as a "fungoid ulcerating growth" metastatic foci were found in the kidneys, both lungs, and multicentrically in the liver. The lymph nodes of the respective organs were affected. Trotter also saw a carcinoma in the lower half of the left lung which had metastasized throughout both lungs as well as to the heart and kidneys.

Two squamous-cell carcinomas of the rumen, one of which had metastasized to a regional lymph node, were described by deKock. Kitt observed an adenocarcinoma of the true stomach (abomasum) of a bovine which must be considered as occurring but rarely. Pfab reported a carcinoma which was situated between two loops of the colon. Metastasis had occurred to the liver.

Murray reported four cases of squamous-cell carcinoma of the rumen and seven of malignant adenoma of the liver. He also mentioned a papilliferous, cystic carcinoma of the udder, an adenocarcinoma of the uterus, and a similar tumor in the testis of a bull. Among Murray's cases was an adenocarcinoma of the bowel and a carcinoma of the base of the horn. Bashford noted that squamous-cell carcinoma of the base of the horn is frequently seen in India in cattle that are used as beasts of burden. Bashford stated that the tumor practically always develops at the base of the right horn, this being the appendage used to attach the animals to the load. Hewlett saw twelve cases of so-called horn-core carcinoma in a period of two years in the hospital of the Bombay Veterinary College. He was unable to examine the animals at necropsy, but noted that as the disease progressed the physical condition of the animals declined. So far as I am aware, this form of the disease has not been reported in America.

A primary adenocarcinoma of the lungs of a cow, with secondary foci in the mediastinal lymph nodes and in both kidneys, was observed by Gilruth, and Moussu reported a case of carcinoma of the tail of an

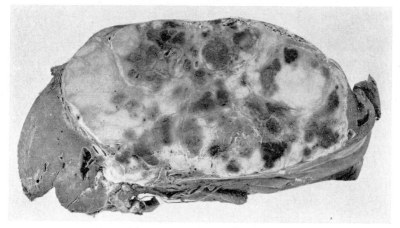

Fig. 141.—Carcinoma of the liver of a bovine.

old cow. The disease continued to progress even after the tail was amputated, and at necropsy the sublumbar lymph nodes were found to be affected. Walter reported carcinoma of the glottis. In Fadyean's five cases the carcinomas originated in the liver, vulva, larynx, skin of the body, and the scrotum. Udall, Fincher, and Cushing reported a case of carcinoma of the cervix of a six-year-old Holstein cow, with metastasis to the lungs and mediastinal lymph nodes.

Carcinomas of cattle may occasionally arise from the epithelium of the biliary tracts or from the parenchymatous hepatic cell (hepatoma) (Fig. 141) the latter variety is the one usually encountered. This form of carcinoma has been studied thoroughly by Trotter,[119, 120] who found 119 cases in examination of 39,704 cattle that had been slaughtered for food. He found primary carcinoma of the liver to be most common in older animals, and that the disease was often associated with various hepatic disturbances, such as chronic venous congestion, cirrhosis, and parasitism.   In one of his cases the affected liver weighed 80 pounds. Most of these tumors are, of course, much smaller.   This form of carcinoma is particularly prone to local metastasis; the occurrence of distant foci is exceptional.   Owing to the highly vascular state of the hepatic tissue, and the tendency of the cells of the tumor to invade the larger veins and to form friable thrombi, distant metastasis more often occurs by way of the blood stream than by way of the lymphatic structures. Metastasis to the lungs, kidneys, and peritoneal surfaces has been noted.

In my series of carcinomas obtained from cattle, the following organs were affected: Uterus, ovary, thyroid gland, gallbladder, vulva, kidney, thymus gland, and skin.   I also observed cases of primary carcinoma of the liver (hepatoma), primary adenocarcinoma of the lungs, and one instance of adenocarcinoma which resembled histologically the thyroid gland in the subcutis of the neck, lateral and just posterior to the first cervical vertebra,[30] and massive carcinoma of the lungs which presented much evidence to substantiate the suggestion that it arose from aberrant thyroid tissue.   The eye and its appendages were the sites of primary origin of twenty-eight of the eighty-nine carcinomas obtained from cattle.

In my series of nineteen tumors of the adrenal glands of cattle, twelve were considered histologically to be carcinomas originating from certain epithelial constituents of the cortex.   The cytologic appearance of adrenal tumors varies greatly and although metastasis was observed in only three of the twelve adrenal carcinomas in the series, all of them were extremely cellular and quite vascular.   The parenchyma of the tumors revealed many immature cells and little if any tendency to encapsulation.   Degeneration of certain parts of the tumor, accompanied by calcification, was commonly seen, but in practically every instance, young, vigorously growing cells were to be found adjacent to the vascular elements of the blood.   Epithelial tumors of the adrenal cortex, which consist of immature cells, should be considered potentially malignant even though demonstrable metastasis has not occurred.   Adrenal carcinomas of cattle have also been reported by Görig, Horne,[54] Holmbo, and Silva.

Carcinoma of the mammary gland, which is of common occurrence in human beings, appears to be extremely rare in the domestic cow. Joest,[61] in an extensive experience, failed to see a case of mammary carcinoma in cattle, and the only references I have found in the literature were cases mentioned by Murray, Sticker, and Cleland, one each.

Cleland's case, in which there was metastasis to the iliac and sublumbar lymph nodes, was described as "a large, scirrhous-looking mass." The photomicrographs which accompany the brief description of this tumor attest to the authenticity of the claim that the neoplasm had its origin from the epithelial cells of the parenchyma of the mammary gland. The neoplastic cells were in irregular nests or pockets, and each group was separated from the others by rather dense strands of fibrous tissue. Without doubt carcinoma of the mammary gland of the cow is extremely rare.

Many of the cases described as instances of carcinoma of the mammary gland are in reality squamous-cell carcinomas which arise in the skin that covers the udder. Drabble,[17] and Drabble and Massy described several cases of this nature, and I observed one such tumor in the material in my collection. These carcinomas often ulcerate, and extensive sloughing of the tissues immediately adjacent to the growth may ensue. The carcinomatous process may extend into the glandular portion of the udder and the disease often extends by metastasis to the supramammary, internal iliac, and sublumbar lymph nodes. Metastasis to the lungs has also been observed.

Carcinoma of the ovary of the cow, which, according to Schlegel, may be solid, cystic, or papillary, not infrequently gives rise to widespread metastasis throughout the abdominal cavity (Fig. 142). Implantations may occur extensively over the surface of both the parietal and visceral peritoneum. Although the regional lymph nodes usually are affected, the liver, spleen, and kidneys, seldom show more than superficial or subserous involvement.

Scholer commented on the rarity of carcinoma of the uterus of cows, and after reviewing briefly the seven cases reported by Guillebeau, described in detail two cases that he observed. Among more than 12,000 cows which were examined at necropsy during a period of two years the tumors occurred in cows aged eight years and ten years, respectively, and apparently originated from the epithelial glands of the uterine mucosa. The growth in each instance was situated in the body of the cornu and extended from the internal orifice anteriorly for a considerable distance. One of the tumors had metastasized to both ovaries, and the other had established secondary foci in one ovary, the kidney, and the liver.

Briefly summarized, it may be said that externally the great majority of carcinomas of cattle occur in the tissues of the orbital region. The skin, particularly that covering the mammary gland, occasionally is the site of primary growths which may infiltrate the mammary gland

and metastasize to the regional lymph nodes. Carcinoma of the parenchyma or of the excretory ducts of the mammary gland rarely occurs.
Internally the majority of the carcinomas have their origin in the cortex
of the adrenal gland, the liver, the ovary, and the mucosa of the rumen.
Infrequently the bile ducts, the urinary bladder, the uterus, the kidneys,
and the lungs may be affected. Carcinoma of the true stomach and
intestines seldom occurs.

Dog.—Because a considerable number of dogs lives to be old, it is
not surprising that the incidence at tumor should be relatively high in

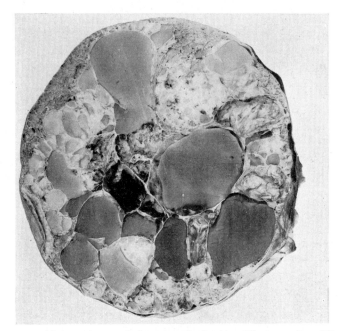

Fig. 142.—Adenocarcinoma of the ovary of a bovine. The tumor is multilocular in
structure. The respective cavities are filled with a mucinous-like fluid, an example of
colloid degeneration.

this species. Goodpasture commented on the paucity of malignant
tumors of young dogs, but expressed the opinion that in the later years
of life the dog, of all the domestic animals, is by far the most prone to
malignant disease. In fact, there is some evidence to indicate that carcinoma occurs more frequently in dogs than in man.

In Murray's series of forty-nine cases of malignant tumors of dogs,
twenty-three were carcinomas. The growths were distributed as follows: Mammary gland, eight cases; pharynx, five; palate, one case;
tongue, one; buccal mucous membrane, one; skin, one; foreleg, one;

liver, one; rectum, one, and anus, three cases. The twenty-three carcinomas reported by Fadyean were primary in the following situations:
Skin, five cases; region of the anus, five; liver, three; mammary gland,
three; prepuce, two; kidney, two; pharynx, one case; orbit, one; and
undetermined, one.

Sticker compiled a series of 766 cases of carcinoma of the dog, in
754 of which organs as follows were affected: Mammary gland, 341
cases; skin, 166; anus, eighty-nine; thyroid gland, thirty-two; liver,
twenty; kidney, nineteen; testis, eighteen; penis, sixteen; prostate
gland and lung, each ten; eye, eight; vagina, six; urinary bladder, six;

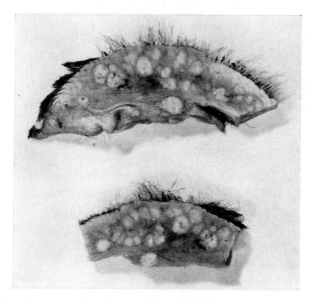

Fig. 143.—Squamous-cell carcinoma of the subcutis of a dog, primary in the skin.

ovary, three; ureter, three; uterus and pancreas, each two cases; parotid
glands, stomach, and nasal passage each one case.

In my series of seventy-eight canine tumors, twenty-eight were true
carcinomas; they were found in organs as follows: Skin, nine cases;
thyroid gland, eight; mammary gland, three; testis, two; ovary, two;
pharynx, gums, and lung, each one case. In one case the primary site
of the tumor was not determined.

Hobday stated that carcinoma in dogs occurs most frequently in
the pharynx, larynx, and mammary gland. He also mentioned the
orbit and lips as favorable sites for the origin of carcinoma in this animal.

Carcinoma seems to have a predilection for the skin of the dog, which
increases as the age of the animal advances (Fig. 143). Lubarsch found

the skin (exclusive of the anus, palpebræ, mamma, penis, and scrotum) affected in 143 cases (23.7 per cent) of a total of 784 cases of carcinoma of the dog. Of 766 cases of primary carcinoma of dogs, compiled by Sticker, 166 (approximately 21.9 per cent) had their origin in the skin proper. Schütz, during a period of fourteen years, found carcinoma present in sixty-nine (5.4 per cent) of the 1,241 dogs examined at necropsy. These were distributed as follows: 20.4 per cent affected the exterior integument; 26.6 per cent affected the urogenital system; 25.8 per cent affected the digestive tract, and 26.6 per cent affected the respiratory tract. Milks reported one case of carcinoma of the skin of an adult male Boston bull terrier. The primary tumor, which may have originated in the sudoriferous gland, was situated at the mesial side of the scapulohumeral joint, with secondary nodules over the region of the thorax and abdomen. At necropsy metastatic tumors were observed in the spleen and liver.

The anal region of dogs not infrequently gives rise to cancerous growths. They may originate in the skin immediately adjacent to the anal opening, or they may grow from the mucosa of the anus or rectum. Benign adenomas not uncommonly arise from the perianal sebaceous glands. Dupas described a malignant epithelial tumor which arose from perianal sebaceous glands. The tumor metastasized to the inferior surface of the caudal appendage, a distance of approximately 10 cm. from the primary growth.

Although data revealing the exact incidence of carcinoma of the thyroid glands of dogs are somewhat meager, Sticker's statistics would indicate that it constitutes somewhat more than 4 per cent of all primary carcinomas of dogs. The disease seems to occur more often in localities in which dogs are most prone to goiter, and in which the thyroid gland experiences benign hyperplasia before malignancy is initiated.

The majority of malignant tumors of the thyroid gland of dogs are carcinomatous. Of the eighty cases summarized by Ewald, sixty-three were carcinomas, six were sarcomas, seven were mixed tumors, and in four cases the exact histologic character of the growths was undetermined. The distribution of metastatic tumors in sixty-two of the cases of malignant growths of the thyroid gland reviewed by Ewald showed that the lungs were involved in thirty-three, the spleen in nine, the kidney in six, the heart and liver each in four, the testis in two, and the skin, adrenal gland, mammary gland, and intestine in one each (Fig. 144).

In a series of 234 thyroid glands obtained from dogs in southern Minnesota, Schlotthauer, McKenney and Caylor found fifty-four which were histologically classified as goitrous. Two (3.7 per cent) of the goiters were definitely carcinomatous, and metastasis had occurred in both cases.

Bartlett reported two cases of adenocarcinoma of the thyroid gland with metastasis to the lungs, and emphasized the significance of goiter in the histogenesis of carcinoma of the thyroid gland. He quoted Marine and Lenhart as follows: "Goiter in some way favors the development of cancer, just as it favors the development of benign tumors. Cancer developing in an otherwise normal gland is extremely

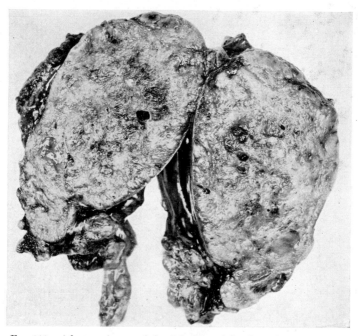

Fig. 144.—Adenocarcinoma of the right lobe of the thyroid gland of a dog.

rare. We have never observed thyroid cancer apart from preëxisting goiter." As further evidence of the influence of goiter on the incidence of carcinoma of the thyroid gland, Bartlett stated that in the vicinity of Chicago, where goiter is very common in dogs, carcinoma of the thyroid gland is common. Wegelin, in a recent paper, recorded a wealth of evidence to show that endemic goiter predisposes to malignant disease of the thyroid gland in both man and animals, and according to Huguenin in Berne, where endemic goiter is extremely prevalent in dogs, carcinoma of the thyroid gland arises in old animals with benign goiters.

Milks and Muldoon reported an unusual case of colloid carcinoma of the thyroid gland with metastasis to the liver and hepatic lymph nodes in a twelve-year-old pointer. Goldberg described a case of carcinoma of the thyroid gland with metastasis to the liver and the hepatic and omental lymph nodes, and a carcinoma of similar character which metastasized to the lungs, liver, pancreas, adrenal gland, and subcutaneous tissue. Mann[79] reported a case of carcinoma of the thyroid gland in the dog associated with spontaneous peptic ulcers, with multiple metastasis in the lungs. In all of my cases of carcinoma of the thyroid gland the lungs were extensively involved (Fig. 145).

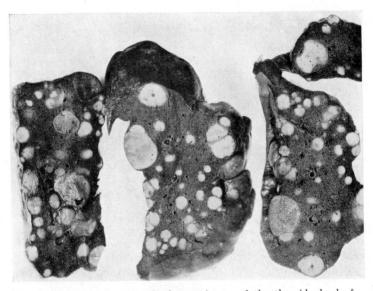

Fig. 145.—Pulmonary metastasis of adenocarcinoma of the thyroid gland of a dog Same case as that represented in Figure 144.

The frequency of involvement of the lung secondary to primary carcinoma of the thyroid gland of the dog should make one cautious in diagnosing primary carcinoma of the lungs of this animal. The lungs should be considered as being primarily involved only when careful search fails to incriminate the thyroid gland as the site of the initial lesion. Primary carcinoma of the liver also frequently metastasizes to the lungs.

Goldberg noted in the literature a report of an adenocarcinoma of the mucous glands of the tracheal wall, which contained spicules of bone. Lewis noted an adenocarcinoma in the undescended testis of a five-year-old fox terrier, and D'Arcy Power[73] mentioned a carcinoma of a dog's tongue (Fig. 146).

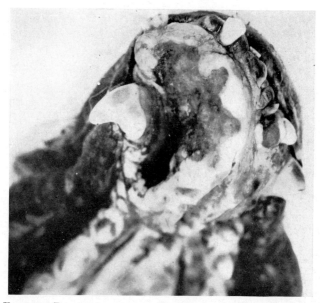

Fig. 146.—Recurrent squamous-cell carcinoma of the mouth of a dog.

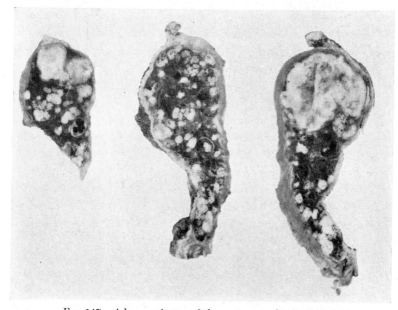

Fig. 147.—Adenocarcinoma of the mammary gland of a dog.

The mammary gland is one of the commonest sites of epithelial neoplasm in the dog, and carcinoma of this gland is often mentioned in the literature (Fig. 147). Murray reported eight cases of mammary carcinoma in a total of forty-nine cases of malignant growth, and in Fadyean's series of twenty-three cases, three of the carcinomas originated in this structure. As I have mentioned, carcinoma of the mammary gland constituted 341 of the 766 cases (approximately 44 per cent) of carcinoma of the dog compiled by Sticker. Mann[78] made a detailed study of mammary carcinoma in an old Scotch collie. The tumor was enlarged and indurated and involved the third mammary gland on the right side, and the axillary lymph node on the same side. The animal refused food and lost weight, and just before death showed evidence of jaundice. Necropsy revealed metastasis in the axillary lymph nodes, lungs, mediastinal lymph nodes, liver, pancreas, one kidney, and one adrenal gland. Mann attempted to transplant the tumor in 134 dogs, without success. Petit found carcinoma of the mammary gland of a bitch; metastasis had occurred to the lungs, liver, and spleen. Fröhner[38] observed a case of carcinoma of the mammary gland of a male dog. In female dogs such lesions may arise from either the epithelium of the skin, the epithelium of the milk ducts, or the parenchymal epithelium of the alveoli. Those which originate from the lining of the milk ducts are, according to Joest,[59] perhaps the most common. Schlotthauer had occasion to observe a squamous-cell carcinoma in the region of the mammary gland of a female mongrel collie, aged eight years. The tumor, which was situated largely in the subcutis, had progressed rapidly and had apparently originated from the skin overlying the mammary gland. The process consisted of multiple foci that extended from the umbilicus to the perineum, and down the mesial aspects of both thighs to the femorotibial joint. Although the mammary gland was invaded by the neoplastic process, metastasis to the internal organs was not apparent. Many of the tumors of the mammary gland of the dog contain sarcomatous neoplastic elements besides those which are purely epithelial. Several tumors of this kind were reported by Ortschild. Retrogressive changes not infrequently occur in mammary carcinomas of the dog, as a consequence of which fibrosis, cystic cavitations, cartilage, and even bone may be present.

Carcinoma of the stomach and of the intestines is one of the rarer manifestations in most of the domesticated mammals, including the dog. Friedberger and Fröhner mentioned one case of carcinoma of the stomach in 70,000 dogs observed. They quoted Eberlein's case of primary carcinoma of the stomach in a dog, and mentioned that Parascandolo is said to have performed gastrectomy on a dog for gastric carcinoma, with good results. Carcinoma of the small intestine of the dog is described by Joest.[60]

Huynen reported a case of carcinoma of the anterior extremity of the urinary bladder of a six-year-old dog. It involved both ureters; the right was entirely obliterated. The right kidney was hydronephrotic and was three times normal size. Little reported carcinoma of the wall of the urinary bladder of an eight-year-old great Dane. Horne[55] described an adenocarcinoma of the prostate gland which metastasized to the lungs. Richter reported carcinoma of the gallbladder of a six- or seven-year-old dog. The growth had infiltrated and penetrated the wall of the gallbladder and involved the liver. Metastasis occurred to the lung, pancreas, and peritoneum. Kitt,[65] and Borrel described primary carcinoma of the pancreas of the dog.

In brief it may be said that the majority of carcinomas affecting the dog arise in the tissues of the integument; those which originate from the tissues of the internal organs are relatively uncommon. The mammary glands and their ducts, and the overlying skin are usually affected. The region of the anus, and the mucosa of the lips, gums, and pharynx are also frequently involved; less frequently, the thyroid gland, the penis, and the testis. Carcinomas of the liver, the kidney, the prostate gland, the ovary, the urinary bladder, and the lungs occasionally are observed. Primary carcinoma of the uterus and vagina is sometimes seen; it is extremely rare in the gastro-intestinal tract.

Swine.—This animal appears to be less frequently affected with carcinoma than any of the other domestic animals. Aside from Sticker's statistics, the literature contains slight mention of carcinoma of swine. In Sticker's series of approximately 1,200 carcinomas from the common domestic animals, twelve occurred in swine. Two were in the skin; one was in the gums; one was in the liver; one was in a mesenteric lymph node (probably secondary) and seven were in the kidney. It is doubtful whether all the renal tumors listed by Sticker were true carcinomas; they may have been embryonal nephromas which are so common in the kidney of this animal.

Wankmüller reported a carcinoma of the milk ducts of the left side of a four-year-old sow. Schaible observed a carcinoma of the mammary gland, and Johne observed a case of carcinoma of the liver.

In my series of seventy-six neoplasms of swine, there were three carcinomas. One tumor apparently had originated in the parenchyma of the mammary gland. The histologic character of the type cell and the general appearance of the growth were suggestive of a carcinoma of mammary origin. The second tumor occurred in the liver, and was considered to be a hepatoma, with early carcinomatous changes. The third tumor involved the skin over the back and sides. It was rather extensive in its distribution, had a scarred appearance, and the precrural and inguinal lymph nodes were involved by metastasis. The primary tumor was cystic and the involved lymph nodes consisted of infiltrating strands of undifferentiated epithelial cells.

Cat.—Judging by the infrequency with which practicing veterinarians see tumors in cats one would be justified in concluding that carcinoma must be rare in this species. However, the literature on comparative pathology contains enough records of cases of carcinoma of cats to lead one to believe that the incidence of the disease in this animal is much higher than is generally believed.

Murray noted seven carcinomas in eleven malignant growths among cats. They originated in situations as follows: Esophagus, one case; mammary gland, four cases; tongue, one case, and anus, one case. In Fadyean's series of sixty-three carcinomas collected from domestic animals over a period of six years there were but two cases of carcinoma of the cat; one of these involved the skin of the shoulder, and the other the tongue. Herzog reported two cases; one affected the ear, and the other, which was an adenocarcinoma, the mammary gland. In Sticker's report of twenty-one carcinomas of the cat, the tumors were distributed as follows: Skin, six cases; mammary gland, five cases; lungs, three cases; liver, two cases, and anus, penis, ovary, tongue, and mediastinum, each one case.

Wooldridge reported carcinoma of the esophagus of a cat, and Goldberg described an adenocarcinoma of the parotid gland of an old Maltese cat. Hobday noted carcinoma of the orbit and tongue. Mann and Brimhall found primary carcinoma of the pancreas with metastasis to the liver in a twelve-year-old castrated cat, and Scott and Moore reported pancreatic carcinoma in an adult male cat; it had metastasized to the duodenum and to the retroperitoneal lymph nodes. Field observed two cases of carcinoma of the mammary glands of cats. The animal in the first case was aged between fifteen and sixteen years. The growth, which was considered to be a scirrhous carcinoma, grew steadily for about six months when the animal was killed because of the development of a severe cough. The internal organs were not examined, but metastasis to the lungs was suspected, since the animal exhibited pronounced respiratory distress. The second case was reported in detail. The mammary nodule was observed for a period of five months, during which time the animal gradually became emaciated, and painful polyuria developed. The animal was killed and metastatic tumors were found in the axillary and inguinal lymph nodes, the peritoneum, and the mesenteric lymph nodes, the spleen, kidneys, lungs, heart, and parietal pleura. Strangely enough the liver was not involved. Johne also reported one case of mammary carcinoma. Roussy and Wolf described a mammary epithelioma, and Petit described a mammary carcinoma in which there were secondary nodules in the sublumbar lymph nodes, abdominal wall, kidneys, spleen, lungs, and costal pleura. Petit observed that the nodules of the pleura and lungs grossly resembled the condition seen in tuberculosis. Another case of carcinoma of the mammary gland, which metastasized to the liver and the lungs, was recorded by Cornil and Petit. My collection of more than 500 tumors of animals did not contain a carcinoma from the cat.

The available data seem to indicate that the majority of carcinomas of the cat affect the respective tissues or organs in order of frequency as follows: Mammary gland, skin, and tongue; cases have occasionally been reported in which the esophagus, the tissues of the eye, the pancreas, the lung, the liver, and the ovary were affected. Carcinoma of the gastro-intestinal tract appears to be extremely rare.

Sheep.—Sheep appear to be relatively immune to carcinomatous proliferation, and there are few references in the literature to carcinoma of this animal. Of Sticker's series of approximately 1,200 carcinomas of the common domestic animals, only seven were from sheep. Five of the seven carcinomas were primary in the liver; one arose in the lung and one was listed as primary in the mesenteric lymph nodes. Hodgson's case of carcinoma of the liver suggests the rarity of the disease of this animal. Only one case of carcinoma was observed in the examination of more than 17,000 carcasses in the public abbatoir at Halifax. Fadyean also recorded cases of two primary hepatic carcinomas in sheep, and Trotter reported the finding of several similar tumors. Six cases of primary carcinoma of the liver of sheep were reported by Frenekl, and Aynaud described a case of primary carcinoma of the lungs. The affected animal was one of a group of sheep suffering from epidemic parasitic bronchitis. Goldberg observed diffuse carcinoma of the turbinated bones in a well-nourished adult ewe, and Eggeling reported carcinoma of the mammary gland.

In my collection of more than 500 neoplasms of lower animals, forty-one were obtained from sheep. Twenty-five (60 per cent) were carcinomas, distributed as follows: Adrenal glands, nine cases; liver, four; lung, three; eye and orbital region, two; skin, two; bile ducts, two; thymus, one case; thyroid gland, one, and in one instance the point of primary origin was undetermined. Six of the adrenal carcinomas were unilateral and three were bilateral. The adrenal growths were cellular and were derived from some portion of the adrenal cortex. Although it was not observed that any of the growths had broken through the capsule of the adrenal gland they were nevertheless destructive in character as could be seen histologically. Mitotic figures were numerous in most of the material, and the neoplastic elements were destroying and replacing a large portion of the normal tissues. Since the cells of adrenal carcinomas frequently invade the blood stream, the presence within the gland of immature, infiltrating neoplastic cells constitutes a possibility for widespread metastasis.

The most common site of carcinoma of sheep is the cortex of the adrenal gland. The liver and the bile ducts also are frequently affected, and occasionally the lung. The digestive tract is seldom if ever affected. Externally, carcinomas sometimes originate from the tissues of the eye and its appendages and from the skin.

Rabbit.—Polson recently reviewed the cases of tumor of rabbits. He found fifty-two such neoplasms recorded in the literature and described fourteen cases of his own. He concluded that the uterus is the most frequent site of tumor, and that the growths of this organ were either adenoma or adenocarcinoma; eight and twenty-one cases, respectively. Other cases described by Polson were adenocarcinoma of the mammary gland, carcinoma of the kidney and carcinoma of the neck. Rusk and Epstein described in detail spontaneous adenocarcinoma of the body of the uterus in a virgin female rabbit aged four and a half years. The tumor extended into the fallopian tubes, bladder, and vaginal walls, and had metastasized to the retroperitoneal mesenteric, mediastinal, and cervical lymph nodes. The liver and lungs were also involved. Attempts to transplant the tumor in six other rabbits were unsuccessful. Polson mentioned Niessen's case of primary carcinoma of the bile ducts, and the cases of Petit, one of which was carcinoma in an accessory pancreas and the other carcinoma of the lungs.

Fowls.—Carcinoma occasionally occurs in chickens, but the most common tumor affecting this species is lymphoblastoma. Adenocarcinoma of the intestine is common (Fig. 148). Six of the fifteen carcinomas in my series of fifty-four tumors of chickens were of this type. The other nine carcinomas of the chicken in my collection occurred as follows: Ovary, three cases; oviduct, two; skin of the region of the neck, two; mucosa of the pharynx, one case, and liver, one. In one case of adenocarcinoma of the intestine, in which metastasis over the surface of the peritoneum, and to the parenchyma of the liver, had taken place, there were also extensive lesions of tuberculosis throughout the spleen and the lungs, in which many acid-fast bacillary forms were demonstrated by appropriate stains.

The intestinal form of the disease apparently runs a more or less protracted course and does not seem to embarrass seriously general health except in the later stages. The tumor early becomes multiple, and often involves the entire abdominal viscera with subserous metastatic implantations. The intestines of chickens seem to be affected with carcinoma much more frequently than the intestines of mammals. In one case I observed an adenocarcinoma of the mucosa of the ileocecal juncture of a two-year-old white Leghorn hen. The tumor was an elongated, roll-like structure about 0.6 cm. in height and occupied about half of the circumference of the lumen. Metastasis had not occurred.

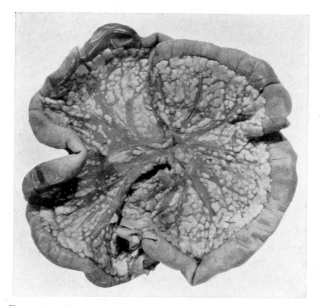

Fig. 148.—Adenocarcinoma involving the mesentery of a chicken.

Ehrenreich and Michaelis recorded in detail two cases of adenocarcinoma of the small intestine of the common fowl. Murray described adenocarcinoma of the small intestine of a grouse, and a columnar-celled carcinoma of the ovary of a canary. Koch, and Pick[94] each reported squamous-cell carcinoma of the floor of the mouth of a chicken. Three cases of adenocarcinoma of the ovaries of hens were described by Bürger, and one case was described by Gordon and Happold. Boynton reported a large squamous-cell carcinoma of the lateral surface of the right leg. Although metastasis was not observed, there were definite, amyloid-like changes in the liver, but the tissue failed to respond to the reactions such as are given by amyloid of human beings.

Fujinami reported thirty-two carcinomas in the common fowl, affecting chiefly the ovary. Joest[61] considered the ovary the most common site of epithelial malignant growths of this animal. In a list of thirty-seven cases reviewed from the literature by Joest and Ernesti, the ovary was the site of primary origin in twenty. Nineteen of the twenty tumors were found in hens and one tumor was found in a wild turkey. Joest and Ernesti also reported nineteen cases of their own, in six of which the carcinomas were primary in the ovary. They found another ovarian carcinoma in a dove. Pentimalli described carcinoma of the ovary in a hen in which there was metastasis to the peritoneum, liver, and spleen. Two hepatic cell carcinomas are also included in Joest and Ernesti's series.

Mathews described six pedunculated carcinomas from the region of the adrenal gland and the ovary of adult hens. The ovary was involved in each instance, but Mathews was unable to determine with certainty the exact anatomic origin of the respective tumors. The tumors were not particularly aggressive, and their histologic aspect was suggestive of the adrenal cortex. Metastasis was limited to the mesentery and the visceral peritoneum.

An unusual form of the disease was reported by Savage. He observed what appeared to be adenocarcinoma of the gallbladder in a three and a half year-old Rhode Island hen. The occurrence of a carcinoma of the gizzard of a domestic hen was recorded by Schöppler. The chicken was aged three years, and at the time of death was in a state of extreme emaciation due to inappetence, which had been observed for four weeks prior to death. At necropsy, a rounded tumor, measuring 2.9 by 3.4 cm. was found involving the mucosa of the stomach. The size and position of the growth had occasioned marked constriction of the pylorus. The unusualness of carcinoma of the gizzard of the domestic hen makes this case noteworthy.

Epidermoid carcinomas of the integument of the feet of certain wild birds recently have been described by Emmel. The tumors, which are of low-grade malignancy, appear as nodular masses, both vertically and dorsally, over the metatarsophalangeal articulation. Emmel reported three cases, two of which occurred in the slate-colored junco (Junco hyemalis hyemalis) and one in a bronze grackle (Quiscalam quiscala æneus).

In Fox's series of forty-four tumors of captive wild birds, almost 25 per cent were true carcinomas, and the highest incidence was shown by parrakeets. One of Fox's cases was a papillary adenocarcinoma of the ovary of a wild turkey. This is of considerable interest because of the paucity in the literature of neoplasms of the turkey.

It is probably correct to assume that the greatest number of carcinomas of the common domestic fowl originate from the tissues of the intestines or from the ovary. Other regions which may occasionally be involved are the liver, oviduct, skin, and the mucosa of the mouth and pharynx. Wild fowl are also susceptible to carcinomatous growths which have an anatomic distribution perhaps comparable to those which affect domestic fowl.

Other species.—The literature seems to show that carcinoma is practically universal in its zoölogic distribution in most of the species of wild animals. A few cases selected at random will suffice to emphasize the wide range of occurrence in the nondomesticated animals.

Fox recorded several cases among which occurred the following: Malignant adenoma of the cervix of the uterus, with metastasis to the lungs in a lioness; adenocarcinoma of the pancreas of an Indian paradoxure; carcinoma of the mammary glands of a black bear, of an opossum and of two white-footed mice; epithelioma of the tongue of a black bear; carcinoma of the liver, with intestinal extension, in an alpaca; carcinoma of the uterus of a wild boar; carcinoma of the lung, with metastasis to the spleen and stomach of a kangaroo, and adenocarcinoma of the uterine body with local extension and metastasis to the liver of a wild boar. Murray quoted Petit, who described squamous-cell carcinoma of the cervix of the uterus of a gazelle; carcinoma of the parotid gland of a jackal, and carcinoma of the thyroid gland of an opossum. Murray also mentioned carcinoma of the mammary gland of an old lioness. Betke reported an interesting case of papillary adenocarcinoma of the cervix in a forty-year-old captive rhinoceros. The growth was associated with a fibromyoma of the uterus. Four cases of carcinoma of fawns were observed by Joest. In two cases the disease was primary in the liver, in one case the uterus was primarily affected, and in another the growth had metastasized to the lungs, but the point of origin was not determined. Scott reported a carcinoma of the tonsil of a female wolf, and Perry reported renal carcinoma of a brown bear which had lived for thirty-four years in a zoo. An adenocarcinoma of the guinea pig, which had its origin from the mucosa of the smaller bronchi or bronchioles, and which metastasized to the liver was described by Goldberg. I have observed a large adenocarcinoma of the thyroid gland of an adult guinea pig which, although locally very destructive, did not metastasize.

The observations of Murray, Plehn, Pick, Gaylord, Gaylord and

Marsh, Takahashi, and others, have definitely established the fact that carcinoma occurs among fishes. The thyroid gland is frequently the site of origin.

Effects on the host.—The maximal effect of a carcinoma on the animal depends on the significance of the tissue primarily occupied by the growth, the anatomic possibilities for early metastasis, the histologic character of the tumor, and its inherent capacity for growth. The latter factor is probably dependent on the autonomy of the carcinoma and on the lack of protective resistance on the part of the noncarcinomatous tissues.

From the time of its inception, a carcinoma is engaged in destruction, and if life is not terminated by some other cause, death as a result of the carcinoma is eventually inevitable. Carcinoma lives at the expense of normal cells which may be injured or entirely destroyed by the pernicious activities of the neoplastic elements. This process may be so rapid as to menace life within a few months, or it may proceed so slowly as to require years to exert a fatal influence.

Unlike nonmalignant epithelial growths, carcinomas commonly spread by the lymph channels and blood stream, and appear as secondary growths in such vital tissues as the lungs, liver, kidneys, spleen, and even the heart. When this occurs the disease is launched on its final phase, with death certain if the disease be permitted to run its course. If carcinomas are situated along the esophagus or intestinal tract they may constitute a serious obstacle to the passage and digestion of food. If they are in the mouth or pharynx, and if they are large enough, they naturally interfere with the proper ingestion of food and water. Those on the alveoli of the molars usually cause loosening of the involved teeth. Those that affect the membrana nictitans and conjunctival mucosa, if undisturbed, may eventually destroy the entire eye and the adjacent bony structures, and metastasis to the regional lymph nodes and lungs is not uncommon. In one case I observed the eye had been destroyed, and in another case only a vestige of the retinal sac and the lens remained. Carcinomas on the penis and prepuce often make urination difficult, and the sexual act is impossible. Involvement of the ovary or the oviduct usually induces cessation of ovulation and subsequent sterility. If the uterus is affected, the usefulness of the animal as a breeder is terminated.

If the heart is involved by metastasis, fatal termination may ensue from cardiac embarrassment. Dyspnea bordering on suffocation may be observed in cases in which the tumor is situated in the larynx, trachea, or lungs. Obviously, the maximal effects will be observed while the animal is exercising. If the exertion is prolonged and strenuous, collapse may occur.

If large vessels are eroded by the carcinomatous process, serious or even fatal hemorrhage may result. In generalized carcinomatosis of the parietal and visceral peritoneum, ascites commonly occurs from the irritation which results from movement of the roughened viscera. This is frequently seen in carcinoma of the intestine of chickens.

The extreme cachexia, frequently a part of the picture in the human being suffering from carcinoma, is not so often observed in lower animals, although it is mentioned in some of the cases reported, particularly those of internal carcinoma. Only rarely is the affected animal permitted to live until the disease has exerted the full measure of its destruction.

The extent to which an animal can be affected with a carcinomatous process with minimal deleterious effect is well exemplified in adenocarcinoma of the intestine of chickens. This form of carcinoma may practically encrust the entire bowel and metastasize to the subserosa of the liver, spleen, and peritoneum, and yet the chicken will often remain in good flesh and give no outward symptoms that might aid one in suspecting the presence of a serious internal neoplasm.

In lower animals the progress of most internal tumors is insidious. and it may be only in the last stages of the disease, when grave systemic disturbances arise, that attention is directed to the possibility of the presence of tumor. Even then the great majority of internal neoplasms are discovered only at necropsy.

Infection, which so often accompanies external neoplasia, is usually present in external carcinoma. Most of the carcinomas of the exterior of the body are subject to more or less trauma, and as soon as the surface is eroded, infection with common pyogenic bacteria results. The tumor soon becomes purulent, foul smelling, and repulsive, and more or less absorption of toxic material must occur. Even many of the internal carcinomas, in situations such as the kidneys, lungs, and intestinal tract, are subject to infection, the effects of which must be given cognizance in estimating the fatal possibilities of a carcinomatous process.

Metastasis and malignancy.—Carcinomas are, with few exceptions, always potentially malignant, although some exhibit this feature more markedly than others.

One does not study these tumors long before realizing that they exert considerably more influence on the surrounding tissues than can be accounted for by simple mechanical interference. Their manner of growth is usually apparent. The majority cause progressive infiltrative destruction of the adjacent tissues, and push their tentacles of growing cells into and along lymph spaces and channels, and even through the walls of blood vessels. When this happens, the growing cells of the tumor are transplanted to virgin fields, where a new program of destructiveness is initiated. Metastasis not infrequently imparts impetus to the transplanted cells, and they proliferate in their new situations with amazing rapidity. After metastasis has occurred, the condition of the affected animal is usually rapidly downward.

Changes in the lymph nodes constitute the most dependable criteria as to whether metastasis has taken place. These structures provide favorable conditions for multiplication of carcinoma cells which may

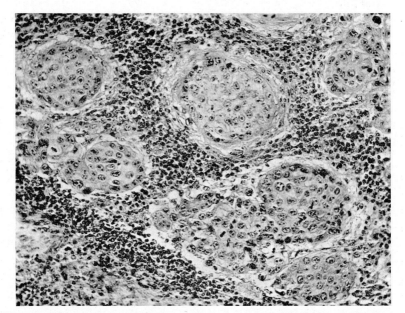

Fig. 149.—Metastatic squamous-cell carcinoma of a mediastinal lymph node of a bovine. The primary growth was in the eye (× 175).

reach them, and the nodes soon become indurated and enlarged (Fig. 149). Metastasis from one lymph node to another of the same chain may occur, until practically all nodes in a given region are involved.

Although the lymph nodes may temporarily impede the progress of the multiplying carcinoma cells, those of the more malignant variety are not long restrained by these structures. Some may break through the capsules of the nodes and infiltrate the adjacent tissues, invading without favor, nerves, blood vessels, and even bone.

Generally speaking, metastasis of carcinomas takes place by way of the lymphatic channels, although a notable exception to this manner of spread is seen in many of the primary hepatic cell carcinomas. Although these tumors do not usually metastasize, occasionally one appears which is capable of vigorous growth and widespread dissemination. On account of the proximity of the proliferating tumor cells to the portal vein and its branches, it frequently happens that the aggressive neoplastic cells break through the walls of the vessel and form thrombi. Since the cells are very friable, some of them become loosened and are swept along with the blood stream, with the resultant establishment of new communities of tumor cells in the lungs. From the lungs, further hematogenous distribution may take place, with possible deposits in the kidneys. The blood vascular system of the thyroid gland and the adrenal gland favor the blood stream as a mode of metastasis in carcinomas of these structures. Carcinoma of the ovary and of the adrenal cortex may establish metastasis throughout the peritoneum by surface implantations.

I have observed invasion of an artery by the carcinomatous cells in a case of metastatic carcinoma of the eye of a cow. In this case the lungs were markedly involved, as were the regional lymph nodes. It seems true that the highly malignant, rapidly growing type of carcinoma spreads by any and all means available, pushing its tentacles of destruction in every direction, now into lymphatics and again into convenient blood vessels. Unfortunately, the individual cells are not strongly bound to each other and since they are relatively small, those that become detached are readily carried along by the blood or lymph stream until they are finally deposited in a lymph node, or reach a terminal blood vessel too small for them to pass through. Although many so transplanted, no doubt, soon perish, some adapt themselves to the new environment and proceed to propagate a new focus of growing carcinoma cells which may be remote from the parent tumor.

Gross characteristics.—These growths are usually diffusely attached to the surrounding tissue and are not encapsulated except in rare instances. If they are external, they commonly present a bleeding, suppurating surface due to the constant trauma and subsequent infection to which they are subject. Their surfaces may be irregularly roughened by ulcerations, and if infected they usually give forth a disagreeable odor. Certain forms, particularly those that are papillary, are divided by deep clefts or convolutions, giving the tumor a cauliflower-like appearance. They vary from flesh pink to grayish-white, depending on the blood supply and their histologic constituents. The size, also, varies from a minute collection of cells barely visible, to masses weighing many pounds. The largest specimens are found in the lungs, liver, thyroid gland, and ovary. Their presence in internal organs is usually characterized by the presence, over the surface, of single or multiple nodules of varying sizes. These nodules are usually firm and grayish-white, by which they are distinguished from the tissues of the involved organs.

Carcinoma of the mucous surfaces is frequently complicated by extensive ulcerations, and the surface may appear ragged and angry. Hemorrhage of varying degree is not uncommon. Gastric, intestinal, and ovarian carcinomas may undergo a peculiar glue-like change, known as colloid degeneration. This occurs as a result of the secretory activity of the neoplastic cells which have retained a certain amount of the functional differentiation that characterizes their progenitors (Fig. 142). Owing to the tendency of the cells to grow in packets, or in an adenomatous fashion, without communications by which the mucinous product of the cells can be eliminated, the secretion continues to increase until practically every cell is filled to saturation. The activity of the cells often continues, as a consequence of which the gelatinous material may cover the entire tumor. Not infrequently, dilated cysts of varying sizes are produced by the activity of the cells, which secrete a substance that has no avenue of escape. Cystic degeneration may take place in cells devoid of secretory functions as a result of retrogressive changes. Colloid carcinomas can readily be recognized from the fact that they are shiny, of semisolid consistence, and of light yellowish color. The texture of the tumor is homogeneous, translucent and gelatinous, and the mass may be very irregular and reveal multiple cysts on cross section.

Microscopic description.—Carcinomas arise from a great variety of epithelial tissues, and it is evident that there should be some differences in their histologic design dependent on the character of the epithelium from which they originate. Since the morphology of the normal epidermis is quite dissimilar to that of the mucosa of the intestinal tract, and the epithelial cells of the thyroid gland are different from those of the uterus, it is not unusual that carcinomas arising from one of these structures should also be histologically dissimilar to those arising from the other. The one feature which different varieties of carcinomas display in common is the infiltrative character of their growth. The degree of invasiveness may vary widely, but this is the one characteristic which all carcinomas possess.

Squamous-cell carcinoma.—Squamous-cell carcinomas originate from the cells of the epidermis, and consequently the majority of carcinomas of the skin are of this character. Most carcinomas of the orbital region, the penis, the vulva, the esophagus, the mouth, the pharynx, and the nasal passages are of squamous-cell type. Histologically, the tumor consists of diffuse collections or compact masses of squamous epithelial cells, irregularly and often incompletely separated by fibrous stroma into nest-like groups, or strand-like processes which infiltrate the adjacent nontumorous tissues (Figs. 150 and 151). The blood channels are found in the fibrous stroma. The epithelial cell which constitutes a squamous-cell carcinoma often varies widely in appearance in different parts of the same tumor, depending on the state of nutrition and certain extraneous factors such as trauma and infection. The cells, for the most part, remain polyhedral, although the morphology of individual cells

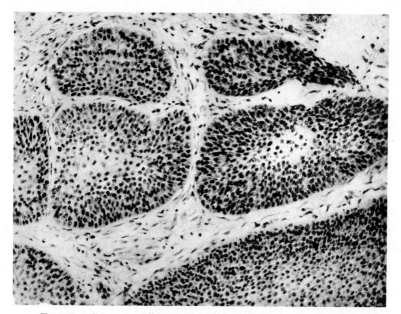

Fig. 150.—Squamous-cell carcinoma of the eyelid of a horse (× 150).

may differ greatly from that of cells of normal squamous epithelium (Fig. 152). Usually the majority of the cells appear immature, and mitotic figures are frequently numerous. Regions of necrosis, often caseous, are frequently observed, especially in cases in which the tumor is large. The necrobiosis is usually due to inadequate nutrition brought about by failure of the blood vascular channels to keep pace with the rapidly growing epithelial cells. Lymphocytes and eosinophils may be present in the meshes of the supporting stroma, and if infection has occurred, polymorphonuclear leukocytes usually can be seen.

The cells of a great many squamous-cell carcinomas tend to exhibit a functional difference comparable to normal cells of the epidermis.

21

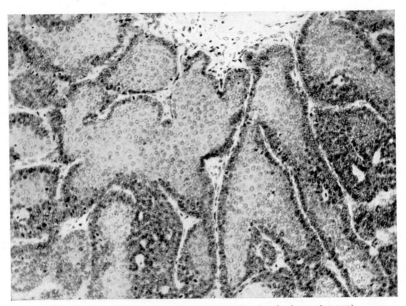

Fig. 151.—Squamous-cell carcinoma of the skin of a horse (× 150).

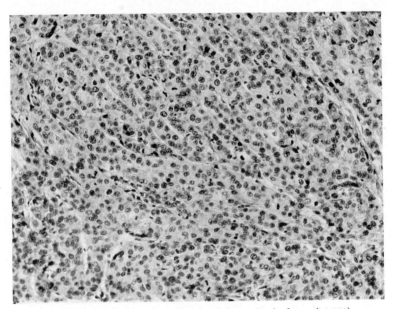

Fig. 152.—Squamous-cell carcinoma of the penis of a horse (× 160).

As a result of this tendency, cornification occurs and intercellular bridges become evident (Fig. 153). In a carcinoma of this kind the cells are frequently arranged in nest-like whorls or in large bulbous masses

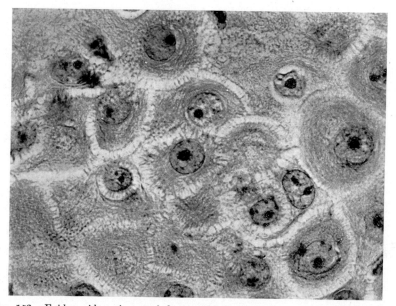

Fig. 153.—Epidermoid carcinoma of the eye of a cow, showing the intercellular bridges (× 860).

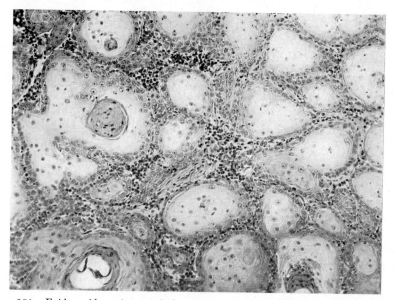

Fig. 154.—Epidermoid carcinoma of the eye of a bovine. Many so-called epithelial "pearls" are apparent (× 120).

(Fig. 154). The cells of the respective groups reveal a tendency toward a concentric type of arrangement and the center usually appears as a compact cellular mass in which definite individual cell outlines are faintly discernible or absent. Remains of atrophic nuclei are sometimes seen. Such a structure usually is somewhat more acidophilic in staining than the elements which constitute the remainder of the cell mass. On account of the peculiar, hyaline appearance of these concentrically disposed groups of cells, such a carcinoma is often designated "pearl-cell carcinoma" (Fig. 155) or epidermoid carcinoma. The formation of these cornified centers is due to inability of the older or cornified cells to be eliminated, as they are eliminated from the surface of normal epidermis. Consequently, the cells, which retain a certain amount of

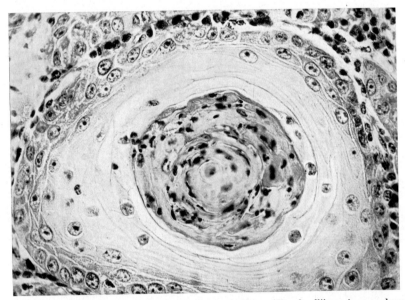

Fig. 155.—Epidermoid carcinoma of the eye of a bovine. "Pearl cell" carcinoma, showing the cornified center of a concentrically arranged group of cells ($\times$ 400).

the functional capacity possessed by their forerunners present a characteristic appearance.

In another subvariety of squamous-cell carcinoma which occasionally arises from the epidermis, and which is called papillary carcinoma, the surface of the growth, grossly, is rough and cauliflower-like. It usually consists of a number of rugæ, or folds of tissue, with deep clefts between them, giving the whole a convoluted appearance. It may be attached to the integument by a pedicle, or over a broad surface at its base. There is no capsule. Microscopically, these tumors consist of a conspicuous core of fibrous connective tissue, from which small papillæ of a similar structure are given off irregularly (Fig. 156). Squamous epithelial cells cover these skeletal papillæ so as completely to fill the spaces between them. In sections obtained from a plane longitudinal to the long axis of the central core, the parenchyma of the tumor is observed as being arranged in finger-like sheets. The epithelial cells of such a tumor frequently grow vigorously, and mitotic figures may be exceedingly numerous. Although these tumors possess most of the histologic features of malignant growths, the outward manner of growth of those that affect the exterior of the body minimizes the possibility of metastasis. Likewise, since the direction of growth is away from the body rather than into or toward it, the extent of the local injury is

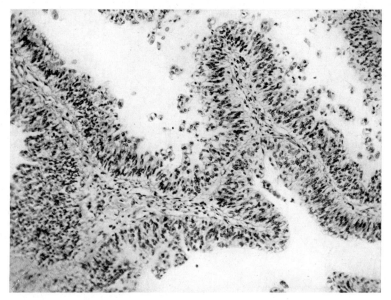

FIG. 156.—Papillary carcinoma of the sinuses of the head of a bovine (× 120).

relatively small compared to the menacing possibilities of a nonpapillary type of squamous-cell carcinoma.

So-called basal-cell carcinoma.—A group of epithelial tumors, whose exact histogenesis is somewhat controversial, is that commonly referred to as basal-cell carcinoma (Fig. 157). Some observers, including Mallory, contend that these tumors arise from the undifferentiated epithelial cells of the matrix from which the hair normally develops, whereas Krompecher derived the type cell from the basal or deepest layer of the stratum germinativum of the epidermis. Although Mallory's view has not been generally accepted, the evidence in support of his contention is impressive. The recognition of the cells of the hair matrix as potential precursors of possible epithelial tumors provides a logical explanation for some of the peculiarities exhibited by certain tumors of the integument which obviously do not arise from the cells of the malpighian layer* (Fig. 158). It does not appear that tumors of the type referred to as basal-cell carcinoma have been recognized often in lower animals. My collection contains three specimens of this kind, two from dogs and one from a horse. One of the former arose in the skin of the face; the other in the skin at the point of the shoulder. The specimen obtained from the horse was in the skin of the tail.

Morphologically, these tumors are subject to some variation even within different fields of the same section. The cells not infrequently

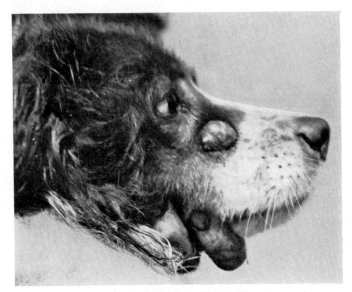

Fig. 157.—So-called basal-cell carcinoma of the skin. The microscopic appearance is shown in Figure 159.

resemble in general the basal cells of the malpighian layer; they are cuboidal or slightly columnar, and have a marked affinity for basic stains. The cytoplasm is slight in amount, and the nucleus appears vesiculated. Nucleoli are not prominent. The cells may exhibit a tendency to arrange themselves in slender, irregularly tortuous columns,

* Since this was written, Haythorn [Am. Jour. Cancer, 15: Suppl., 1969–2000 (July), 1931] has published the results of a detailed study of 144 noncornifying tumors from human beings of the so-called basal-cell type. One hundred thirty-nine of these were considered to be typical hair matrix carcinomas. He concluded that the anatomic distribution and the histopathology of these tumors support the contention that the basal-cell carcinomas arise from the elements of the hair matrix and not directly from the basal cells of the rete malpighii.

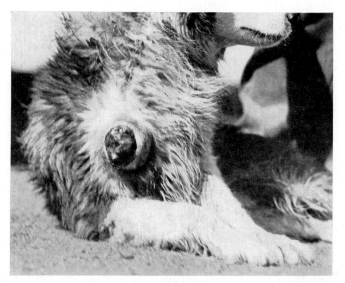

FIG. 158.—Carcinoma of the hair matrix. Microscopic appearance is shown in Figure 160.

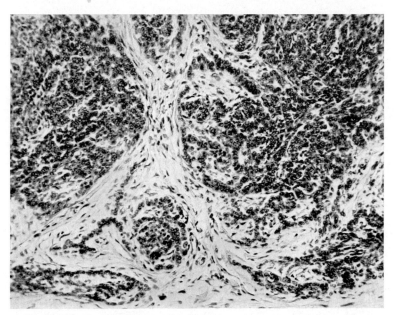

FIG. 159.—So-called basal-cell carcinoma of the skin of a dog. Same case as that represented in Figure 157.

many of which eventually fuse to produce diffuse collections of closely packed cells, with a minimal amount of stroma (Figs. 159 and 160). The cells of the deeper portions of the larger accumulations are not uncommonly fusiform, and assume a concentric arrangement. The cells at the peripheral line of contact with the stroma may reveal a pigment content not unlike those of the normal hair matrix. An adenomatous appearance is sometimes imparted to certain of these growths by the occurrence of lumens of various dimensions. These occur through the retrogressive softening and eventual disappearance of groups of tumor cells or of portions of the stroma, as a consequence of which a zone of peripheral cells, often several layers thick, remains (Fig. 161).

A moderate number of mitotic figures usually can be seen. In one specimen that I examined from a dog, many of the connective tissue cells of the stroma were also undergoing mitotic division. Although I

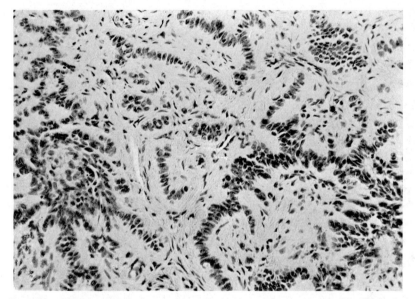

Fig. 160.—Carcinoma of the hair matrix. Same case as that represented in Figure 158.

failed to find epithelial pearls, intercellular bridges could be definitely seen in sections prepared from one of the specimens.

The growth is usually covered by taut, pink skin, practically devoid of hair, and attached by a rather broad base, constituting a firm, nodular elevation which frequently ulcerates. The rate of growth is usually slow, and distant metastasis seldom occurs. These are probably the least malignant of all carcinomas affecting lower animals.

Carcinoma may also originate from the epithelial cells of the alveoli of sebaceous glands, and from the epithelial elements of the sweat glands. Benign tumors, such as adenoma sebaceum, are not uncommonly seen, particularly in the dog, but malignant epithelial tumors derived from the sebaceous glands rarely occur. Likewise, malignant tumor of a sweat gland is uncommon. In my series of neoplasms I observed only one specimen which may have had its origin from this source. This occurred in the skin of a sheep, and metastasis had taken place to a near-by regional lymph node. The adenomatous and more or less cystic character of the tumor suggested origin in a sweat gland.

Carcinomas exceptionally may arise from the epiblastic cells of the enamel. These are only locally destructive and are designated adamantinoma. A few examples of this tumor as it affects animals have been reviewed by Fölger.

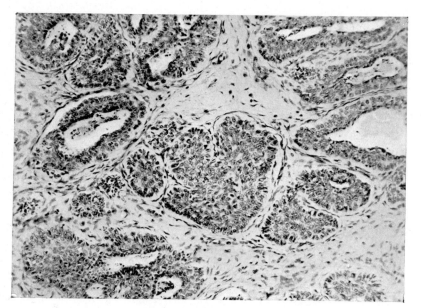

FIG. 161.—Carcinoma of the hair matrix of a horse.

Adenocarcinoma.—The epithelial cells of these tumors assume a gland-like arrangement. The mimicry is seldom complete, and one of the most characteristic features of these tumors is the extreme variation in their structure, which is due in part to the type of epithelium which constitutes the parenchyma, to the character of the structure from which the tumor originated, and to the degree of differentiation exhibited by the carcinomatous cells. The majority of adenocarcinomas arise from such structures as the thyroid gland, the mucosa of the gastro-intestinal tract, the ducts and alveoli of the mammary glands, the bile ducts, the prostate gland, the kidneys, the uterus, and certain glandular structures of the mucous lining of the respiratory tract.

Microscopically, an adenocarcinoma consists of epithelial cells, cuboidal to columnar in type, arranged in an alveolar or duct-like fashion. They are destructive, and they infiltrate surrounding tissues. The cells rest on a fibrous stroma of variable dimensions, which carries the blood vessels (Fig. 162). The epithelial cells may occur in single layers, or they may be heaped up until several indistinct layers become evident. If there is a tendency to produce alveolar-like spaces, these often become filled to capacity with the parenchymatous cells of the tumor. A tortuous, duct-like structure is commonly seen, and papillary projections of epithelial cells often characterize some of these tumors (Figs. 163 and 164). Others, in which the cells retain some degree of the functional

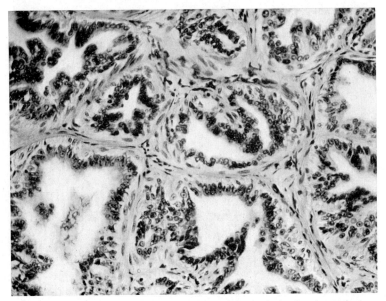

Fig. 162.—Adenocarcinoma of the mammary gland of a dog (× 220).

propensities possessed by the parent growths frequently develop cystic cavitations of variable sizes. The gelatinous or mucoid contents of these spaces represent the secretory activity of the carcinomatous cells (colloid carcinoma, page 320). Occasionally, an adenocarcinoma experiences a change in structure due to the rapid proliferation of immature cells. In such a tumor, diffuse sheets, or solid nests, of cells with no tendency toward formation of alveolus or lumen, may result although the parent growth was typically adenomatous. Such changes are not uncommon in secondary foci which have resulted as a consequence of metastasis.

Besides cystic degeneration which may overtake some adenocarcinomas, evidence of pyogenic infection is often seen. The open spaces

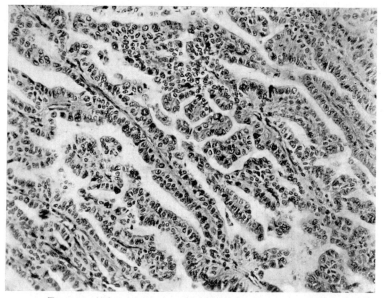

Fig. 163.—Adenocarcinoma of the kidney of a bovine (× 150).

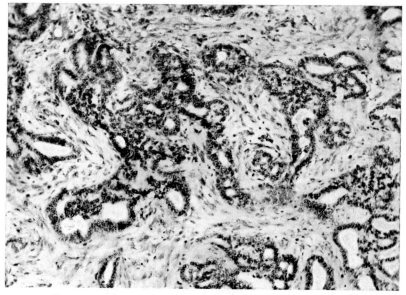

Fig. 164.—Adenocarcinoma of the intestine of a chicken (× 170).

of the tumor become filled with inflammatory exudate, and polymorphonuclear leukocytes are often numerous.

Liver-cell carcinoma (malignant hepatoma).—The specialized epithelial cells of the parenchyma of the liver often give rise to carcinoma. These are most frequently seen in dogs, cattle, and sheep. Grossly these tumors often present a rather striking appearance, due to their size and multiplicity. Their microscopic appearance is unusual. The parenchyma of the tumor consists of irregular collections of closely packed, large, polyhedral cells which stain strongly acidophilic. The cells which have an infiltrative tendency possess a significant resemblance, in many respects, to hepatic cells, but lack an orderly anatomic arrangement (Fig. 165). It is not unusual to observe fields in which can be

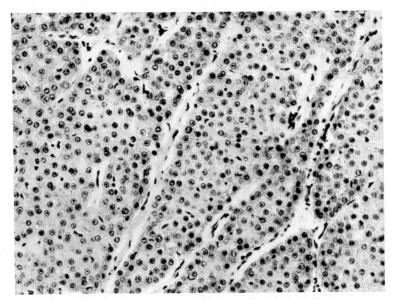

Fig. 165.—Hepatic cell carcinoma of a bovine (× 220).

seen what seems to be the transformation of morphologically normal hepatic cells to neoplastic elements. Although practically imperceptible, close examination will disclose the gradual zone of transition.* The cells of hepatomas possess a minutely granular cytoplasm, and the nuclei are rather large and contain prominent nucleoli. Mitotic figures may be few or numerous. Cystic cavitations often form, and extravasations of blood, resulting in large areas of free blood in direct contact with the cells of the tumor may occur. Capillaries may be distributed among the cells of the growth, but bile ducts are not demonstrable. Hepatic cell carcinoma of lower animals is not viciously malignant.

* A similar phenomenon of direct carcinomatous transformation of the hepatic cells was observed by Oertel in a case of multiple carcinoma of the liver of a human being.

It is true that occasionally widespread metastasis may ensue, but as a rule the tumors are limited to the organ responsible for their histogenesis. The immature character of the type cell, and the generous and often intimate blood supply of many of the tumors, would be expected to favor metastasis. Why more of them do not metastasize widely is not apparent.

Other types.—Malignant epithelial neoplasms are often encountered in situations such as the ovary and the adrenal cortex, which are devoid of many of the qualifying characteristics possessed by the other carcinomas described (Fig. 166). They may consist of very immature or

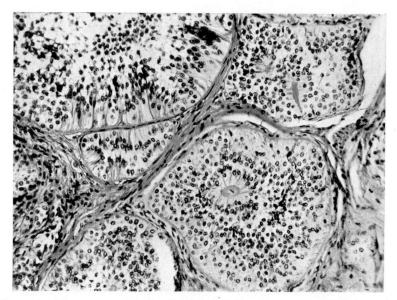

Fig. 166.—Metastasis to a lymph node of an ovarian carcinoma of a bovine (× 150).

undifferentiated types of epithelial cells, disposed in diffuse sheets or of closely packed masses of cells irregularly separated into indefinite units by variable amounts of fibrous connective tissue. The epithelial character of these growths is usually evident from the relation of the cells of the parenchyma to the element of the stroma, and, further, by the fact that their origin usually can be traced to some structure possessing epithelial tissues (Fig. 167).

Carcinomas with excessive production of fibrous connective tissue in the stroma as a consequence of which the growth assumes a firm, compact character, are sometimes designated scirrhous carcinoma whereas those of soft consistence due to the relatively large amount of parenchymatous elements and a minimum of stroma are called medullary carcinoma. These terms should be restricted to clinical use.

Anaplasia.—Carcinomas arising from the same anatomic situation and possessing identical cellular elements are subject to marked variation in their microscopic appearance, due to fundamental differences of cellular differentiation. Clinically, it has also been observed that all carcinomas do not exhibit the same degree of malignancy although they may be composed of the same histologic elements. Broders has utilized these biologic differences as the basis for a classification of malignant growths. He has contended that the malignancy of carcinoma is de-

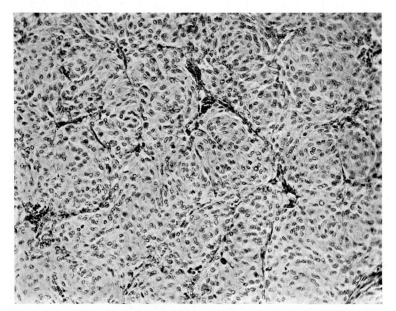

Fig. 167.—Carcinoma of the adrenal cortex of a sheep (× 150).

pendent on the extent to which the cells of the growth resemble the normal parent cells of the tissue from which they originate. On this basis, he would classify as Grade 1, carcinomas in which about a fourth of the cells are undifferentiated or immature in appearance and in which the remaining three-fourths of the cells have characteristics in common with the cells of the normal tissues from which they arise; these are least malignant. Carcinoma graded 4 is the type in which none of the cells is differentiated or resembles cells of the parent tissue, but instead, many of the cells contain deeply staining nucleoli, irregular mitotic figures, and other embryonic features; these are most malignant. Carcinomas graded 2 and 3 hold intermediate positions.

Although anaplasia as a clue to the prognosis of carcinoma of human beings may be of great practical significance, the usefulness of the principle in the field of veterinary practice has not been demonstrated. Tumors of animals apparently exhibit the same cytologic variations as do tumors of man, but for practical and economic reasons their treatment has not attained the refinement justifiable in human practice.

Clinical considerations.—In the treatment of carcinoma, the veterinarian has not kept pace with the physician. Too often the lesion is considered hopeless after a cursory examination, and a valuable work animal or dairy animal is either permitted to live until it dies as a result of the disease, or more often it is slaughtered in the hope that something may be salvaged. Again, the victim may be a valuable and much esteemed pet which may be condemned to early death without the benefit of the treatment that would probably be accorded a human being suffering from a similar tumor. It is not assumed that animals should be given the elaborate and expensive therapeutic assistance often brought to the aid of human beings suffering from carcinoma, yet a better understanding of the general pathologic considerations of carcinoma as it affects lower animals would be beneficial, even though it resulted in palliative treatment only. Not all carcinomas are necessarily fatal, and in many cases proper treatment may not only prolong life, but apparently cures may be obtained in selected cases by appropriate means.

The rational treatment of carcinoma, like the rational treatment of any disease, depends largely on a correct diagnosis. Simply to designate a given condition as tumor or carcinoma, is as unsatisfactory as referring to all acute abdominal disorders which result in pain as colic. Unfortunately, the diagnosis of internal neoplasms of animals had not achieved the refinement of technic practiced in the diagnosis of neoplasms of human beings, and, as a consequence, many benign and malignant tumors which involve the internal structures of animals are usually not discovered until after death. Even if they were suspected, their inoperability in the larger species is apparent, and although operation may occasionally be resorted to for relief of an internal tumor of smaller animals, the surgeon is much handicapped by the inability of the animal to coöperate, for on such assistance success or failure so often depends. From a practical standpoint little relief can be offered in cases in which the animal is suffering from internal neoplasm even if an accurate diagnosis is made. However, a considerable number of tumors affecting the exterior of the body is amenable to some form of treatment.

Much can be determined concerning the true nature of a tumor by careful study of its gross appearance; it is highly desirable, however, whenever possible, to remove a small piece of the growth for histologic examination. This procedure, known as biopsy, usually can be carried out without pain to the animal, or if it is desired, removal can follow the injection of a small amount of a suitable local anesthetic. If the tissue is placed immediately in a 10 per cent solution of formalin and forwarded to the pathologist, a diagnosis usually can be obtained within a few days. When the exact nature of the tumor is determined, its subsequent treatment can be outlined.

In considering the prognosis of carcinomas it should be recognized that they exhibit many degrees or grades of malignancy. Some grow slowly, with little tendency to invade the surrounding tissues, and others grow vigorously with early metastasis to adjacent lymph nodes and organs. Little can be done, when metastasis has occurred, and one is justified in recommending the humane disposal of the animal.

The early operative removal of a carcinoma of low-grade of malignancy, such as a so-called basal-cell carcinoma, should always be attempted, provided, of course, the value of the animal is such as to warrant the procedure. Even if the tumor is moderately malignant and if metastasis has not occurred, it is often possible to give temporary relief by early treatment, and a valuable work animal or breeding animal may remain in service several months longer than would have been possible without operative interference. Cases of carcinoma of the eye of cattle have been noted, in which surgical intervention eliminated demonstrable evidence of the growth for as long as three years, although probably the disease was not eradicated. Although it is true that results of this sort are exceptional, it is also true that treatment of the disease is not entirely futile. The possibility of cure following early recognition of carcinoma is sufficiently promising to warrant a serious attempt to remove the growth by carefully planned and selected procedures, and thus to give the maximal possibility for success. To offer less, constitutes professional negligence. The use of pastes, ointments, and other empiric agents cannot be recommended.

Much of real value results from the treatment of certain malignant growths in human beings by roentgen rays and radium, but these agents have been tried in treatment of only a few animals. The work that has been done indicates that these agents are valuable aids in the treatment of selected cases. To those interested in this form of treatment of carcinoma, the observations of Little should be considered. For a period of several years Little had the opportunity to study the effect of radium emanation on malignant growths of horses and dogs. In some instances complete cure was effected; the best results were obtained with a combination of irradiation and surgical procedures. Sarcomas and carcinomas responded to the treatment, and Little concluded that many of the malignant tumors of horses and dogs respond to radium emanation more readily than similar tumors of man.

Briefly it may be said that for the average practitioner of veterinary medicine the best chance for success in treating carcinomatous growths is to detect them early in the course of the disease, determine their exact nature by microscopic examination if possible, and if the site of the tumor is suitable for operation, and if metastasis has not occurred, removal, by surgical means, of all the tumorous tissue.

BIBLIOGRAPHY

1. Aynaud, M.: Origine vermineuse du cancer pulmonaire de la brebis. Compt.-rend. Soc. de biol., **95**: 1540–1542 (Dec. 31), 1926.

2. Ball, V. and Lombard, C.: Cancer de la vessie. Epithéliome intermédiaire ou dyskératosique propagé à l'utérus chez une jument. Bull. de l'Assn. franç. p. l'etude du cancer, **15**: 301–304, 1926. Abstr. in: Cancer Rev., **2**: 306 (July), 1927.

3. Bartlett, F. K.: Multiple primary malignant tumors with a report of two cases in dogs. Arch. Int. Med., **13**: 624–639 (April), 1914.

4. Bashford, E. F.: The ethnological distribution of cancer. Third Scientific Report on the Investigations of the Imperial Cancer Research Fund, London, 1–40, 1908.

5. Betke, R.: Multiple Tumoren bei einem Nashorn. Frankfurter Ztschr. f. Path., **6**: 19–26, 1911.

6. Borrel: Quoted by Wolff, Jacob: Die Lehre von der Krebskrankheit. Jena, Gustav Fischer, 1913, **3**: p. 221.

7. Boynton, F. N.: A study of a malignant tumor in the domestic fowl, with an attempt at transplantation, and with special reference to amyloia-like changes occurring in the liver. Contribution to medical research. Ann Arbor, Michigan, George Wahr, 1903, pp. 535–540.

8. Broders, A. C.: Squamous-cell epithelioma of the lip. A study of five hundred and thirty-seven cases. Jour. Am. Med. Assn., **74**: 656–664 (March 6), 1920.

9. Broders, A. C.: The grading of carcinoma. Minnesota Med., **8**: 726–730 (Dec.), 1925.

10. Bürger, Max: Untersuchungen über das Hühnersarkom (Peyton Rous). Ztschr. f. Krebsforsch, **14**: 526–542, 1914.

11. Cadiot and Almy: Quoted by French, Cecil: Surgical diseases and surgery of the dog. Chicago, A. Eger, 1923, p. 383.

12. Cleland, J. B.: Some examples of malignant disease in animals. Jour. Comp. Path. and Therap., **21**: 243, 1908.

13. Cornil, V. and Petit, G.: Épithéliome à cellules cylindriques de la mamelle, généralise au poumon et au foie, chez une chatte. Bull. et mém. Soc. anat. de Par., **81**: 208–211 (March), 1906.

14. Crocker, W. J.: Three thousand autopsies. Cornell Vet., **9**: 142–161 (Jan.), 1919.

15. Cunningham, E.: Cancer cases. Jour. Comp. Path. and Therap., **16**: 163–169, 1903.

16. Davis, C. L. and Leeper, R. B.: Personal communication to the author.

17. Drabble, J.: Cancer of udders of cows. Jour. Comp. Path. and Therap., **42**: 40–44 (March 30), 1929.

18. Drabble, J.: Skin cancer in cattle. Australian Vet. Jour., **5**: 71–76, 1929.

19. Drabble, J. and Massy, A. E.: Cancer in the udder of a cow. Jour. Comp. Path. and Therap., **39**: 247–250, 1926.

20. Dupas: Epithelioma of the perineal glands in the dog. Abstract: Vet. Jour., **85**: 276–278 (June), 1929.

21. Eberlein: Primäres Karzinom der Klitoris beim Pferde. Monatschr. f. prakt. Tierh., **10**: 14, 1899.

22. Editorial: Cancer in horses. Am. Vet. Rev., **44**: 299–300 (Dec.), 1913.

23. Eggeling: Quoted by Joest.

24. Ehlers: Adenocarcinoma in the colon of a horse. Abstract: Am. Vet. Rev., **25**: 219, 1901–1902.

25. Ehrenreich, M.: Wietere Mitteilungen über das Vorkommen maligner Tumoren bei Huhner. Med. Klin., **3**: 614–615 (May 26), 1907.

26. Ehrenreich, M. and Michaelis, L.: Ueber tumoren bei Hühnern. Ztschr. f. Krebsforsch., **4**: 586–591, 1906.

27. Emmel, M. W.: Epidermoid cancers on the feet of wild birds. Jour. Am. Vet. Med. Assn., **77**: 641–644 (Nov.), 1930.

28. Ewald, Otto: Ueber maligne Hundestrumen nebst Bemerkungen über die sekretorische Tätigheit der Schilddrüse. Ztschr. f. Krebsforsch., **15**: 85–110, 1915–1916.

29. Fadyean, J. M.: The occurrence of cancer in the lower animals. Practitioner, **62**: 456–462 (April), 1899.

30. Feldman, W. H.: An adenocarcinoma resembling the thyroid gland in a bovine. Am. Jour. Path., **1**: 281–284 (May), 1925.

31. Field, Eva H.: A contribution to the study of malignant growths in the lower animals. Jour. Am. Med. Assn., **23**: 982–985 (Dec. 29), 1894.

32. Fölger, A. F.: Geschwülste bei Tieren. Ergebn. d. all. Path. u. path. Anat., **18**: 372–676, 1917.

33. Fox, Herbert: Disease in captive wild mammals and birds; incidence, description, comparison. Philadelphia, J. B. Lippincott Co., 1923, 665 pp.

34. Frenkel, H. S.: Primary carcinoma of liver of sheep. Over primaire bloedvormende gezwellen in de Lever van het schapp. Med. Vet., Utrecht, 1927, 100 pp.

35. Friedberger, Franz and Fröhner, Eugen: Veterinary pathology. London, Hurst and Blackett, **1**: 182, 1908.

36. Fröhner: Hundert weitere Geschwulste beim Pferde. Monatschr. f. prakt. Thierh., **13**: 138, 1902.

37. Fröhner, E.: Carcinoma of the adrenal gland in the horse, with hemorrhage into the abdominal cavity. Monatschr. f. prakt. Tierh., **27**: 102, 1916. Abstr. in: Jour. Am. Vet. Med. Assn., **49**: 533–534 (July), 1916.

38. Fröhner: Quoted by Müller, Georg and Glass, Alex.: Diseases of the dog and their treatment. Chicago, A. Eger, 1926, p. 339.

39. Fröhner: Quoted by Goodpasture.

40. Fujinami: Quoted by Baird, A. I.: Spontaneous epithelioma of the fowl. Jour. Cancer Res., **2**: 103–106 (Jan.), 1917.

41. Gaylord, H. R.: Further observations on so-called carcinoma of the thyroid in fish. Jour. Cancer Res., **1**: 197–204 (April), 1916.

42. Gaylord, H. R. and Marsh, M. C.: Carcinoma of the thyroid in the Salmonoid fishes. Bull. Bureau of Fisheries, vol. 32 (1912). Document No. 790, Washington, Government Printing Office, 1914, 524 pp.

43. Gilruth, J. A.: Adeno-carcinomata of the lungs with secondary growths in a cow. Abstract: Am. Vet. Rev., **38**: 401–402 (Dec.), 1910.

44. Goldberg, S. A.: The occurrence of epithelial tumors in the domesticated animals. Jour. Am. Vet. Med. Assn., **58**: 47–63 (Oct.), 1920.

45. Goodpasture, E. W.: An anatomical study of senescence in dogs with especial reference to the relation of cellular changes of age to tumors. Jour. Med. Res., **38**: 127–189 (May), 1918.

46. Gordon, J. and Happold, F. C.: Adenocarcinoma of the ovary in a hen. Jour. Path. and Bacteriol., **30**: 573, 1927.

47. Görig: Primäres Karzinom der Nebenniere bei einer Kuh. Deutsch. tierärztl. Wchnschr., **4**: 305, 1896.

48. Grüttner, F.: Gallenganskarzinom beim Pferde. Ztschr. f. Fleisch. u. Milchhyg., **37**: 294, 1927.

49. Herzog, M.: Cancer in domestic animals. Illinois Med. Jour., **20**: 387–390 (Dec.), 1911.

50. Hewlett, K.: Cancer of the horn-core of cattle. Jour. Comp. Path. and Therap., **18**: 161–163, 1905.

51. Hobday, F. T. G.: Surgical diseases of the dog and cat. Chicago, Chicago Medical Book Co., 1925.

52. Hodgson, J. F.: A case of cystic cancer of the liver in a sheep. Jour. Comp. Path. and Therap., **16**: 269–270, 1903.

53. Holmbo, F. V.: Quoted by Fölger.

54. Horne: Sur les tumeurs cancéreuses primitives des capsules surrénales du bœuf. Rev. gén. de Méd. Vétér., **6**: 62, 1905.

55. Horne: Quoted by Fölger.

56. Huguenin: Quoted by Wegelin.

57. Hutchinson, Woods: Studies in human and comparative pathology. London, H. J. Glaisher, 1901, p. 258.

58. Huynen, E.: Hydronephrosis caused by vesical cancer in a dog. Abstract: Am. Vet. Rev., **41**: 610–611 (Aug.), 1912.

59. Joest, Ernst: Handbuch der speziellen pathologischen Anatomie der Haustiere. Berlin, 1925, **4**: pp. 93 and 166.

60. Joest, Ernst: Handbuch der speziellen pathologischen Anatomie der Haustiere. Berlin, 1926, **1**: pp. 755–759.

61. Joest, Ernst: Ueber Bosartige Geschwulste der Tiere. Zweifel-Payr Klinik der Bosartige Geschwülste. Leipzig, S. Hirzel, **3**: 592–628, 1927.

62. Joest, E. and Ernesti, S.: Untersuchungen über spontane Geschwülste bei Vögeln mit besonderer Berüchsichtigung des Haushuhns. Ztschr. f. Krebsforsch., **15**: 1–75, 1915–1916.

63. Johne: Quoted by Fölger.

64. Kitt, Theodor: Text-book of comparative general pathology. Chicago, Chicago Medical Book Co., 1906, p. 405.

65. Kitt, T.: Quoted by Wolff, Jacob: Die Lehre von der Krebskrankheit. Jena, Gustave Fischer, 1913, **3**: p. 221.

66. Kitt, Theodor: Quoted by Joest.[59]

67. Koch, Max: Demonstration einiger Geschwülste bei Tieren. Verhandl. d. deutsch. path. Gesellsch., **7**: 136–147, 1904.

68. de Kock, G.: Two cases of squamous-cell carcinoma (cancroid) in the rumen of bovines. Thirteenth and fourteenth reports of the director of Veterinary Education and Research, October, 1928.

69. Krammell, D.: A case of cancer of the stomach in the horse. Berlin Tier. Wchnschr., 259, 1919. Abstr. in: Jour. Am. Vet. Med. Assn., **60**: 334, 1921–1922.

70. Krompecher, E.: Der drüsenartige Oberflächenepithelkrebs. Carcinoma epitheliale adenoides. Beitr. z. path. Anat. u. z. allg. Path., **28**: 1–41, 1900; Der Basalzellenkrebs, Jena, 1903.

71. Law, James: Text-book of veterinary medicine. Ed. 3, Ithaca, New York, 1911, p. 372.

72. Lewis, J. C.: Adeno-carcinoma in undescended testicle. Abstract: Jour. Am. Vet. Med. Assn., **49**: 538–539 (July), 1916.

73. Lingual cancer. Abstract: Jour. Am. Vet. Med. Assn., **55**: 322–323 (June), 1919.

74. Little, G. W.: Some studies in the behavior of malignant growths in dogs and horses. Jour. Am. Vet. Med. Assn., **71**: 171–188 (May), 1927.

75. Loeb, Leo: Ueber das endemische Vorkommen des Krebses beim Tiere. Centralbl. f. Bakt., Orig., **37**: 235–245, 1904.

76. Lubarsch: Quoted by Olt: Cancer in domestic animals. Jour. Comp. Path. and Therap., **18**: 278–279, 1905.

77. Mallory, F. B.: The principles of pathologic histology, Philadelphia, W. B. Saunders Co., 1914, p. 371; Recent progress in the microscopic anatomy and differentiation of cancer. Jour. Am. Med. Assn., **55**: 1513–1516 (Oct. 29), 1910.

78. Mann, F. C.: Attempts to obtain a transplantable tumor in the higher species of animals. Jour. Cancer Res., **4**: 331–347 (Oct.), 1919.

79. Mann, F. C.: A case of spontaneous acute and subacute peptic ulcers and carcinoma of the thyroid in a dog. Jour. Lab. and Clin. Med., **6**: 213–217 (Jan.), 1921.

80. Mann, F. C. and Brimhall, S. D.: Pathologic conditions noted in laboratory animals. Case Report. Jour. Am. Vet. Med. Assn., **52**: 195–204 (Nov.), 1917.

81. Mathews, F. P. and Walkey, F. L.: Hypernephromas in the common fowl. Jour. Am. Vet. Med. Assn., **77**: 218–224 (Aug.), 1930.

82. Milks, H. J.: Carcinoma of the skin. Cornell Vet., **9**: 49, 1919.

83. Milks, H. J. and Muldoon, W. E.: Colloid carcinoma. Cornell Vet., **7**: 146, 1917.

84. Moussu, G.: Cancer of the tail. Abstract: Jour. Am. Vet. Med. Assn., **49**: 715–716, 1916.

85. Multiple epithelioma. Vet. Med., **17**: 26–27 (Jan.), 1922.

86. Murray, J. A.: The zoölogical distribution of cancer. Third Scientific Report on the Investigations of the Imperial Cancer Research Fund, London, 1908, pp. 41–60.

87. Oertel: Quoted by Adami, J. G.: The principles of pathology. Ed. 2, Philadelphia, Lea & Febiger, 1910, **1**: p. 836.

88. Ortschild, J. F.: A report of eight cases of canine neoplasm. Bull. Johns Hopkins Hosp., **16**: 186–196 (May), 1905.

89. Pentimalli, F.: Ueber die Geschwülste bei Hühnern. I. Allgemeine Morphologie der spontanen und der transplantablen Hühnergeschwülste. Ztschr. f. Krebsforsch., **15**: 111–153, 1915–1916.

90. Perry, C. B.: Renal carcinoma in a brown bear. Jour. Comp. Path. and Therap., **42**: 133 (June 29), 1929.

91. Petit, G.: Generalization of carcinoma of the mammary gland in the bitch and cat. Rec. de Méd. Vét., **16**: 63–64, 1903.

92. Pfab: Karzinom des Darmes und der Leber beim Rinde. Wchnschr. f. Tierh., 797, 1909.

93. Pfeiffer, W.: Karzinom der Schildrüse beim Pferde, mit Metastasebildung in sämtlichen Halslymphdrüsen und den Lungen. Monatschr. f. prakt. Tierh., **10**: 149, 1899.

94. Pick, L.: Zur Frage vom Vorkommen des Carcinoms bei Vögeln: Grosser Plattenepithelkrebs des Mundhöhlenbodens bei einem Huhn. Berl. klin. Wchnschr., **40**: 669–670 (July 20), 1903.

95. Pick, L.: Der Schilddrüsenkrebs der Salmoniden (Edelfische). Berl. klin. Wchnschr., **2**: 1435–1440 (Nov. 13), 1905.

96. Plehn, Marianne: Bösartiger Kropf (Adeno-Carcinom der Thyroidea) bei Salmoniden. Allg. Fischerei-Zeitung., 117–118 (April 1), 1902.

97. Polson, C. J.: Tumours of the rabbit. Jour. Path. and Bacteriol., **30**: 603–614, 1927.

98. Quentin: Generalized cancer of the pancreas, with perforation of the stomach. Rec. Med. Vet., **95**: 290–296, 1919. Abstr. in: Jour. Am. Vet. Med. Assn., **57**: 189–190 (May), 1920.

99. Richter, J.: Carcinom der Gallenblase beim Hunde. Ztschr. f. Thiermed., **8**: 115, 1904.

100. Roussy, Gustave and Wolf, Maurice: Le cancer chez les animaux. Ann, de méd., **8**: 462–492 (Dec.), 1920.

101. Rusk, G. Y. and Epstein, Norman: Adenocarcinoma of the uterus in a rabbit. Am. Jour. Path., **3**: 235–240 (May), 1927.

102. Savage, A.: Adenocarcinoma of gallbladder in a hen. Cornell Vet., **16**: 67, 1926.

103. Schaible: Quoted by Fölger.

104. Scheidt: Quoted by Fölger.

105. Schlegel: Quoted by Joest.[58]

106. Schlotthauer, C. F.: The incidence and types of disease of the thyroid gland of adult horses. Jour. Am. Vet. Med. Assn., **78**: 211–218 (Feb.), 1931.

107. Schlotthauer, C. F., McKenney, F. D. and Caylor, H. D.: The incidence of goiter and other lesions of the thyroid gland in dogs of southern Minnesota. Jour. Am. Vet. Med. Assn., **76**: 811–819 (June), 1930.

108. Scholer, P. T.: Zur Kenntnis der Uteruscarcinome beim Rind. Ztschr. f. Krebsforsch., **15**: 193–211, 1915–1916.

109. Schöppler, Herrmann: Carcinoma ventriculi cylindrocellulare beim Haushuhn. Ztschr. f. Krebsforsch., **13**: 332–335, 1913.

110. Schütz: Über Vorkommen des Carcinoms bei Thieren. Deutsch. med. Wchnschr., **27**: 240, 1901.

111. Scott, Ernest and Moore, R. A.: A case of pancreatic carcinoma in a cat. Jour. Cancer Rev., **11**: 152–157 (June), 1927.

112. Scott, H.: Carcinoma of the tonsil in a common wolf. Proc. Zoöl. Soc. of London, 1918, pp. 43–47.

113. Semmer: Quoted by Goodpasture.

114. Siedamgrotzky: Quoted by Joest.[59]

115. Silva, P.: Primitives Karzinom einer Nebenniere bei iner Kuh. Tierärztl. Zentralbl., **35**: 415, 1912.

116. Sticker, Anton: Ueber den Krebs der Thiere insbesondere über die Empfänglichkeit der verschiedenen Hausthierarten und über die Unterschiede des Thier- und Menschenkrebses. Arch. f. klin. Chir., **65**: 616–696; 1023–1087, 1902.

117. Takahashi, Keizo: Studie über die Fischgeschwülste. Ztschr. f. Krebsforsch., **29**: 1–73, 1929.

118. Trotter, A. M.: Six cases of carcinoma of the ox. Jour. Comp. Path. and Therap., **16**: 244–252, 1903.

119. Trotter, A. M.: Primary adenocarcinoma of the liver. Jour. Comp. Path. and Therap., **17**: 129–140, 1904.

120. Trotter, A. M.: Supplementary note on adeno-carcinoma of the liver. Jour. Comp. Path. and Therap., **18**: 143, 1905.

121. Trotter, I. M.: Malignant diseases in bovines. Am. Vet. Rev., **39**: 365–368 (July) 1911.

122. Udall, D. H., Fincher, M. G. and Cushing, E. R.: Cancer of the cervix in a cow. Cornell Vet., **16**: 230–231, (July), 1926.

123. Udall, D. H., Fincher, M. G. and Gibbons, E. V.: Cancer of the duodenum in a horse. Cornell Vet., **16**: 299 (July), 1926.

124. Voges, O.: Panophthalmia bovina carcinomatosa. Zentralbl. f. Bakt., Orig., **31**: 142–145, 1902.

125. Walter, F. A.: Carcinoma of glottis in cow. Jour. Am. Vet. Med. Assn., **50:** 733 (Feb.), 1917.

126. Wankmüller: Karzinom am Gesäuge des Schweines. Wchnschr. f. Tierh., **46:** 600, 1902.

127. Wegelin, C.: Malignant disease of the thyroid gland and its relations to goitre in man and animals. Cancer Rev., **3:** 297–313 (July), 1928.

128. Wooldridge, C. H.: Carcinoma of the œsophagus in a cat. Abstract: Am. Vet. Rev., **43:** 96 (April), 1913.

129. Woundenberg, N. P.: Über Vergrösserung der Schilddrüse bei Haustieren. Virchow's Arch. f. path. Anat. u. Physiol., **196:** 107–126 (April 1), 1909.

CHAPTER XX

TRANSMISSIBLE LYMPHOSARCOMA OF DOGS

DEFINITION AND TERMS

Transmissible lymphosarcoma is composed of lymphoid cells. The growth exhibits a predilection for the genital organs of dogs, and is readily transmissible by contact. The tumor has been the subject of much investigation and is commonly referred to in the literature as infectious sarcoma of dogs. Among veterinarians it is known as "venereal granuloma," "canine condyloma," and "venereal lymphosarcoma." The condition seems to be universal in distribution. Seligmann mentioned that the disease was endemic in New Guinea before the advent of the white man, and hence was not dependent for its appearance on imported dogs.

HISTOGENESIS

Practically all investigators who have studied this tumor have attempted to classify the type cell, and, although a few of the early observers thought the tumor was carcinoma composed of epithelial cells, the opinion of the majority is that the growth probably originates from certain mesenchymal elements and should be considered sarcoma. Although definite proof is lacking, the evidence seems to favor derivation of the tumor from undifferentiated cells of the lymphocytic series. The cells, however, are perhaps larger and more uniform in size than those of the usual lymphoblastoma, and an intercellular reticulum has not been observed. Furthermore, the facts that the tumor is readily transmissible, is slightly malignant, and is peculiar to dogs, constitute characteristics that are at variance with the majority of lymphoid tumors. The designation of the growth as lymphosarcoma is made for morphologic reasons only, and it is perhaps proper to say that the exact histogenesis of the type cell has not been conclusively determined.

INCIDENCE

Among eighty-one neoplasms of dogs that I examined, seven (8.6 per cent) were considered histologically to be transmissible lymphosarcomas. Suggestive of the frequent occurrence of the disease is the statement of Beebe and Ewing that they had no difficulty in securing numerous cases in New York City. The condition is often seen in kennels which house large numbers of dogs, and occasionally it is seen not associated with kennel life.

OCCURRENCE AND POINTS OF ORIGIN

Practically all observers agree that the primary lesion is usually the penis or the vagina, although Beebe and Ewing were of the opinion that in both sexes isolated tumors may occur anywhere over the body (Fig. 168). Three of the tumors in my series were found in the vaginal vault; one tumor was embedded in the connective tissue, between the

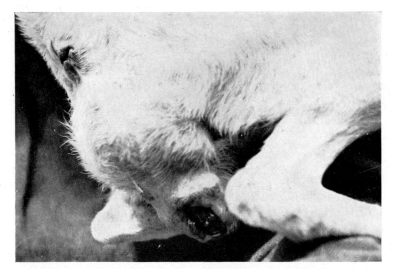

FIG. 168.—Transmissible lymphosarcoma. The mass completely fills the vaginal vault, causing protrusion of the affected parts.

penis and the wall of the abdomen, and in one instance two tumors, morphologically identical, appeared respectively in the orbital space and under the skin of the frontal region of a mongrel aged four to five months.[8] In two cases the tumors were confined to the superficial tissues of the neck and the prepectoral region. In the absence of evidence pointing to the origin of these extragenital tumors, through contact with animals possessing similar growths, they must be considered of spontaneous origin. Judged by the observations of others, the occurrence of tumors of this nature, apart from the genitalia, are unusual (Fig. 169).

In England the disease has commonly affected animals of the bulldog breed, but it has been observed in St. Bernards, terriers, poodles, and pugs. Although it is contended that the higher bred animals are most susceptible, it is my belief that breed is no protection. Perhaps the disease appears to be more common in pure-bred animals than in mongrels, because the former more often have the benefit of veterinary service, and consequently the disease is more likely to be recognized.

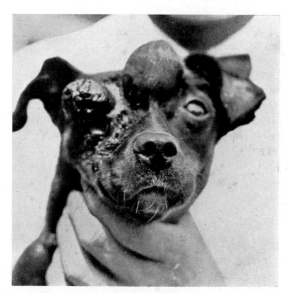

FIG. 169.—Transmissible lymphosarcomas. Multiple nodules of the same histologic structure as those that affect the genital apparatus.

All of the dogs I observed that were affected with this tumor were mongrels.

METASTASIS AND MALIGNANCY

The failure of the tumor seriously to influence the well-being of the affected animal is a notable feature in many cases. Occasionally it produces metastatic foci in the near-by or distant tissues, but it is very unusual for the tumor to display a metastatic distribution in keeping with the evidences of malignancy exhibited by the cytologic characteristics of the primary growths. The tumor lacks many of the malignant qualities one might properly ascribe to other growths possessing similar structural elements, and it is seldom that death results as a direct consequence of the neoplasm. I have had under observation for more than four years a mongrel terrier that had a large, transmissible lymphosarcoma of the vagina for almost three years. The tumor gradually diminished in size, and finally disappeared. At present the vaginal passage, although somewhat eroded, is free of tumorous tissue, and metastasis is not demonstrable. The general health of the animal appears to be excellent. The fact that many of these tumors can be extirpated surgically and do not recur is further evidence of their more or less benign clinical course, notwithstanding the fact that they have all the microscopic appearances of malignancy. This fact alone places the growth in a unique position among other neoplastic diseases.

GROSS CHARACTERISTICS

In the vagina, in the early stages, the process appears as a single, or rarely multiple, nodular, or papillary elevation in the mucosa. The

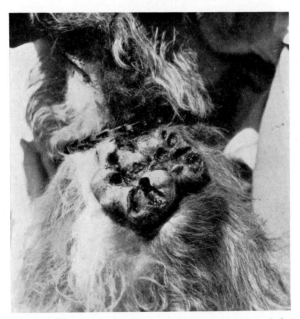

Fig. 170.—Transmissible lymphosarcoma of the subcutaneous tissues of the neck. There are ulcerations on the surface of the tumor.

growth seems to have its inception in the submucosa of the dorsal portion, and the expansion caused by increased growth frequently stretches the mucosa to a thin sheet, which may rupture and permit the growth to extend into the vaginal vault as a roughened, ulcerated, friable mass. Growths of the penis are frequently multiple, and may appear as firm, raised, nodular, fleshy masses of variable size, situated anywhere over the glans penis. Masses may also occur in the loose tissues of the sheath, and may extend to the perineum and the scrotum. Those on the penis begin, as Smith and Washbourn have stated: "As small, glistening elevations, about the size of millet seeds, mostly transparent but sometimes blood-stained."

As the growths become larger and more subject to trauma, hemorrhage frequently occurs. This is often associated with superficial infection, so that the affected parts give off a bloody, serous, or purulent discharge that may have an offensive odor. The large and more superficial masses are prone to ulcerate, and large portions of the tumor may slough, to be followed by eventual disappearance of the growths. The extragenital growths I have observed appeared first as small, firm, slightly elevated masses in the subcutis. If the skin eventually was penetrated, the tumor assumed a pink, irregularly lobulated contour, devoid of a capsular covering (Fig. 170).

A great many transmissible lymphosarcomas are characterized by a tendency to break down after some months of progression, and on incision it is not uncommon for semipurulent fluid to escape.

MICROSCOPIC DESCRIPTION

The histologic characteristics of transmissible lymphosarcoma are fairly consistent. The tumor is extremely cellular, and consists of closely

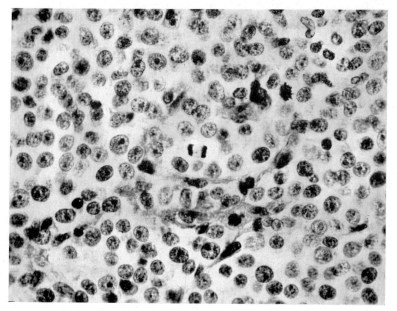

FIG. 171.—Transmissible lymphosarcoma, vaginal tumor (× 660).

arranged, rather large, irregularly shaped cells that are inclined to be spherical or polyhedral (Fig. 171). The cytoplasm of the neoplastic cells is finely granular, and although in most instances it is basophilic or moderately acidophilic in its staining reaction, it is not uncommon to find cells in which the cytoplasm exhibits but little tendency to stain, and appears pale or even clear (Fig. 172). The nuclei which take the basic stain represent about half of the cellular bulk, and possess a large number of coarse, chromatin granules. A prominent, somewhat eccentrically situated nucleolus is present in the majority of cells. Mitosis is a striking feature of the microscopic picture, and several phases of this phenomenon often can be seen in a single field. The evidence of

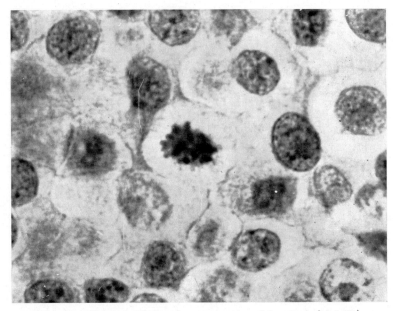

FIG. 172.—Transmissible lymphosarcoma, one cell in mitosis ($\times$ 2,000).

cellular progression is impressive, and suggests the potential malignancy of these tumors.

The continuity of the closely packed cells is frequently interrupted by strands of fibrous tissue of variable thickness, which sometimes assume an alveolar arrangement and which support the numerous blood vessels of the growth (Fig. 173). Aside from these fibrous elements, an intercellular reticulum or stroma has not been demonstrated. Free blood is commonly observed in contact with large numbers of the tumor cells, and some of the more superficial vessels may become thrombosed.

The growing propensities of the cells is further indicated by the locally invasive nature of the growth, although it is not unusual to observe, particularly in the extragenital specimens, a definite increase

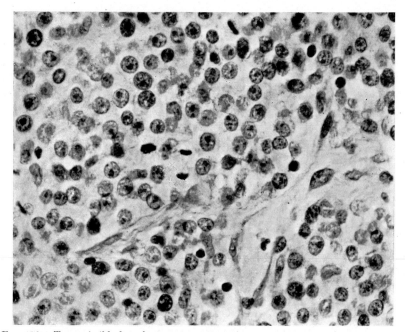

FIG. 173.—Transmissible lymphosarcoma, tumor of eye, same case as that represented in Figure 169 (× 660).

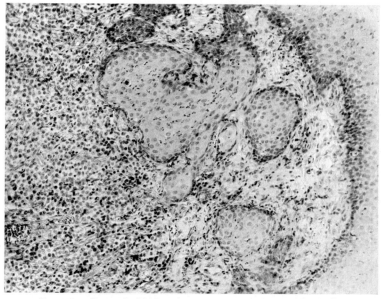

FIG. 174.—Transmissible lymphosarcoma, vaginal tumor (× 150).

of the fibrous connective tissue in immediate contact with the tumor cells (Fig. 174).

TRANSMISSION

One of the most noteworthy features of this neoplasm is the facility with which it is transmitted to other dogs by natural or artificial means. This quality has prompted a considerable number of transmission experiments, the more important of which are summarized, beginning on page 351.

The ease with which the tumor cells can be successfully transplanted to a normal dog during copulation makes the existence of the disease in breeding kennels serious. The disease is as readily transferred from the female to the male as from the male to the female. The affected male is the greater menace, however, since, if used extensively for breeding, he is likely to inoculate a large number of bitches, and these in turn become a focus of transmissibility to other males. There is no evidence that transmission is likely to occur spontaneously from tumors situated extragenitally, although the possibility must be conceded.

Experimental transmission can be accomplished in a large percentage of the recipients by the simple procedure of introducing into the subcutis, with a sterile trocar and cannula, a small disk of fresh tumor tissue. Sepsis should be avoided. Transmission is dependent on the growth and multiplication of the intact tumor cells that have been transferred from the body of the donor to the body of the recipient. Filtrates free of cells are impotent.

These tumors are often erroneously referred to as infectious sarcoma or infectious lymphosarcoma. There is no reason to assume that a specific infectious agent is responsible for their causation, or that they are transmissible for the same reason. They apparently are transmissible because the transplanted or inoculated cells are able to grow in the tissues of the recipient, and not because of transference of a separate infectious substance in the strict bacteriologic sense.

CLINICAL CONSIDERATIONS

Transmissible lymphosarcomas of the genitalia seldom are recognized early, because the tumor is usually in a situation that is ordinarily hidden from view. The initial stage of the growth is frequently accompanied by a catarrhal inflammation of the involved mucosa, and if the growth is near the urethral orifice, the animal may experience some difficulty and pain in urinating. The affected part may give forth a serous or purulent discharge that may result in examination and discovery of the neoplasm. Since the growth is friable and generously supplied with blood, hemorrhage is common even though the mass is small. Hemorrhage in either sex after copulation, painful copulation, or failure to mate, are factors of significance in suggesting the presence of a transmissible lymphosarcoma of the penis or vagina. Digital examination of the vagina and manual exposure of the penis usually will enable one to detect growths if present.

An affected animal should not be used for breeding purposes. In fact, isolation of an animal which possesses a tumor of this kind would be desirable.

The manner in which a great many of these tumors respond to surgical intervention lends encouragement to the belief that surgical removal should be attempted whenever practical. Tumors of the penis, unless they are very numerous, and tumors situated near the vulva, in the vagina, are frequently amenable to operation. If the entire vaginal vault is occupied, or if the tumor involves the os uteri, or the cervix, removal is not advisable.

The operation often can be satisfactorily carried out under local anesthesia, but it is best done with the animal completely anesthetized. In removing the tumors, it is imperative to excise a liberal margin of the surrounding tissue in order to obtain all of the growth. Unless this is done, recurrence may be expected. Contraindications to operation would be extensive local involvement of situations not readily accessible, and metastasis.

Even though the disease may have attained what is considered an inoperable stage, if the general condition of the dog is maintained, spontaneous disappearance of the growth may take place. In fact, spontaneous recovery is not uncommon, and recovery seems to be associated with sufficient immunity to enable the animal to resist successfully the development of other tumors of the same kind.

INVESTIGATIONAL STUDIES

Nowinsky is given credit for the first published observations on this tumor. He reported a transplantable neoplasm which was removed from the vagina of a bitch and which recurred after three months. He diagnosed the tumor as myxosarcoma. It was successfully transplanted subcutaneously into three puppies, aged eight days, fourteen days, and two months, respectively. Metastasis was not observed. Nowinsky's report was published in 1877.

Wehr reported successful transplantation of the tumor which he considered a carcinoma. Geissler also considered the growth to be a carcinoma, although Hansemann, in discussing Geissler's paper, was of the opinion that the tumor was not a carcinoma.

Duplay and Cazin were the first to suggest the possible inflammatory nature of the growth, although in one of the animals which bore successful transplantation of the tumor, metastasis to one testis was noted. Bashford, Murray, and Cramer, after a careful study of the disease, denied that it was neoplastic, and although they admitted that there was histologic resemblance between this growth and round-cell sarcoma, they concluded that "these tumors of the vagina and penis of the dog are connective tissue reactions to a living virus which has not yet been demonstrated."

In a series of papers dealing with this tumor, Smith and Washbourn[13, 14, 15] described an instance in which twelve bitches were served by a dog affected with a tumor on the penis. Vaginal tumors developed in eleven. Three of the bitches with the transplanted vaginal growths were served by a second male on whose penis a tumor developed subsequently. The second male, in turn, served two unaffected bitches, and a vaginal tumor developed in one. Smith and Washbourn also recorded a case in which a healthy dog was permitted to serve a bitch with a vaginal tumor and, in spite of the fact that the penis was frequently washed after coitus, a number of small growths developed on the part. These observers noted that transplanted growths were visible within one week after inoculation. They looked like vesicles, but when they were pricked they proved to be solid. In three instances Smith and Washbourn found the inguinal lymph nodes invaded with metastatic tumor cells, and metastasis was present in the liver and spleen of one dog. They considered that the highly bred and more sensitive dogs, and dogs in poor general condition, offered more favorable environmental conditions for the growth of the tumor than were offered by the mongrel type or those that are well nourished. They noted spontaneous recovery, with immunity to subsequent exposures, in several instances.

From the results obtained in a series of inoculation experiments, and from a general study of the disease, Smith and Washbourn noted that death may occur from "cachexia or from kidney disease, the result of obstruction of the ureters or from septic poisoning owing to sloughing of the growth." They concluded: (1) The tumors are infectious round-cell sarcoma; (2) they can be transplanted from the genitalia, where they naturally occur, to the subcutaneous tissues of dogs; (3) they can be transplanted from the subcutaneous transplants in like manner, through a series of dogs; (4) their spontaneous disappearance may occur with or without ulceration; (5) death may occur from metastatic deposits in the viscera, and (6) if the tumor disappears, the animal is then immune to subsequent inoculation.

Sticker,[16, 17, 18] who considered the growth to be round-cell sarcoma, made several significant observations concerning its physiologic and pathologic aspects. He noted that successful transplants were possible in the spleen, bone, and peritoneum, as well as in the skin. He was able also to secure successful transplants in two of three foxes which were used, but he was not successful with cats, rabbits, guinea pigs, or mice. In 16 per cent of all dogs with transplanted tumors in Sticker's series, the growths disappeared spontaneously, and these animals were immune to reinoculation. Sticker experimented with the viability of the tumor cells, and found them resistant to extremes of temperature. They remained viable after twenty-four hours of exposure to a temperature of $-14°$ C. and after two hours of exposure to $50°$ C. On the other hand, attempts failed to produce growths from cells which were kept at $-11°$ C. for twenty-five days and from cells which had been subjected to crushing. Neither did growths result from filtered or centrifuged emulsions of cells.

White's observations concerning the contagiousness and malignancy of the tumor are of interest. Two pure-bred bull bitches were served by an apparently healthy male, and vaginal tumors developed in both shortly after whelping. In one, a mammary growth also appeared. Both bitches were operated on, and after removal of the tumors they recovered completely. They remained well, were bred twice afterward, and each gave birth to normal litters. The male used to breed the first two bitches also served four other females, in all of which growths developed, and from the results of which they died. One of the first two bitches was served by three other males, and all died of the disease.

White believed that these growths have several features in common with infectious diseases, but he concluded that the growths which occur following inoculation have their origin from the transplanted cells and not from a separate infective agent. White also pointed out certain differences between the tumor and the usual forms of sarcoma. He mentioned the marked contagiousness of the venereal growths, and the relatively mild malignancy of the majority of these tumors, in that they show little tendency to infiltrate the surrounding tissues and do not often metastasize.

Beebe and Ewing undertook to show, by experiments with transplantation, the exact manner of origin of the tumors which resulted. They transplanted small grafts of tumorous tissues subcutaneously,

23

and made histologic studies of excised portions at intervals of one to twenty-one days. This was done in an attempt to determine "whether the growth comes from the proliferation of the transplanted cells, or by stimulation of the surrounding tissue cells as maintained by Bashford, Murray, and Cramer." Beebe and Ewing found that all the tumor cells in transplants do not die; some at the periphery remain alive. These undergo mitosis, and "leave no doubt that the transplanted cells give rise to the tumor." Concerning the nature of the disease, these writers were "forced to conclude that the infectious lymphosarcoma of dogs is a true malignant neoplasm." They admitted, however, their inability to determine the exact tissue cells involved in the histogenesis of the tumor. At the time of Beebe and Ewing's report, the tumor with which they had worked was in its fifth generation, and thirty-five tumors had developed in twenty-nine dogs.

Wade also conducted a rather exhaustive investigation of the disease, during the course of which he successfully inoculated two fox cubs. The animals became much emaciated and died, after the tumors had attained the size of about 2 by 1 cm.

Rabbits, rats, and guinea pigs resisted transplantation of the tumor, and six dogs that had recovered spontaneously from previous successful inoculations apparently were immune to attempts at reinoculation. Wade observed interstitial nephritis in many successfully inoculated dogs, and he thought this lesion represented the effect of a soluble toxin from the tumor cells; this constituted the strongest evidence advanced up to that time in favor of the disease being an infective granuloma and not a true neoplasm. It was Wade's opinion that the growths, which occurred as a result of inoculation of tissue, had their origin in part from the vigorously dividing peripheral cells of the tissue which was introduced, and in part from the surrounding connective tissue fibroblasts which become altered in the process of repair and assume an immature, sarcomatous nature. He therefore considered the growth to be an infective sarcoma, a tumor belonging "to the borderline between the infective granulomas and the true neoplasms." Those tumors which arise after natural infection, Wade believed to consist of cells derived entirely from the tissue of the host.

In another report, by Beebe, the correctness of considering these growths to be of an infectious nature was questioned. Beebe felt that evidence in support of the action of microörganisms in their genesis was lacking, and brought out the fact that successful transfer of the tumor had been accomplished only by means of a living tumor cell. Beebe again expressed his belief in the true neoplastic nature of the process.

Crile and Beebe subscribed to the view that these growths are neoplastic: "From the total available evidence, we are convinced that the process is a true tumor." They made some extremely significant observations concerning the curative value of blood from animals that had recovered spontaneously. In brief, they effected direct transfusion of whole blood from an animal that had recovered spontaneously, and therefore was immune, to an animal with an actively growing tumor. Of ten tumorous dogs that were the recipients of transfused blood, seven were cured, and in two the transfusion apparently produced marked inhibition or regression of the growth. Crile and Beebe did not think the protective or curative properties that were exhibited were analogous to bacterial immunity; nevertheless, they thought that there was a specific factor capable of rendering an affected animal passively immune.

Two other papers that have to do with the use of certain biologic products in the treatment of these tumors were written by Bergell and Sticker, and by Beebe and Tracy. Bergell and Sticker, by injection of a specific hepatic ferment, were able to cause the tumor to disappear completely in cases in which spontaneous recovery was unlikely. In one case, with metastasis to lymph nodes, injection of the hepatic ferment caused regression which extended to the involved node. Following the injection the tumors became cystic, with marked phagocytic action by macrophages, and, in place of the numerous mitotic figures which characterize the tumor in its progressive stage, the injected tumor was devoid of mitotic figures. Beebe and Tracy demonstrated the destructive influence of certain bacterial toxins on the tumor. Tumors at a distance from the injected growth regressed simultaneously with those injected. In one instance, an animal with four transplanted tumors received four injections at a considerable distance from the growths, and six weeks after the first injection the tumors had completely disappeared. The authors were not convinced that the effect produced was peculiar to the bacterial toxin used, since they closed by saying, "It seems possible . . . that an equal bulk of any toxic organism would exert a similar destructive action."

Novak and Craig recently reported a case, and after reviewing the literature they concluded that the weight of evidence seemed to substantiate the contention of Beebe and Ewing that these growths are true tumors and not inflammatory granulomas.*

* In unpublished data, Mann recorded the successful transference of a transmissible lymphosarcoma through the fortieth generation, using hundreds of dogs in the experiment. The neoplasm remained consistent throughout.

BIBLIOGRAPHY

1. Bashford, E. F., Murray, J. A. and Cramer, W.: Comparison between the transmission of an infective granuloma of the dog and carcinoma of the mouse. Scientific Rep. Invest. Imp. Cancer Research Fund, 1905, No. 2, pp. 33–37.

2. Beebe, S. P.: The growth of lymphosarcoma in dogs. Jour. Am. Med. Assn., **49:** 1492–1493 (Nov. 2), 1907.

3. Beebe, S. P. and Ewing, James: A study of the so-called infectious lymphosarcoma of dogs. Jour. Med. Res., **15:** 209–227 (Sept.), 1906.

4. Beebe, S. P. and Tracy, Martha: The treatment of experimental tumors with bacterial toxins. Jour. Am. Med. Assn., **49:** 1493–1498 (Nov. 2), 1907.

5. Bergell, Peter and Sticker, Anton: Ueber Pathogenese und über den spezifischen Abbau der Krebsgeschwülste. Deutsch. med. Wchnschr., **2:** 1521–1522, 1907.

6. Crile, G. W. and Beebe, S. P.: Transfusion of blood in the transplantable lymphosarcoma of dogs. Jour. Med. Res., **18:** 385–405 (June), 1908.

7. Duplay and Cazin: Quoted by Woglom, W. H.: Studies in cancer. Transmissible lymphosarcoma of the dog. New York, Crocker Research Fund, Columbia University Press, 1913, **1,** pp. 227–236.

8. Feldman, W. H.: So-called infectious sarcoma of the dog in an unusual anatomic situation. Am. Jour. Path., **5:** 183–194 (March), 1929.

9. Geissler: Gelungene Carcinomubertragung beim Hunde. Verhandl. d. deutsch. Gesellsch. f. Chir., **24:** 20–23, 1895.

10. Novak, Emil and Craig, R. G.: Infectious sarcoma ("venereal granuloma") of the vagina in dogs. Arch. Path. and Lab. Med., **3:** 193–202 (Feb.), 1927.

11. Nowinsky: Quoted by Sticker.

12. Seligmann, C. G.: On the occurrence of new growths among the natives of British New Guinea. Third Scientific Rep. Invest. Imp. Cancer Research Fund, 1908, pp. 26–40.

13. Smith, G. B. and Washbourn, J. W.: Infective venereal tumors in dogs. Tr. Path. Soc. London, **48:** 310–323, 1897.

14. Smith, G. B. and Washbourn, J. W.: Infective sarcomata in dogs. Brit. Med. Jour., **2:** 1807–1810 (Dec. 17), 1898.

15. Smith, G. B. and Washbourn, J. W.: Infective sarcomata in dogs. Brit. Med. Jour., **2:** 1346–1347 (Nov. 11), 1899.

16. Sticker, Anton: Transplantables Lymphosarcom des Hundes. Ztschr. f. Krebsforsch., **1:** 413–444, 1904.

17. Sticker, Anton: Infectiöse und krebsige Geschwülste an den äussern Geschlechtsorganen des Hundes. Arch. f. klin. Chir., **78:** 773–800, 1906.

18. Sticker: Quoted by Woglom, W. H.: Studies in cancer. Transmissible lymphosarcoma of the dog. New York, Crocker Research Fund, Columbia University Press, 1913, **1,** pp. 227–236.

19. Wade, Henry: An experimental investigation of infective sarcoma of the dog, with a consideration of its relationship to cancer. Jour. Path. and Bacteriol., **12:** 384–425, 1908.

20. Wehr: Weitere Mitteilungen über die positiven Ergebnisse der Carcinomueberimpfungen von Hund auf Hund. Arch. f. klin. Chir., **39:** 226–228, 1889.

21. White, C. P.: Contagious growth in dogs. Brit. Med. Jour., **2:** 176–177 (July 19), 1902.

CHAPTER XXI

EMBRYONAL NEPHROMA

DEFINITION AND TERMINOLOGY

Embryonal nephroma usually originates in the kidney, as a consequence of some congenital mishap, from multipotent, undifferentiated, nephrogenic cells. It has been given many names: Adenoma sarcomatode, adenomyosarcoma, sarcocarcinoma, sarcoadenoma, rhabdomyoadenosarcoma, and adenosarcoma; the last is the term most commonly used by comparative pathologists and by meat inspectors. Each term represents an attempt to create a nomenclature that would express the dominating structural elements of the particular tumor under consideration and was perhaps fittingly applied to the particular tumor that happened to be the object of a given author's description. The structural variation of different tumors and of different portions of the same tumor justifies the use of a term that is applicable to all tumors that arise from the elements of the primitive nephrogenic tissue, regardless of the degree of differentiation; therefore the name embryonal nephroma seems appropriate.

The disease in swine was first described by Day,[3] in 1907, who pointed out the embryogenic and morphologic relationship of the neoplasm, as it occurs in swine, to the so-called Wilms' tumor of children, which was originally described by Birch-Hirschfeld. Further studies have strengthened this opinion; and it is now generally agreed that these embryonic tumors of the kidneys of lower animals are analogous to if not identical with those of children.

HISTOGENESIS

Many hypotheses have been offered in explanation of the histogenesis of these growths. Although hypotheses differ in many respects, it seems to be agreed that they develop as a result of some congenital mishap. The exact nature of the anomaly is not yet determined, although there is suggestive evidence that it may be the result of fetal rest or fetal displacement.

Wollstein, in a recent paper in which she accepted Wilms' point of view, presented a logical explanation of the origin of these tumors: "As to the origin of these renal neoplasms it seems probable that they all come from the same type of embryonal cell, but that they come from the cell at different stages of its differentiation and consequently of its potency. The more embryonic and less differentiated the cells from which the tumor originates, the more complicated will its structure be because of the multipotency of the undifferentiated mesodermal cells. Thus for the rhabdomyoadenosarcomas it seems simple to presuppose a parent cell with an inherent ability to give rise to striated muscle, supporting tissues and kidney elements, since these are all mesodermal in origin and closely approximated in the young embryo, and the inclusion of such early cells within the developing kidney is possible. This was Wilms' view. It seems the only way to account for the striated muscle tumors, for striated muscle cannot develop from unstriated muscle, and so metaplasia gives no adequate explanation of these growths. The presence of cartilage and bone in the mixed tumors is also explained. For the less complex tumors two possible origins suggest themselves. Either the parent cells are more differentiated, of later origin, and so have the potentiality only of the renal and supporting tissue elements or the cells of the early renal blastoma are adequate for the development of the tumors containing only kidney elements like tubules, connective tissue, and unstriated muscle. Again, growths with more embryonal epithelial elements may take their origin from an earlier cell of the renal blastoma than that which gives rise to the more adenomatous forms, when the cells have reached the stage of differentiation of renal tubular epithelium. Since these neoplasms are not all alike, but only closely related, there seems no special reason why a single origin must be involved for them as a group."

The foregoing would seem to explain the derivation of those tumors which occur, as the majority do, within the substance of the kidney proper. An occasional tumor of this kind is found entirely separate from the kidney, and its histogenesis may be explained on the basis of so-called fetal rests derived from the remains of the wolffian body. These fetal rests probably result from failure of certain portions of the mesonephron to be utilized in the development of the permanent kidney. Instead of undergoing retrogression, the unused cells continue to grow but without the guiding influences of normal tissues, and an unrestrained focus of immature elements with neoplastic possibilities results.

INCIDENCE

Embryonal nephroma is by no means common although it is often observed in slaughtering establishments where large numbers of swine are examined; it probably does not occur on the average oftener than once in every 40,000 to 50,000 carcasses examined. This is without question the most common tumor of swine, but there is reason to believe that it is more likely to develop in chickens than in other species.

Day[4] observed forty-seven renal tumors of this kind among ninety-three tumors of swine, and in my collection of 536 tumors from animals fifty-two (9.6 per cent) were embryonal nephromas. These were distributed among the respective species as follows:

Among eighty-six tumors of swine, there were forty-six embryonal nephromas; among fifty-five tumors of chickens there were five embryonal nephromas, and among 230 tumors of cattle, there was one embryonal nephroma.

Polson found in the literature mention of fifty-two tumors of rabbits, to which he added records of fourteen. Among the sixty-six neoplasms seven were composed of embryonic renal tissue.* Mathews reported the occurrence of twelve tumors that were encountered in five years, at necropsy of approximately 2,000 chickens, an incidence of 0.6 per cent.

OCCURRENCE

Forty-three of the forty-six embryonal nephromas in my series that were obtained from swine were situated in the kidney. In three cases the tumors were entirely separate from the kidneys; two of the growths occupied a lumbar position posterior to the kidney, and one growth was just anterior to this organ. In cases in which the tumors were extranephric, the kidneys were without demonstrable involvement. In rabbits, the tumors have been attached to the kidney or have definitely involved it, whereas those in chickens have shown more or less variation in this regard (Fig. 175). The twelve tumors of chickens reported by Mathews were attached to the periosteum of the spinal column dorsal to the kidney and separated from the organ by a capsule of fibrous connective tissue. The two tumors reported by McKenney were situated within the kidney, and skeletal attachment was not discernible. Those I have observed were likewise definitely a part of the kidney, and apparently originated within it (Fig. 176). The majority of the tumors are unilateral, but eight of the forty-six tumors of swine that I observed were bilateral.

Both sexes are equally affected in all species. Thirty swine in my series in which the ages were known, varied in age from eight to thirty-six months, with an average age of seventeen months. Kinsley reported

---

* These included in addition to one case described by Polson, one described by Lubarsch, one by Nürnberger, two by Bell and Henrici, one by Scott, and one by Dible.

an embryonal nephroma in a gilt aged from four to six months. The large tumor had practically replaced the renal tissue and perhaps was

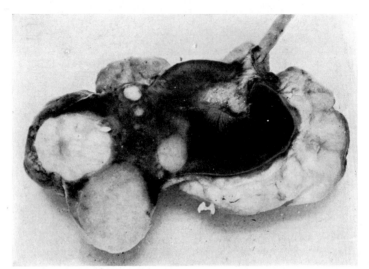

Fig. 175.—Embryonal nephroma of the kidney of a rabbit. Photograph obtained through the courtesy of Dr. Cyril Polson of Manchester, England.

well established at the time of birth. The chickens with tumors of this kind have varied in age from three months to two and a half years.

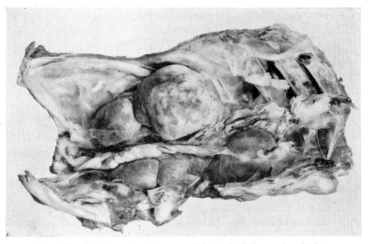

Fig. 176.—Embryonal nephroma of the right kidney of a chicken.

In Mathews' series nine of the chickens were aged from nine to twenty-four months before symptoms of the disease were observed.

The histogenesis of embryonal nephroma is of such a character as to provide possibilities for their early development, and it is probable that if affected swine were necropsied after the first few months of life, gross evidence of the tumors would be discernible in the majority of instances. In fact it is not unlikely that occasionally embryonal nephroma may acquire demonstrable proportions during the uterine residence of the fetus.

The one tumor which I obtained from the bovine species was found at necropsy in the right kidney of a six-year-old grade cow that had been slaughtered for food. The mass weighed approximately 2 kg. and had metastasized to the adjacent lymph nodes and, to a slight extent, to the lungs.

Whether breed has any influence on the occurrence of such tumors is problematic. There is no evidence that they appear with greater frequency in any particular breed of swine, although ten of Mathews' series of twelve tumors were obtained from chickens of the Barred Rock breed. Mathews was inclined to believe that this breed showed particular predisposition for the development of neoplasia, and that breed was therefore of significance in their occurrence. However, data seem to be inadequate to determine this question, at least so far as embryonal renal tumors are concerned.

EFFECTS ON THE HOST

Such tumors seldom provoke recognizable symptoms. Even when large tumors are found at necropsy symptoms of sufficient magnitude to command attention are usually absent. The larger tumors must interfere to some extent at least with the proper functioning of the various abdominal organs by encroaching on the space ordinarily occupied by the abdominal viscera, and it is reasonable to assume that the affected animal experiences sensations of discomfort as a consequence. The horizontal posture of such animals as the hog and the rabbit, and the subsequent pendulous condition of the abdomen, provide a circumstance that enables large neoplastic growths of the kidney to escape detection during life. The upright posture of human beings and the anatomic configuration of the abdomen reveal the presence of the tumors rather early in life, and before they become unusually large.

If the involvement is limited to one kidney, gradual compensatory hypertrophy of the unaffected organ will probably occur. In instances of bilateral renal involvement, the encroachment and destruction of renal tissue might be expected to cause serious renal insufficiency. This phase of the disease, for obvious reasons, has not been studied.

The fact that the majority of embryonal nephromas are found in animals which have been slaughtered for food probably accounts for the failure to observe symptoms which might be expected from tumors of this nature. If all animals which had these tumors were permitted to live out their natural span of life it is reasonable to presume that objective symptoms would arise in the majority of instances, particularly if metastasis had occurred.

METASTASIS AND MALIGNANCY

Although embryonal nephromas are capable of a pernicious, advancing type of growth so far as the renal substance is concerned, metastasis to the regional lymph nodes, or to distant organs, is relatively infrequent. Day observed metastasis in two of the eight cases in swine and metastatic dissemination had occurred from three of the forty-six tumors in my collection. In Day's cases metastasis in one instance was to the lung; in the other, the sublumbar lymph nodes were affected secondarily. The renal and sublumbar lymph nodes were invaded in one of my cases, the liver in another, and the lung in addition to the renal and sublumbar lymph nodes in the third. The only case reported of metastasis in chickens was one of those in Mathews' series. The animal was a male Barred Rock aged somewhat more than two years. Besides the primary growth in the left kidney metastatic foci were present in the muscles of the left thigh, the left lung, and the right kidney. In the one bovine case that I observed metastasis was noted in the adjacent renal lymph node, and to a slight extent in the lungs. Metastasis from tumors of rabbits has not been reported.

It seems unusual that tumors possessing such potentialities for mischief should metastasize so infrequently. The effects of the neoplasm on the adjacent renal tissue is commonly profound; yet the growth seldom extends beyond its capsular covering. Although locally tumors of this character must be considered malignant, they are generally benign so far as effects on the animal as a whole is concerned. The physical condition of forty-one hogs affected with embryonal nephroma in my series was as follows: Good in thirty cases; fair in seven; poor in one case, and cachectic in one. In the three cases in which metastasis had occurred the physical condition was good.

Metastasis is apparently dependent on the growing propensities of the elements constituting the tumor and their inherent capacity to invade the blood and lymph vessels rather than on the duration of the neoplastic process. Metastasis will occur early if the cells of the tumor have the ability to invade the surrounding tissue and to prosper and multiply in distant situations, whereas tumors that lack these qualities remain localized within the encapsulated neoplastic focus. The ages of two of the swine in my series in which secondary foci had been established were eight months and twelve months, respectively; the third was considered aged. No doubt, if it were possible to ascertain the presence of these embryonal renal tumors and to affect their surgical removal, the likelihood of recurrence or the appearance of subsequent metastasis would be remote. The majority continue as localized growths, and metastasis is the exception rather than the rule.

GROSS APPEARANCE

The appearance of embryonal nephromas is subject to much variation, although the majority consist of rather bulky masses of grayish-

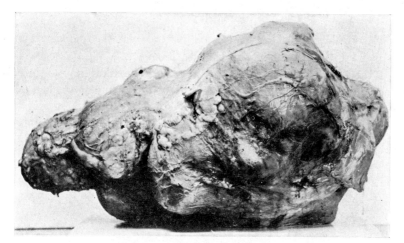

Fig. 177.—Embryonal nephroma of the kidney of a hog.

white tissue, oval, elongated, or irregular, frequently with deep lobulations (Fig. 177). The growth may be so extensive as practically to obliterate the renal tissue or it may consist of one or several neoplastic foci that extend from the surface of the kidney through the entire cortex (Fig. 178). Growths that affect the kidney may involve any part of the organ, although they appear to arise more frequently at the extremities rather than at the hilum. Solitary nodules measuring from 1 to 5 cm. in diameter are sometimes seen on the surface of the involved kidney, and occasionally multiple excrescences of neoplastic tissue cover a portion of its surface (Fig. 179).

If the interior of the large tumors is exposed by incision, the multiple, lobulated character of the growths, and not infrequently large cystic cavitations, are exposed (Fig. 180). Many of the cysts contain a

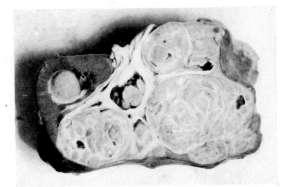

Fig. 178.—Embryonal nephroma of the kidney of a hog.

semiclear fluid resembling urine and some a somewhat purulent foul-smelling substance that may be tinged with blood.

If the tumor is unusually large, much retrogression may be in evidence, and large areas of friable, or broken down, spongy tissue, with

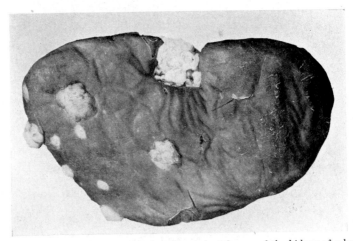

Fig. 179.—Multiple tumorous foci, embryonal nephroma of the kidney of a hog.

extravasation of blood is not uncommon. The tissue may also show considerable serous infiltration, which extends in some instances to the adjacent striated musculature.

Except in the early stages, a capsule usually can be demonstrated.

This may be delicate and of paper thinness or rough, resilient and fibrous, measuring several centimeters in thickness.

Embryonal nephromas vary from small foci, barely visible to the eye, to huge masses weighing many kilograms. Although the average tumor weighs from 0.5 kg. to 2 or 3 kg. specimens weighing more than

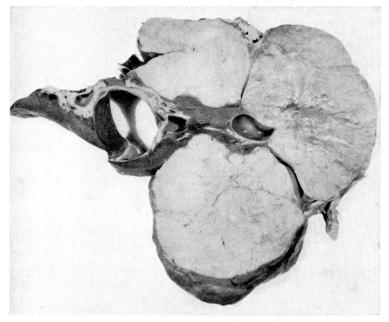

FIG. 180.—Embryonal nephroma of the kidney of a hog. There is evidence of extensive replacement of the nephric tissue, and one large cyst.

30 kg. have been reported. The largest tumor in my collection weighed a little more than 25 kg.

MICROSCOPIC DESCRIPTION

The multipotency of elements making up a typical embryonal nephroma is usually apparent on microscopic examination. The growth consists of cellular parenchyma, which is irregularly interrupted by well defined septums of adult connective tissue in which are numerous, ill-formed blood channels (Fig. 181). From the large septums smaller strands, given off in haphazard fashion, pass into the more cellular portions, eventually to become lost in the structural complexity. The parenchyma exhibits wide variation in design and cellular constituence, depending on the degree of differentiation achieved by the respective elements. The cells may be spherical or oval units, which on the one

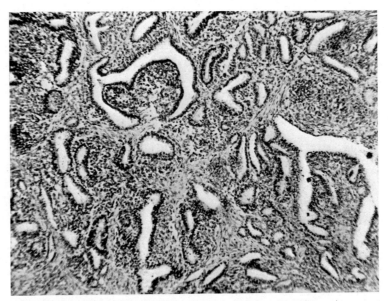

Fig. 181.—Embryonal nephroma of the kidney of a hog (× 110).

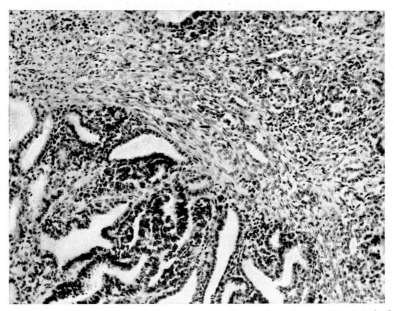

Fig. 182.—Extranephric embryonal nephroma of a hog, with both sarcomatous and adenomatous types of structure (× 180).

hand merge almost imperceptibly into collections of immature, spindleshaped cells that have a definite sarcomatous appearance; on the other

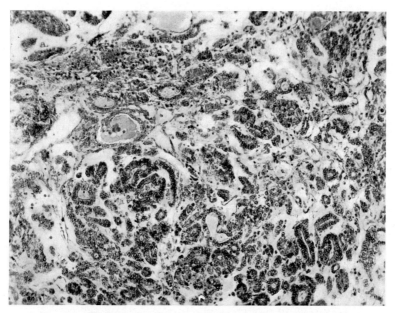

FIG. 183.—Embryonal nephroma of the kidney of a chicken (× 150).

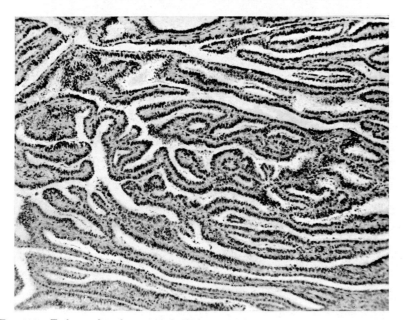

FIG. 184.—Embryonal nephroma of the kidney of a hog in which an epithelial type of architecture prevails (× 120).

hand, they form irregular, adenomatous, tubular-like structures not unlike epithelial elements (Figs. 182 and 183). Usually the irregular, epithelial,

tubular-like structures are numerous, and an occasional tumor is encountered in which the epithelial elements predominate to such a degree that it is difficult to demonstrate sarcomatous cells (Fig. 184).
The cells which line the irregular, tortuous, duct-like structures often
exhibit a tendency to project into the lumens in a papillary fashion,
that frequently gives the structure an intricate, bizarre appearance
(Fig. 185). Rarely a tumor is found that is characterized by the predominance of cells which reveal marked sarcomatous tendencies. These
are more common in chickens (Figs. 186 and 187). I have observed a
few embryonal nephromas, in which, in the cells of the parenchyma,

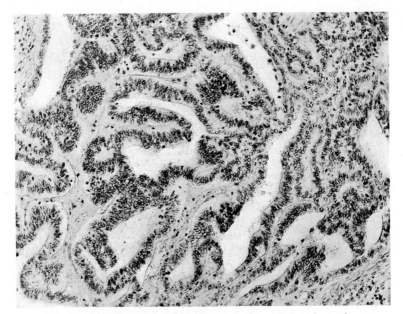

Fig. 185.—Embryonal nephroma of the kidney of a hog (× 150).

differentiation was not demonstable. The parenchyma consisted of
diffuse, compact accumulations of oval or spherical cells, with prominent
nuclei separated into groups of variable proportions by broad, connective tissue trabeculæ (Fig. 188).

The varied potencies of the type cell responsible for this tumor provide possibilities for the development of tissue, that has little if any resemblance to the parent cell. Smooth and striated muscle, cartilage,
and even bone may be encountered rarely.

Some interesting attempts of the cells to attain the differentiation
observed in certain specialized structures of the kidney sometimes can
be seen. Peculiar, tuft-like arrangements of the parenchyma, suggestive

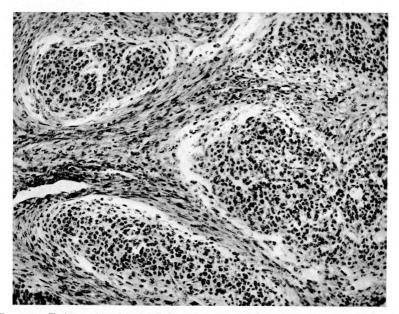

Fig. 186.—Embryonal nephroma of the kidney of a chicken. There are several nests of undifferentiated cells (× 180).

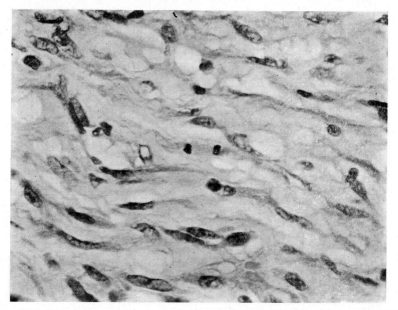

Fig. 187.—Sarcomatous portion of embryonal nephroma of the kidney of a hog (× 660).

of a renal corpuscle, may occur. The mimicry is never complete. Capillary vessels are absent; the structure consists only of convolutions of

24

flattened, epithelial-like cells, and fibrous stroma, within a cavity which is lined with a continuation of the small, flattened cells that constitute the tuft-like portion (Fig. 189).

The epithelial cells which line the alveolar, or tubular-like structure vary from cuboid to columnar, and the gradual transition of one to the other, within the same tubule, can often be seen in the same microscopic field. Mitotic division is usually prominent, particularly in the highly cellular, intertubular portions, although this phenomenon is commonly displayed by the lining cells of the duct or alveolar-like structure. Many of the growths reveal considerable extrasvacular blood in direct

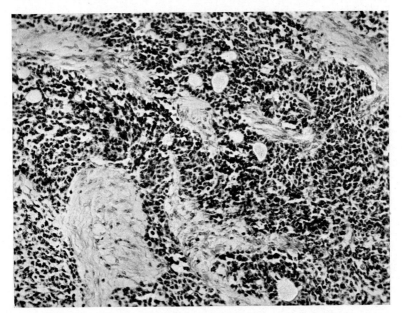

Fig. 188.—Embryonal nephroma of the kidney of a cow (× 150).

contact with the cells of the parenchyma, and thrombosis of some of the larger vessels occasionally occurs.

Cystic cavities that may be present are usually lined with a single layer of cuboidal epithelial cells. The spaces are often filled with a homogenous substance which stains pink with eosin, and which resembles, to some extent, epithelial hyalin, although the color reaction with van Gieson's stain is not entirely typical for this material.

Areas of hydropic degeneration, associated with necrosis of the tumor cells, are occasionally encountered. Ample blood supply is insured by the many vessels which run in the connective-tissue stroma, and by the capillary structures which can sometimes be seen in the midst of the highly cellular parenchyma. In a tumor of the kidney of a swine that I examined, an enormous amount of hyalinized collagen had encroached on and replaced much of the parenchymatous elements of the tumor.

In the later stages of the disease the tumor may extend by infiltration into the substance of the adjacent kidney, particularly in chickens, but such occurrence is rare. Usually a formidable zone of fibrous connective tissue is present between the parenchyma of the kidney and the neoplastic elements, which provides an effective barrier against the invasive tendencies of the tumor. Except in the early stages of the proc-

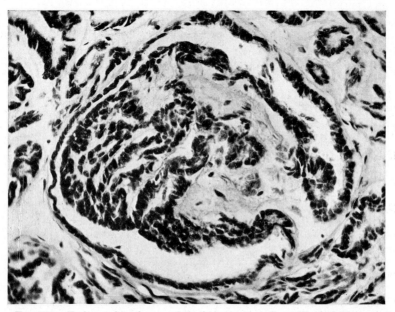

Fig. 189.—Embryonal nephroma of the kidney of a swine. The tuft-like convolutions of flattened cells, which give the structure a glomerular-like appearance, can be seen (× 400).

ess, destruction and replacement of the nephric tissue is usually brought about through gradual, progressive expansion of the growth. The structure of the kidney is reduced in amount as a consequence of pressure atrophy and other retrograde influences.

The sequence of events is better understood when one keeps in mind the genesis of these tumors. They arise not from the elements of the postnatal kidney but from certain cells that have persisted from an early developmental period of fetal life. As such they behave in a manner quite unlike cells of adult tissues that may suddenly suffer a loss of restraint and assume the characteristics of neoplasia.

CLINICAL CONSIDERATIONS

The relative infrequency of embryonal nephromas, and the fact that they are seldom if ever diagnosed in life of animals, make these growths of little significance to the clinician. They are primarily of interest to the meat inspector and to the student of comparative pathology.

BIBLIOGRAPHY

1. Bell, E. T. and Henrici, A. T.: Renal tumors in the rabbit. Jour. Cancer Res., 1: 157–168 (April), 1916.

2. Birch-Hirschfeld, F. V.: Beiträge zur pathologischen Anatomie der Nierengeschwülste. Sarkomatöse Drüsengeschwulst der Niere im Kindesalter (Embryonales Adenosarkom). Beitr. z. path. Anat. u. z. allg. Path., 24: 343–362, 1898.

3. Day, L. E.: Embryonal adenosarcoma of the kidney of swine. Twenty-fourth annual report of the Bureau of Animal Industry, Washington, D. C., 1907, pp. 247–257.

4. Day, L. E.: Quoted by Slye, Maud, Holmes, Harriet F. and Wells, H. G.: Primary spontaneous tumors in the kidney and adrenal of mice. VII. Jour. Cancer Res., 6: 305–336 (Oct.), 1921.

5. Dible: Quoted by Polson.

6. Kinsley, A. T.: An interesting case of adenosarcoma of a gilt. Vet. Med., 25: 362, 1930.

7. Lubarsch, O.: Ueber einen grossen Nierentumor beim Kaninchen. Centralbl. f. allg. Path. u. path. Anat., 16: 342–345 (May 15), 1905.

8. McKenney, F. D.: Embryonal nephroma in the chicken; report of two cases. Am. Jour. Cancer, 15: 122–128 (Jan.), 1931.

9. Mathews, F. P.: Adenosarcomata of the kidneys of chickens. Jour. Am. Vet. Med. Assn., 74: 238–246 (Jan.), 1929.

10. Nürnberger, Ludwig: Über einen Tumor in der Kaninchenniere vom Typus der embryonalen Drüsengeschwülste des Menschen. Beitr. z. path. Anat. u. z. allg. Path., 52: 523–539, 1912.

11. Polson, C. J.: Tumours of the rabbit. Jour. Path. and Bacteriol., 30: 603–614, 1927.

12. Scott, Ernest: Tumors of the kidney in rabbits. Jour. Cancer Res., 2: 367–372 (July), 1917.

13. Wilms, Max: Die Mischgeschwulste der Niere. Leipzig, 1899.

14. Wollstein, Martha: Renal neoplasms in young children. Arch. Path. and Lab. Med., 3: 1–13 (Jan.), 1927.

CHAPTER XXII

EXPERIMENTALLY TRANSMISSIBLE TUMORS*

Very early in the scientific attack on the problem of malignant tumors, investigators attempted to demonstrate the transmissibility of various kinds of tumors from the host to other animals of the same or closely related species. Although a great many successful transplantations have been recorded when the recipient was of the same species as the donor, the recorded "takes," when animals of heterologous species were used, have been few indeed. Because of the universal use of mice and rats in laboratories of biologic research, and their relatively brief span of life, these animals have been used extensively in experimental transmission of neoplasms. The further fact that mice and rats are subject to a considerable number of spontaneous neoplasms makes them particularly desirable for work of this kind.

One of the earliest attempts to transplant tumors from one animal to another was that of Nowinsky, who, in 1876, successfully transmitted a tumor from the vagina of a bitch to the subcutaneous tissues of three puppies. In 1889, Hanau effected the first transfer of a carcinoma within animals of the same species. The donor was an old rat with carcinoma of the vulva. Small portions of the tumor were placed under the skin of the scrotum of two rats, and in both multiple tumors eventually developed which were similar in their histologic details to the vaginal tumor.

Pfeiffer, in 1890, reported the transference of a pigmented carcinoma of a mouse to other animals of the same species, and in the same year von Eiselsberg reported the successful transplantation of a sarcoma, consisting of spindle-shaped cells obtained from a rat. Bits of the original growth from the periosteum of the scapula were inoculated into the mesenteric tissue of two rats, and in one of the rats which died five months after the inoculation, a nodular mass was found at the point of transplantation, which was histologically the same as the original tumor.

---

* In the preparation of the first portion of this chapter, free use has been made of Woglom's comprehensive review entitled "The Study of Experimental Cancer," Columbia University Press, 1913. Those interested in transmissible tumors should consult this résumé of the experimental investigation which is remarkably complete up to 1913.

Morau, although one of the earlier workers with transplantable tumors, made some extremely interesting and valuable observations. From a tumor which occurred in the axilla of a white mouse, a large number of subsequent transmissions were obtained in a period of three years. Morau was of the opinion that the development of the tumors was dependent, to a considerable degree, on the heredity of the recipients, and that trauma appeared to aggravate metastasis. Their growth in immature animals resulted in a decrease in the virulence of the tumor. Tumors that did not ulcerate did not contain demonstrable microorganisms.

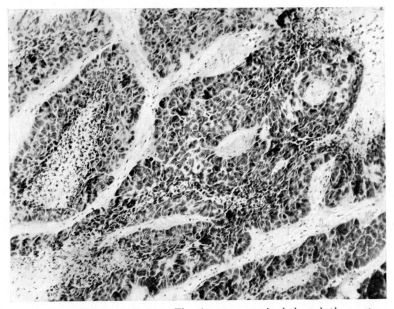

Fig. 190.—Jensen mouse carcinoma. The tissue was received through the courtesy of Dr. J. A. Murray of the Imperial Cancer Research Fund, London (× 150).

Firket, in 1892, reported a series of successful transplantations of a spindle-cell sarcoma of a rat, and although takes were secured in rats, they were not successful in guinea pigs.

Another spindle-cell sarcoma of the rat, which was perpetuated to the eighth generation, was reported by Velich. Inoculations were attempted by many different methods, and it was noted that cell-free fluids derived from the tumor did not initiate growths at the point of inoculation. Likewise, the blood from an incised tumor failed to produce subsequent growths. Attempts to inoculate guinea pigs failed, and gradual diminution of the tumor's virulence was noted throughout the course of the experiments.

Loeb,[16, 17] in 1901, described his work with a sarcoma of the thyroid gland of the rat which he was able to propagate through forty generations, when infection made further transmission impossible. Metastasis was not observed, although there was evidence of growth following contact inoculation from intraperitoneal implantations.

Jensen, in 1903, described a transplantable carcinoma which originated in the skin of a mouse (Fig. 190). He was able to transmit this through nineteen generations. Takes were successful in approximately 50 per cent of the animals, and in no instance were metastatic foci

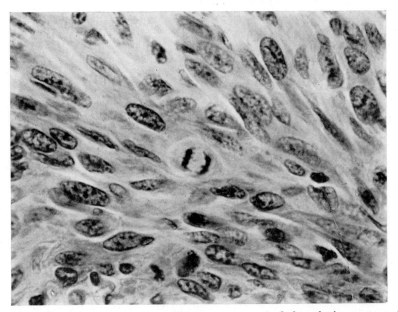

Fig. 191.—Jensen rat sarcoma. The tissue was received through the courtesy of Dr. William H. Woglom, Institute of Cancer Research, Columbia University, New York (× 950).

demonstrated. Jensen, in 1907, reported two other transplantable neoplasms which he obtained from two rats. The tumors, which were spindle-cell sarcomas, would not at first grow in wild rats, but they occasionally developed in laboratory strains of European brown and white rats (Fig. 191). Flexner and Jobling were able, however, to pass the tumors through several generations of American rats, from rats with tumors which they received from Jensen in Europe. Jensen noted a gradual increase in the number of successful takes in the successive generations, until finally tumors resulted in from 85 to 100 per cent of the inoculated recipients.

Many other successful homologous transplantations were made but the foregoing constitutes a brief summary of the more important earlier observations of this phase of research. On account of the large amount of work done, and its relation to the biologic aspects of neoplasia in general, three other types of transmissible tumors will be considered a little more in detail.

THE FLEXNER-JOBLING RAT TUMOR

This tumor has been the subject of considerable investigation[5-8] in white rats. Because the percentage of takes following transplantation is unusually high, this tumor is still propagated by many laboratories and has proved extremely valuable in certain phases of cancer research and allied problems.

The original growth occurred in the seminal vesicle of a white rat which had died spontaneously. The tumor was considered to be a mixed-cell sarcoma; it was about 2 cm. in diameter and was readily transplanted to a series of white rats by subcutaneous and intraperitoneal inoculations. Although metastasis had not occurred in the rat with the original tumor, it was very striking in the inoculated animals which died as a result of the tumor's growth. The metastatic growths were both large and numerous. In one rat which had been given intraperitoneal injections, the secondary growths appeared in the ribs and intercostal muscles, as well as in the lungs, pericardium, and myocardium.

The tumors obtained from the earlier series of inoculations were histologically sarcomatous, and according to Flexner and Jobling were "made up of spindle-shaped and polygonal cells, the latter being often of large size with lobed or irregular nuclei. Intercellular substance is present and it is in places fibrillated."

Up to the fifth generation metastatic growths were in the lungs and kidneys, but at the fifth generation in one series of transplantations metastasis was first noticed in the regional lymph nodes. In this particular series metastasis by way of the lymphatic system became progressively more common and more widely disseminated.

Coincidental with the change in the metastatic behavior of the tumor was the remarkable transition which took place in its histologic morphology. It gradually lost its sarcomatous tendencies and became adenomatous, and exhibited the capacity to invade nearby and distant lymph nodes. In attempting an explanation for the adenomatous transformation which became apparent in this tumor, Flexner and

Jobling noticed that these changes occurred in tumors which had been transplanted beneath the skin; consequently, the epithelial cells were considered as having arisen from elements present in the graft. The original material was carefully restudied, and unmistakable evidence of epithelial overgrowth was found in several places. It was concluded that carcinomatous elements were present in the original tumor, which was probably teratoma, but that these had been held somewhat in restraint by the vigorously growing sarcomatous portions of the tumor, which dominated the picture until the fifth generation. The change in

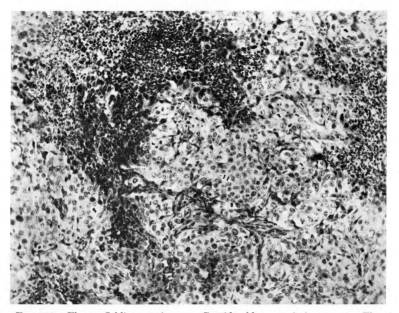

Fig. 192.—Flexner-Jobling carcinoma. Considerable necrosis is present. The tissue was obtained in 1929 from a rat into which the tumor had been experimentally introduced ($\times$ 120).

the nature of the structural elements, which was first noticed in one series of transplants, gradually become evident in all, and the tumor is now considered to be an adenocarcinoma, although a glandular type of structure is not always apparent. Extensive necrosis is common in the larger tumors (Fig. 192).

Tumors failed to occur from the injected filtered emulsions of tumor cells, and even strained emulsions of tumor cells, in a solution of sodium chloride, did not initiate growths. Bacterial cultures could not be obtained from nonulcerated tumors. Solutions of sodium chloride reacted unfavorably to the tumor cells, as did exposure to direct sunlight.

THE TRANSMISSIBLE LYMPHOSARCOMA OF DOGS

Full consideration of this subject is given in Chapter XX (page 351).

THE ROUS CHICKEN SARCOMA

Considering the relatively high incidence of neoplasms in chickens, and the wide variety of tumors in the common fowl, it is perhaps not surprising that a tumor of remarkable transmissible possibilities should be encountered in this species. Rous, in 1910,[27, 28] reported the finding of a chicken tumor that could be transplanted to other birds of the same breed, and from which a cell-free "causative agent" could be separated by filtration through a Berkefeld filter. This tumor was the inspiration for a great amount of subsequent[20, 29-36] research by Rous and his collaborators, as a consequence of which much has been learned concerning the physiologic and pathologic features of this unusual tumor.

The original tumor occurred spontaneously in a strong, young, pure-bred barred Plymouth Rock hen. The mass, which involved the tissues of the side of the right breast, became evident when the hen was aged fifteen months. Under ether anesthesia the tumor was removed and bits of neoplastic tissue were transplanted into the peritoneal cavity of the host, and in a like manner into two other hens from the same setting of eggs. Thirty-five days later the original chicken was dead as a result of intraperitoneal growths, and a large nodule had developed in the breast of one of the other chickens. Rous considered the original tumor and the subsequent inoculation growths to represent a spindle-cell sarcoma. The tumor exhibited an infiltrative, destructive type of growth. Metastically the tumor showed a striking predilection for the lungs, and it was suggested that the origin of the pulmonary tumors was from tumor cell emboli which had been filtered out of the blood by the capillaries of the lungs, thus emphasizing the importance of the blood stream in the metastatic distribution of the tumor. The malignancy of the tumor increased, and its rate of growth was much accelerated in the later generations of its transmissible existence.

Further transplantation experiments demonstrated that the tumor thrived best in the closely related chickens of the pure-bred stock in which the original tumor appeared. The number of successful takes even in the closely related original stock was only moderate at first, but later successful inoculations occurred in a large percentage of the animals used. It was always necessary, however, to use pure-bred, light barred Plymouth Rock hens, since the tumor maintained a stubborn reluctance to thrive in chickens of other breeds. Young birds appeared more susceptible to the tumor's growth than the older, more mature chickens. It was not possible to secure successful transplantations in guinea pigs or pigeons, and a chicken once negative to transplantation remained so.

When grafts of tumor cells were introduced into the tissues of naturally immune chickens, a tremendous lymphocytic reaction occurred in the immediate zone surrounding the transplanted cells, but general lymphocytosis was not observed. Repeated bacteriologic examinations of tissue from the tumor gave consistently negative results. Special stains, or dark field illumination, failed to reveal an organized substance that might be considered an etiologic factor in genesis of the tumor.

By far the most interesting features of the Rous neoplasm was the presence of a "causative agent" which could be separated from the tumor cells by filtration, and which was capable of producing tumors histologically not unlike those developing from tissue grafts. It was found that the specific tumor-inciting substance would pass through a No. 5 medium Berkefeld filter impermeable to Bacillus prodigiosus but would not pass through a Chamberland filter. The substance retained its activity in dried tissue for seven months, and for one month in 50 per cent solution of glycerin. Freezing and thawing, repeated many times, did not destroy it, but it did not survive boiling, and it became inactive after contact with 0.5 per cent phenol (carbolic acid).

Observations suggested to Rous and his associates the possible influence of injury to or derangement of cells on the growth of the resultant tumor following injection of the filtrate. In order to test this hypothesis they introduced a large quantity of active filtrate into one side of the breast, and an equal quantity of filtrate, to which had been added a small amount of sterile, washed, diatomaceous earth, was injected into the other side of the breast. The tumors resulting from the filtrate plus the diatomaceous earth were diffuse masses; those from the filtrate alone appeared as small, discrete nodules in the track of the injecting needle. In another experiment, filtrate only was introduced into the blood stream of seventeen chickens and tumor developed in four; three in the ovaries and one in the liver. This would indicate that the tumors had predilection for injured or deranged tissue, since the ovary suffers a certain amount of trauma daily, and it was felt that, perhaps, focal derangement was present in the liver. In another series of twenty chickens, tumor filtrate and diatomaceous earth was injected into the blood stream, and growths developed in seven.

The tumor could be transplanted to the developing embryos of barred Plymouth Rocks, and to the eggs of pigeons or ducks, by bits of tumor tissue or by the cell-free filtrate. Of 147 chicken eggs that were inoculated, results were successful in 108. In the nine incubating pigeon eggs injected, positive results were observed in four, and tumors developed in six of the sixteen duck embryos inoculated.

The investigators were unable to demonstrate that the tumor could be made to appear in susceptible chickens by contagion or infection, in the usual sense of these terms. During a period of three years, 1,200 chickens, some affected with the tumor, were kept in close quarters. In no instance did a spontaneous tumor of this variety develop, notwithstanding the fact that many were fed the fresh, tumorous tissue, and that many were probably contaminated with the dried tissue containing the viable causative agent.

That the Rous sarcoma is unique and uncommon among neoplasms of chickens is suggested by the attempts of Rous and his coworkers to obtain other spontaneous cases of the disease. From a New York concern dealing in live poultry, twenty-seven chicken tumors were acquired in seven months. Attempts were made to transplant each of the tumors, and in two the transplantations were successful. Histologically, neither of these resembled the original sarcoma described by Rous.

A tremendous amount of work has been done by others in the attempt to elucidate the exact nature of the tumor-inducing agent of the so-called Rous sarcoma.* It is entirely beyond the scope of this work to give a review of all the contributions dealing with this problem, but brief mention should be made of the more recent work of Nakohara and that of Ragnotti. The former reported that the ability of the dry tissue of the tumor to induce new growths in the recipient was seriously impaired if the tissue was previously subjected to grinding in a mortar; he pointed out the improbability of injuring a chemical substance by this means. He concluded that the transmission of the sarcoma depends on a foreign body, probably the sarcoma cell itself. Ragnotti's work confirmed the previous observations of Rous that the blood of chickens affected with the Rous sarcoma frequently contains the etiologic agent, so that the growth can be transmitted by injections of blood. The causative agent may be present in the plasma, in the erythrocytes or in the leukocytes, but the monocyte did not seem to be concerned. If blood which contains the tumor-inducing element is allowed to clot, the fibrin is frequently found to contain the etiologic substance.

Whether the etiologic agent of the sarcoma described by Rous is

---

* For a review of the exhaustive studies of Carrell and others on the nature of the infective agent of the Rous tumor the reader is referred to the monograph by McGowan.

in the nature of a living virus that is capable of being separated from the cells of the tumor, or whether the growth-stimulating agent is specific and noncellular, is problematic and as yet undetermined. The entire phenomenon pertaining to the Rous sarcoma is so unique, that one must be cautious in subscribing to definite conclusions concerning it. Suffice to say that the nature of the growth-inciting element has not been established. Many of the attempts to explain the phenomenon have been philosophic descriptions of what occurs rather than an elucidation of the factor which initiated the process.

OTHER EXPERIMENTS

A transplantable fibrosarcoma was obtained from the mesentery of a white Leghorn hen by Begg.[1, 2] Early in the experimental existence of the tumor growth was slow, and eight generations were reached only after three years. In the eighth generation the tumor assumed a softer consistence and exhibited a tendency to grow rapidly. It was demonstrated that the tumor could be propagated by free-cell filtrates, and by material that had been dried in a vacuum over phosphorus pentoxide for five days.

Richter and MacDowell[25, 26] observed the frequent occurrence of lymphoid leukemia in a particular strain of mice which had been inbred by brother and sister matings for many years. Death from leukemia occurred most frequently when animals were aged more than eight months. Emulsions prepared from lesions of animals that died spontaneously of the disease failed to transmit leukemia to several strains of mice in which leukemia had not been observed spontaneously, but intraperitoneal or subcutaneous inoculation of young mice of the highly inbred strain in which leukemia occurred with great frequency at a later age, resulted in rapid development of the disease.

Furth and Strumia, however, succeeded in transmitting leukemia of mice, by intravenous inoculation of suspensions of tissue, to strains of mice in which spontaneous leukemia had not been known to occur. The relationship to leukemia of neoplasia, and the opportunity provided for the study of the various aspects of the disease, make these observations of no little significance.

Except in a limited sense, heterologous transplantations of tumorous material usually have failed. Funk, however, was able to transmit a mouse tumor to rats in several instances during a series of experiments in which the influence of diet on resultant growths is suggested. Sixty rats were injected with Ehrlich's chondroma of the mouse, after which they were divided. Lot 1 was fed the ordinary ration, and lot 2, in addition to the ordinary ration, was fed twice daily with fresh tumor tissue which was excised from mice with experimentally produced tumors of the same variety used to inoculate the rats. The growth of the tumors succeeded best in rats which received the tumor diet in addition to the regular food. In the group that received only the regular ration, only one small tumor was found, and in the group which received the tumor tissue, in addition to the regular food, tumors developed in six.

In a second experiment, twenty rats were inoculated with chondroma from a mouse which had been inoculated from a rat, with a successful take in the first experiment. These rats were also divided into lots: Those in one lot were fed the ordinary ration, and those in the other were given the ordinary food with tumor tissue. In the lot which received the tumor tissue two tumors developed; none developed in the controls.

These experiments indicate that by feeding tumor tissue to animals of alien species, some may be rendered more favorable to the growth of this particular tumor. Although at first sufficient growth occurred to provide material for further inoculations, growth eventually failed as the mechanism of resistance increased in effectiveness. Funk's experiments, although ingenious and of considerable interest, cannot be accepted as evidence that successful heterologous transplantation of neoplasm has been accomplished. The progressiveness of the takes were too transitory. This fact, and the reduced vitality of the transplanted tissues, indicate failure of the inoculated cells to overcome the racial inhibition of the recipients, and to eastblish an autonomous existence such as characterizes successful transplantation between two individuals of the same species.

Considering the availability of material it is not surprising that many attempts have been made to effect transmission to animals of neoplastic material from man. Many species have been used, but in general attempts have failed. Occasionally, growth of the transplanted fragment may occur in certain species for a short period. The work of Jobling, in this respect, is of much interest. Several monkeys (Macacus rhesus) were inoculated subcutaneously with portions of a particularly malignant teratoma, consisting of cartilage, glandular epithelium, and cellular stroma removed from "the right lower quadrant of the pelvis" of a fourteen-year-old white girl. Rats and mice were also inoculated but the transplants failed to increase in size in any of the animals, and eventually disappeared. In one series of experiments, however, in some of the monkeys inoculated it was found that although the epithelial elements of the tumor had disappeared, the cartilaginous elements had remained alive for sixteen days, with active mitosis at the end of that period, during which the cartilaginous portions of the graft had increased markedly in size.

In view of the complete failure of any portions of the grafts from tumor of man to grow in rats and mice, and the somewhat different results in monkeys, which bear a close biologic relationship to man, Jobling felt justified in concluding that "tumor transplantations between heterologous species is absolutely impossible." In his opinion the failure of the transplanted cells to grow results from "the want of a special and peculiar nutriment which the foreign host cannot supply, although a sufficient quantity is carried along at the time of inoculation to enable foreign tumor cells to survive for a period."

What appears to have been the successful transplantation of a tumor between animals of different species was reported in 1929 by Fujinami and Hatano. These workers transplanted to the tissues of a duck a myxosarcoma obtained from a chicken, and thus obtained a transmissible tumor in the former species which was successfully transferable from duck to duck in almost 100 per cent of the attempts. It was observed that the tumor grew more rapidly in ducks than in chickens, and would cause the death of the ducks in from fourteen to twenty days.

At the time of the report, the tumors had been transmitted through forty generations and could be retransplanted to chickens even after a residence of several generations in ducks. Transplantation was consummated by the growth and proliferation in the tissues of the recipient of the inoculated cells obtained from the tumor of the donor.

Attesting to the marked vitality of the tumor observed by Fujinami and Hatano was the finding that growth would result following reinoculation into chickens after the graft had resided for as much as fifteen days in the subcutaneous tissue of a guinea pig, whereas in the tissues of the toad it survived for as long as thirty-five days.

In view of the failure of practically all previous attempts to achieve heterotransplantation of a neoplasm, the striking results of Fujinami and Hatano are difficult to explain. It is perhaps of some significance that transplantation was possible in such closely related species as the chicken and the duck. It is reasonable to assume that there exists a less formidable resistance, when two such species are concerned, than exists between mammal and fowl, or in some instances between two species of mammals. Although the close relationship of the species may have constituted a contributory influence in the successful results obtained, it is not unlikely that the nature of the neoplasm was of primary importance in determining the ability of the growth to prosper in an alien environment.

Aside from any biologic peculiarities which might prevent the transplanted cells of a tumor from joining with the tissues of the host, the conditions attendant on their presence in foreign soil are sufficient explanation for the failure of many attempts at transplantation.

When one considers the tremendous local reaction provoked in the tissues by the presence of foreign material, such as a graft of tumor cells in transplantation experiments, it is at once apparent how extraordinary it must be for such an inoculated bit of tissue to grow. The trauma incidental to insertion of the graft, although minimized as much as possible, results in a break in the continuity of the skin and of the subcutaneous tissues in which the transplanted fragment of tumor is placed. This promotes some response on the part of the reparative force of the body, which is often vigorous, particularly if infection has occurred at the time of injury. The reaction of the host's tissues are further stimulated by contact with the inoculated material, which must, from the first, be considered a foreign body, possessing, perhaps, as an inherent part of its cellular constituents, certain properties which antagonize the protective and reparative factors of the host in such a way as to initiate maximal reaction. As a consequence, many or all of the transplanted cells are likely to perish before satisfactory nutritional contacts can be made with the surrounding tissue of the host. Conditions must be favorable indeed if a transplant is to succeed, for the natural reaction of the adjacent tissues is to cause solution or digestion of the inoculated material, and failing in this, to provide a fibrous capsule protecting and separating the bodily tissue from it. For the injected cells to survive in the face of the inevitable protest instituted by the host's tissues, and eventually to perfect contacts insuring sustenance for its future growth, is truly a remarkable phenomenon. As a demonstration of the ability of organized matter to adapt itself to an artificial environment, it is, to say the least, unique.

TECHNIC OF TRANSPLANTATION OF TUMORS

For inoculation of animals with tumor cells in transmission experiments, there are at least three methods of choice. An emulsion containing the tumor cells may be injected with a hypodermic syringe; a small slice of tumor tissue may be inserted under the skin, through an incision, or small pieces of the tumorous tissue may be deposited in the tissues of the recipient by the use of a trocar and cannula. Ordinarily, the latter method is to be preferred, and although a long, 16 or 18 gauge hypodermic needle and a wire stylet may be used with good results, it is desirable when possible to use a trocar and cannula for most work of this nature (Fig. 193).

Every precaution must be taken to insure asepsis throughout the entire procedure, for if infection occurs, transplantation usually fails. The shorter the interval between the time when the tissue is removed from the donor and the time when it is placed in the tissues of the recipient, the better are the chances for success. Inoculations are usually

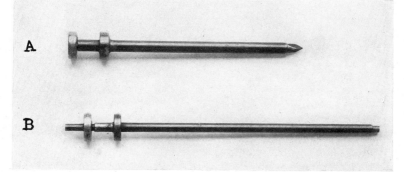

Fig. 193.—Apparatus used in transplantation of tumor; *A*, large trocar and cannula for perforating the skin; *B*, smaller trocar and cannula used to introduce the fragments of tissue into the recipient by way of the larger cannula.

made into the subcutaneous tissues of the abdomen or sternal regions, although other regions may be utilized with equal satisfaction.

BIBLIOGRAPHY

1. Begg, A. M.: A transplantable fibrosarcoma of the fowl. Brit. Jour. Exper. Path., **8:** 147–148 (May), 1927.

2. Begg, A. M.: A filtrable fibrosarcoma of the fowl. Brit. Jour. Exper. Path., **10:** 322–326 (Nov.), 1929.

3. Eiselsberg, A. F. V.: Ueber einen Fall von erfolgreicher Transplantation eines Fibrosarkoms bei Ratten. Wien. klin. Wchnschr., **3:** 927–928 (Nov.), 1890.

4. Firket: Quoted by Flexner and Jobling.[8]

5. Flexner, Simon and Jobling, J. W.: Remarks on and exhibition of specimens of a metastasizing sarcoma of the rat. Proc. Soc. Exper. Biol. and Med., **4:** 12, 1906–1907.

6. Flexner, Simon and Jobling, J. W.: Metaplasia and metastasis of a rat tumor. Proc. Soc. Exper. Biol. and Med., **5:** 52–53, 1907–1908.

7. Flexner, Simon and Jobling, J. W.: Further notes on a rat tumor. Proc. Soc. Exper. Biol. and Med., **5:** 91–92, 1907–1908.

8. Flexner, Simon and Jobling, J. W.: Studies upon a transplantable rat tumor. Monographs of the Rockefeller Institute for Medical Research, **1:** 1–51, 1910–1912.

9. Fujinami, A. and Hatano, S.: Contribution of the pathology of heterotransplantation of tumor. A duck sarcoma from chicken sarcoma. Abstract. Gann., **23**: 65–75 (Aug.), 1929.

10. Funk, Casimir: The transplantation of tumors to foreign species. Jour. Exper. Med., **21**: 571–573 (June), 1915.

11. Furth, J. and Strumia, M.: Observations on the transmissibility of lymphoid leucemia of mice. Proc. Soc. Exper. Biol. and Med., **27**: 834–838 (May), 1930.

12. Hanau, Arthur: Erfolgreiche experimentelle Uebertragung von Carcinom. Fortschr. d. Med., **7**: 321–339 (May), 1889.

13. Jensen, C. O.: Experimentelle Untersuchungen über Krebs bei Mäusen. Centralbl. f. Bakteriol., **34**: 28–34 ;122–143, 1903.

14. Jensen, C. O.: Uebertragbare Rattensarkome. Ztschr. f. Krebsforsch., **7**: 45–54, 1909.

15. Jobling, J. W.: Transplantation experiments in Macacus rhesus with a carcinomatous teratoma from man. Monographs of the Rockefeller Institute for Medical Research, **1–4**: 120–130, 1910–1912.

16. Loeb, Leo: On transplantation of tumors. Jour. Med. Res., **6**: 28–38 (July), 1901.

17. Loeb, Leo: Further investigation in transplantation of tumors. Jour. Med. Res., **8**: 44–73 (June), 1902.

18. McGowan, J. P.: On Rous, leucotic and allied tumours in the fowl. New York, The MacMillan Company, 1928, p. 77.

19. Morau: Quoted by Woglom, W. H.: The study of experimental cancer. New York, Columbia University Press, 1913, p. 54.

20. Murphy, J. B. and Rous, Peyton: The behavior of chicken sarcoma implanted in the developing embryo. Jour. Exper. Med., **15**: 119–132 (Feb.), 1912.

21. Nakahara, W.: The nature of the entity transmitting chicken sarcoma, as evidenced by experiments on desiccated sarcoma tissue. Gann., **22**: 1–9 (March), 1928.

22. Nowinsky: Quoted by Sticker, Anton: Infectiöse und krebsige Geschwülste an den äusseren Geschlechtsorganen des Hundes. Arch. f. klin. Chir., **78**: 773–800, 1906.

23. Pfeiffer: Quoted by Woglom, W. H.: The study of experimental cancer. New York, Columbia University Press, 1913, p. 53.

24. Ragnotti, Ercole: Über die Infektiositat des Blutes von mit Roussarkom behafteten Hühneren. Ztschr. f. Kresbforsch., **29**: 510–515, 1929.

25. Richter, M. N. and MacDowell, E. C.: The experimental transmission of leukemia in mice. Proc. Soc. Exper. Biol. and Med., **26**: 362–364 (Feb.), 1929.

26. Richter, M. N. and MacDowell, E. C.: Studies on leukemia in mice. I. The experimental transmission of leukemia. Jour. Exper. Med., **51**: 659–673 (April), 1930.

27. Rous, Peyton: A transmissible avian neoplasm (sarcoma of the common fowl). Jour. Exper. Med., **12**: 696–705 (Sept.), 1910.

28. Rous, Peyton: Metastatic and tumor immunity. Jour. Am. Med. Assn., **55**: 1805 (Nov. 19), 1910.

29. Rous, Peyton: Transmission of a malignant new growth by means of a cell-free filtrate. Jour. Am. Med. Assn., **56**: 198 (Jan. 21), 1911.

30. Rous, Peyton: A sarcoma of the fowl transmissible by an agent separable from the tumor cells. Jour. Exper. Med., **13**: 397–409 (April), 1911.

31. Rous, Peyton: An avian tumor in its relation to the tumor problem. Proc. Am. Phil. Soc., **51**: 201–205, 1912.

32. Rous, Peyton and Murphy, J. B.: Tumor implantation in the developing embryo. Jour. Am. Med. Assn., **56**: 741–742 (March 11), 1911.

33. Rous, Peyton and Murphy, J. B.: The histological signs of resistance to a transmissible sarcoma of the fowl. Jour. Exper. Med., **15**: 270–286 (March), 1912.

34. Rous, Peyton and Murphy, J. B.: The nature of the filterable agent causing a sarcoma of the fowl. Jour. Am. Med. Assn., **58**: 1938 (June 22), 1912.

35. Rous, Peyton, Murphy, J. B. and Tytler, W. H.: The rôle of injury in the production of a chicken sarcoma by a filterable agent. Jour. Am. Med. Assn., **58**: 1751–1752 (June 8), 1912.

36. Rous, Peyton, Murphy, J. B. and Tytler, W. H.: The relation between a chicken sarcoma's behavior and the growth's filterable cause. Jour. Am. Med. Assn., **58**: 1840–1841 (June 15), 1912.

37. Velich, A.: Beitrag zur Frage nach des Uebertragbarkeit des Sarkoms. Wien. med. Bl., **21**: 711–729, 1898.

CHAPTER XXIII

PRESERVATION OF PATHOLOGIC MATERIAL

SELECTION AND FIXATION OF TUMOROUS TISSUES FOR MICROSCOPIC
EXAMINATION

Except for the few workers who are equipped to handle fresh, frozen sections, fixation must be resorted to in order to secure microscopic preparations for diagnosis and study.

Perhaps the most serviceable of all fixation fluids is a simple solution of one part of formaldehyde 40 per cent, and nine parts of water. This is generally known as "10 per cent formalin solution." It is desirable to prepare a gallon or more of this solution, and to add an excess of calcium carbonate to neutralize any tendency of the fluid to become acid. The solution should be kept in a tightly stoppered, metal, glass, or earthenware, container, and transferred to smaller receptacles as needed.

Although formalin is a fairly satisfactory fixative for most tissues, it cannot be recommended for tumors consisting of lymphoid elements, such as lymphoblastomas, on account of the shrinkage that occurs after embedding in paraffin. For these tumors Zenker's solution is preferable. This is made as follows:

Potassium bichromate	2.5 gm.
Mercuric chloride	5 gm.
Water	100 c.c.

The solution of the mercuric chloride and potassium bichromate is effected by the aid of heat. Glacial acetic acid, 5 per cent, is added to a given quantity of the stock solution just before use. The glacial acetic acid is not essential, however, and is often omitted.

The tissue to be fixed should be cut in thin strips, preferably not more than 0.5 c.c. thick. The amount of fixative fluid should exceed by ten times the volume of the tissue to be fixed. Unsatisfactory results are obtained if many pieces of tissue are crowded into a small container and space for only a minimal amount of fluid remains. It usually requires from eighteen to thirty-six hours to obtain complete fixation by the use of 10 per cent formalin solution although the tissues may be left in this mixture indefinitely without seriously impairing their staining capacity, if the presence of formic acid is precluded by the addition of calcium carbonate to the stock solution.

Tissues placed in Zenker's fluid are usually fixed after twelve to twenty-four hours and should then be removed from the fixative solution and washed in running water for twelve to twenty-four hours, after which they may be preserved indefinitely in 80 per cent ethyl alcohol.

If the material is properly selected and immediately fixed in one of the fluids designed for this purpose the tissue may be shipped any distance to the pathologic laboratory, where a diagnosis usually can be given within one to a few days after receipt of the material.

If biopsy is to be made, it may be necessary to inject about the region of the growth a suitable local anesthetic substance, and means should be provided to control the hemorrhage which not uncommonly ensues following incision of a particularly vascular tumor. With as little manipulation as possible, a small, wedge-shaped piece of tissue should be removed with a very sharp knife. Regions of necrosis are to be avoided, and care should be taken to cut deep enough to pass well beyond any outer covering or capsule that may be present. Many of the tumors of the exterior of the body are covered with skin, and others frequently possess variable amounts of encrusted blood clots and scab tissue which may complicate the securing of that portion of the growth desired for microscopic examination.

PREPARATION OF MATERIAL FOR MUSEUM PURPOSES

If the tissue is obtained at necropsy all unnecessary incisions should be avoided in order that unusual specimens may be acceptable for museum purposes. The dearth of really worthwhile specimens of the various types of neoplasms in the pathologic museums of most veterinary colleges is lamentable. The situation could be appreciably benefited if those who encounter suitable material could be prevailed on to present tissues to institutions in which museum collections are being neglected. Perhaps if an aggressive interest in the furtherance of the museum idea were evinced by clinicians and meat inspectors, the pathologists, and others responsible for the present deplorable state of the pathologic museums in many of our teaching institutions, could be persuaded to assume an active interest and a sympathetic attitude toward this necessary adjuvant to the sound teaching of many of the fundamental as well as clinical aspects of veterinary medicine.

The difficulty of properly preserving pathologic material for museum use has constituted a formidable barrier to many whose routine brings them in daily contact with lesions of disease, and who might be interested in the improvement of museum facilities. Practitioners and those engaged in meat inspection are permitted to observe a practically inexhaustible supply of specimens, many of which would be ideal for teaching purposes, but because of lack of knowledge as to the proper means of preserving the material, little of it finds its way to the museum.

The preparation of specimens for museum display is not a complicated process, and knowledge of the essentials is easy to grasp.

A large container, of sufficient size to hold at least 5 gallons of fixative fluid should be secured. A 10-gallon earthenware crock is satisfactory, or a discarded pickle keg of a capacity of 10 gallons will serve admirably. A cover for the container should be provided. Although ordinary 10 per cent solution of formaldehyde similar to that used in fixing tissues for microscopic study may be utilized for the preservation of tissues for purposes of display, certain other mixtures are preferable on account of the preservation of natural color which follows their use. The more desirable museum preparations are those in which the natural colors of the living tissues have been faithfully retained, and this is possible only if tissues that have been properly fixed in a fluid especially designed with this in mind. The following, recommended by Lundquist, is excellent:

Potassium acetate	425 gm.
Potassium nitrate	225 gm.
Chloral hydrate	400 gm.
Formaldehyde (40 per cent gas)	2,225 c.c.
Water	20,000 c.c.

This formula yields somewhat more than 5 gallons of preservative and will keep satisfactorily for a long time if placed in a tightly stoppered bottle.

Specimens intended for preservation should be no larger than is necessary to include the essential features of the lesions which may be present. Attempts to fix huge masses of tissue usually result unsatisfactorily. The nonessential parts of the specimen should be trimmed away, and if the specimen is unusually large, incisions should be made deeply into the tissue on the side opposite the part which possesses the most desirable features for exhibition. Specimens that would otherwise be splendid if not remarkable are not infrequently ruined for museum purposes because of the indiscriminate use of the knife. If a lesion must be incised, the break in continuity should be to one side or opposite the exposed salient features.

Before the specimen is placed in the preserving fluid, a small bit of tissue should be removed from the more typical part of the lesion and placed in 10 per cent formalin solution or in Zenker's fluid for microscopic study as directed. The slower fixation which ensues in the museum preservative fluid is not conducive to satisfactory histologic preparation. Neither is the chemical make-up of the fluid used so satisfactory for the latter purpose.

Specimens should never be crowded together in the fixative fluid, but should be so oriented as to permit free contact with the fluid over the entire contour of the specimen. There should be approximately ten times as much fluid present as the volume displayed by the tissue being fixed.

Thin pieces of tissues may be satisfactorily fixed after twenty-four to forty-eight hours, but for larger specimens several days to weeks may be necessary. Fixation is complete when the tissue feels firm to the touch, and a thin, blood-like fluid does not exude from a freshly cut surface.

After fixation is accomplished, the specimens must be washed in running water for eight to twelve hours to eliminate all traces of formaldehyde. The tissue can then be trimmed further, and if cut surfaces are to be exposed when the specimen is exhibited, a fresh, clean surface should be made with a long and very sharp knife. An uneven surface, due to ridges and knife marks, seriously detracts from the attractiveness of the final product, and should be avoided.

As a final preservative, the specimens may be placed in a fluid composed of the following:

Potassium acetate	100 gm.
Chloral hydrate	50 gm.
Glycerine	100 c.c.
Water	1,000 c.c.

It is usually advantageous to use two changes of this solution, permitting the tissues to remain in the first for twelve hours before transferring them to the fresh, unused fluid which is to be the final preservative. The fluid should be filtered through paper before it is used and a few crystals of thymol should be added to check the growth of molds.

The specimens may be displayed in museum jars, of which there are many types, or the watch glass method of Day may be utilized.

On account of the high capillarity of glycerine, preservative fluids containing this substance are objectionable in the preparation of watch glass mounts. For this procedure the fluid suggested by Frost, as modified by Klotz and MacLachlan is useful. It consists of the following:

Cane sugar... 1,750 gm.
Potassium acetate....................................... 80 gm.
Chloral hydrate... 40 gm.
Water to which has been added thymol to saturation.......... 4,000 c.c.

The solution must be filtered before it is used.

Of first importance in the securing of pathologic material intended for histologic study, or for museum purposes, is the placing of the tissue in the fixative fluid immediately after its removal from the body, and in the case of necropsy, as soon after the death of the animal as possible.

Material that has undergone postmortem changes is useless for subsequent microscopic study. Good results can be expected only when the material is obtained perfectly fresh and small portions of the tissue are placed immediately in an abundance of the fixative fluid of choice. Tissues intended for microscopic study should never be placed for preservation in borax. Although this agent inhibits to some extent putrefaction of the tissues at the surface of the specimen, it penetrates poorly, and has no fixative capacity whatever.

If many specimens are placed in the same container, some system of numbering to insure future identification is necessary. For this purpose brass or celloidin tags, properly stamped with steel dies, and affixed with strong linen thread, do very well.

BIBLIOGRAPHY

1. Day, L. E.: An improved method for mounting museum specimens. Jour. Am. Vet. Med. Assn., **44**: 66–71, 1913–1914.

2. Feldman, W. H.: A modification of Day's method for mounting museum specimens under watch glasses and a means for their display. Internat. Assn. Med. Mus. Bull. **11**: 18–24 (May 4), 1925.

3. Klotz, Oskar and MacLachlan, W. W. G.: A modified Jores' method for the preservation of colors in gross specimens. Internat. Assn. Med. Mus. Bull. **5**: 59–60 (June 1), 1915.

4. Lundquist, Richard: A proposed modification of the Kaiserling method for preserving gross specimens. Internat. Assn. Med. Mus. Bull. **11**: 16–18 (May 4), 1925.

BIBLIOGRAPHIC INDEX

INDEX OF SUBJECTS